Common Pitfalls in Sleep Medicine

D1484705

Common Pitfalls in Sleep Medicine: Case-Based Learning

Edited by

Ronald D. Chervin, MD, MS

Professor of Neurology
Michael S. Aldrich Collegiate Professor of Sleep Medicine
Director, Sleep Disorders Center
University of Michigan, Ann Arbor, MI, USA

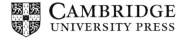

CAMBRIDGE
UNIVERSITY PRESS

CAMBRIDGE
UNIVERSITY PRESS

University Printing House, Cambridge CB2 8BS, United Kingdom

Published in the United States of America by Cambridge University Press, New York

Cambridge University Press is part of the University of Cambridge.

It furthers the University's mission by disseminating knowledge in the pursuit of education, learning, and research at the highest international levels of excellence.

www.cambridge.org
Information on this title: www.cambridge.org/9781107611535

© Cambridge University Press 2014

First published 2014

Printed in the United Kingdom by Clays, St Ives plc

A catalogue record for this publication is available from the British Library

Library of Congress Cataloging-in-Publication Data
Common pitfalls in sleep medicine : case-based learning / edited by Ronald D. Chervin.
    p. ; cm.
Includes bibliographical references and index.
ISBN 978-1-107-61153-5 (Paperback)
I. Chervin, Ronald D., editor of compilation.
[DNLM: 1. Sleep Disorders–diagnosis–Case Reports.   2. Sleep Disorders–therapy–Case Reports. WL 108]
RC547
616.8'498–dc23   2013036058

ISBN 978-1-107-61153-5 Paperback

Contents

Contributors

J. Todd Arnedt, PhD
Associate Professor of Psychiatry and Neurology
Director, Behavioral Sleep Medicine Program
Sleep Disorders Center
University of Michigan, Ann Arbor, MI, USA

Sharon Aronovich, DMD
Assistant Professor
Assistant Program Director, Oral & Maxillofacial Surgery
University of Michigan, Ann Arbor, MI, USA

Alon Y. Avidan, MD, MPH
Professor of Neurology
Director, UCLA Sleep Disorders Center
Director, UCLA Neurology Clinic
UCLA School of Medicine, Los Angeles, CA, USA

Alp Sinan Baran, MD
Associate Professor of Psychiatry
Medical Director, Sleep Disorders Clinic
University of Michigan, Ann Arbor, MI, USA

Johnathan Barkham, MD
Clinical Instructor of Sleep Medicine and Internal Medicine
Veterans Administration Ann Arbor Healthcare System
University of Michigan, Ann Arbor, MI, USA

Lizabeth Binns, PA-C
Physician Assistant
Sleep Disorders Center and Department of Neurology
University of Michigan, Ann Arbor, MI, USA

Tiffany J. Braley, MD, MS
Assistant Professor of Neurology

Multiple Sclerosis and Sleep Disorders Centers
University of Michigan, Ann Arbor, MI, USA

Devin Brown, MD, MS
Associate Professor of Neurology
Associate Director, Stroke Program
University of Michigan, Ann Arbor, MI, USA

Paul R. Carney, MD
Professor of Pediatrics, Neurology, Neuroscience, and
Biomedical Engineering
Wilder Chair for Epilepsy Research
Chief of Pediatric Neurology
Director of the Comprehensive Pediatric Epilepsy Program
University of Florida and McKnight Brain Institute
Gainesville, FL, USA

Philip Cheng, MS
PhD Candidate, Clinical Psychology
University of Michigan, Ann Arbor, MI, USA

Ronald D. Chervin, MD, MS
Professor of Neurology
Michael S. Aldrich Collegiate Professor of Sleep Medicine
Director, Sleep Disorders Center
University of Michigan, Ann Arbor, MI, USA

Naricha Chirakalwasan, MD
Director, International Sleep Medicine Fellowship
Pulmonary and Critical Care Division,
Department of Medicine, Faculty of Medicine,
Chulalongkorn University
Excellence Center for Sleep Disorders,
King Chulalongkorn Memorial Hospital
Thai Red Cross Society
Bangkok, Thailand

Wattanachai Chotinaiwattarakul, MD
Assistant Professor
Siriraj Sleep Center and Division of Neurology
Department of Medicine, Faculty of Medicine,
Mahidol University and Siriraj Hospital
Bangkok, Thailand

Deirdre A. Conroy, PhD
Associate Professor of Psychiatry

Clinical Director, Behavioral Sleep Medicine Program
University of Michigan, Ann Arbor, MI, USA

Charles R. Davies, MD, PhD
Neurologist, Department of Neurology
Carle Physician Group
Clinical Instructor, College of Medicine,
University of Illinois, Urbana, IL, USA

Dawn Dore-Stites, PhD
Assistant Professor of Pediatrics
Division of Child Behavioral Health
University of Michigan, Ann Arbor, MI, USA

Alan S. Eiser, PhD
Clinical Lecturer, Department of Neurology
Adjunct Clinical Lecturer, Department of Psychiatry
Sleep Disorders Center
University of Michigan, Ann Arbor, MI, USA

Todd Favorite, PhD
Assistant Professor of Psychiatry
Director, Psychological Clinic
Attending Clinical Psychology, PTSD Clinical Team
Ann Arbor Veterans Health System
University of Michigan, Ann Arbor, MI, USA

Barbara T. Felt, MD
Professor of Pediatrics
Section Head, Developmental-Behavioral Pediatrics
Division of Child Behavioral Health
University of Michigan, Ann Arbor, MI, USA

James D. Geyer, MD
Director, Sleep Medicine and Behavioral Sleep Medicine
University of Alabama, Tuscaloosa, AL, USA

Jennifer R. Goldschmied, MS
PhD Candidate, Clinical Psychology
University of Michigan, Ann Arbor, MI, USA

Cathy A. Goldstein, MD
Assistant Professor of Neurology
Sleep Disorders Center
University of Michigan, Ann Arbor, MI, USA

John J. Harrington, MD, MPH
Associate Professor of Medicine
Division of Pulmonary, Critical Care and Sleep Medicine
Sleep and Behavioral Health Sciences Section
National Jewish Health
University of Colorado, Denver, CO, USA

Fauziya Hassan, MD, MS
Assistant Professor of Pediatrics
Sleep Disorders Center and Division of Pediatric Pulmonary Medicine
University of Michigan, Ann Arbor, MI, USA

Judith L. Heidebrink, MD, MS
Associate Professor of Neurology
Richard D. and Katherine M. O'Connor Research Professor of Alzheimer's Disease
Veterans Administration Ann Arbor Healthcare System
University of Michigan, Ann Arbor, MI, USA

Joseph I. Helman, DMD
Professor, Department of Dentistry
Professor, Department of Surgery
Section Head, Oral and Maxillofacial Surgery
C. J. Lyons Endowed Chair
University of Michigan, Ann Arbor, MI, USA

Shelley Hershner, MD
Assistant Professor of Neurology
Sleep Disorders Center
University of Michigan, Ann Arbor, MI, USA

Timothy F. Hoban, MD
Professor of Pediatrics and Neurology
Director, Pediatric Sleep Medicine Program
Sleep Disorders Center and Division of Pediatric Neurology
University of Michigan, Ann Arbor, MI, USA

Edward D. Huntley, PhD
Postdoctoral Psychology Fellow
Department of Psychiatry
University of Michigan, Ann Arbor, MI, USA

Rahul K. Kakkar, MD
Chief Executive Officer, Nidra Sleep Institute
Staff Sleep Specialist

North Florida/South Georgia Veterans Health System
Jacksonville, FL, USA

Douglas Kirsch, MD
Associate Neurologist, Brigham and Women's Hospital
Clinical Instructor, Harvard Medical School
Boston, MA, USA

Raman K. Malhotra, MD
Assistant Professor of Neurology
Director, Sleep Medicine Fellowship
Co-Director, Sleep Disorders Center
Saint Louis University, St Louis, MO, USA

Beth A. Malow, MD, MS
Professor of Neurology and Pediatrics
Burry Chair in Cognitive Childhood Development
Director, Sleep Disorders Division
Vanderbilt University, Nashville, TN, USA

Lauren O'Connell, MD
Fellow, Section of Developmental-Behavioral Pediatrics
Division of Child Behavioral Health
Department of Pediatrics
University of Michigan, Ann Arbor, MI, USA

Shalini Paruthi, MD
Assistant Professor of Pediatrics and Internal Medicine
Director, Pediatric Sleep and Research Center
Cardinal Glennon Children's Medical Center
Saint Louis University, St Louis, MO, USA

Meredith D. Peters, MD
Internist, IHA Pulmonary, Critical Care and Sleep Consultants
Ann Arbor, MI, USA

Scott M. Pickett, PhD
Assistant Professor of Psychology
Oakland University, Rochester, MI, USA

Satya Krishna Ramachandran, MD
Assistant Professor of Anesthesiology
Director, Quality Assurance
University of Michigan, Ann Arbor, MI, USA

Fouad Reda, MD
Assistant Professor of Psychiatry
Director of Insomnia Clinic
Sleep Disorders Center
Department of Neurology and Psychiatry
Saint Louis University, St Louis, MO, USA

Daniel I. Rifkin, MD
Clinical Assistant Professor of Neurology
Medical Director, Sleep Medicine Centers of Western
New York
University at Buffalo NY, USA

Emerson Robinson, DDS, MPH
Emeritus Professor of Dentistry
School of Dentistry
University of Michigan, Ann Arbor, MI, USA

Helena M. Schotland, MD
Assistant Professor of Medicine
Division of Pulmonary and Critical Care Medicine
Sleep Disorders Center
University of Michigan, Ann Arbor, MI, USA

Q. Afifa Shamim-Uzzaman, MD
Assistant Professor of Internal Medicine
Director, Ann Arbor Veterans Administration Sleep Disorders
Program
University of Michigan, Ann Arbor, MI, USA

Anita Valanju Shelgikar, MD
Assistant Professor of Neurology
Director, Sleep Medicine Fellowship
Sleep Disorders Center
University of Michigan, Ann Arbor, MI, USA

Renée A. Shellhaas, MD, MS
Assistant Professor of Pediatrics
Division of Pediatric Neurology
University of Michigan, Ann Arbor, MI, USA

Jeffrey J. Stanley, MD
Assistant Professor of Otolaryngology – Head and Neck
Surgery
Assistant Professor of Neurology
Director, Alternatives to CPAP Program

Sleep Disorders Center
University of Michigan, Ann Arbor, MI, USA

Leslie M. Swanson, PhD
Assistant Professor of Psychiatry
University of Michigan, Ann Arbor, MI, USA

Mihai C. Teodorescu, MD, MS
Associate Professor, Division of Allergy, Pulmonary and
Critical Care Medicine
Director, James B. Skatrud Pulmonary/Sleep Research
Laboratory
William S. Middleton Memorial Veteran's Hospital
Center for Sleep Medicine and Sleep Research
University of Wisconsin, Madison, WI, USA

Mihai C. Teodorescu, MD
Assistant Professor
Division of Geriatrics and Gerontology
University of Wisconsin, Madison, WI, USA

Sheila C. Tsai, MD
Associate Professor of Medicine
Division of Pulmonary, Critical Care, and Sleep Medicine
Director, Sleep Medicine Fellowship
National Jewish Health
University of Colorado, Denver, CO, USA

Katherine Wilson, MD, MS
Pediatrician, IHA Pulmonary, Critical Care and Sleep
Consultants
Ann Arbor, MI, USA

Michael E. Yurcheshen, MD
Associate Professor of Neurology and Medicine
University of Rochester School of Medicine and Dentistry
URMC Sleep Disorders Center
Rochester, NY, USA

Sarah Nath Zallek, MD
Clinical Associate Professor of Neurology
University of Illinois College of Medicine at Peoria
Medical Director, Illinois Neurological Institute Sleep Center
Director, Illinois Neurological Institute
Neurology Clinical Affairs, Peoria, IL, USA

Preface

Sleep problems are among the most common complaints that patients bring to their clinicians. However, few medical schools or postgraduate training programs devote more than a few hours to this topic, and sleep disorders tend to remain unaddressed for many years before they are diagnosed. Unrecognized sleep disorders can shorten lives, promote hypertension, diminish glucose control, exacerbate metabolic syndrome, increase overall medical care costs, impair cognition, cause motor vehicle crashes, reduce workplace productivity, and greatly diminish quality of life. Nonetheless, learning sleep medicine by reading a textbook remains unrealistic for many busy clinicians. In contrast, this edition in the Pitfalls case-based teaching series is designed to be more readable, easily assimilated, and memorable. Whether read cover-to-cover or selectively as needed in the context of daily practice, this volume is designed as a more enjoyable opportunity to learn how to investigate and manage common sleep problems that are encountered, whether recognized or not, by nearly every clinician who sees patients.

This book is for practicing physicians, fellows, residents, allied health professionals, and students with interest in conditions that affect sleep, daytime alertness, and circadian rhythms. The material covered should be particularly useful for clinicians in neurology, internal medicine, pulmonary medicine, family medicine, pediatrics, psychiatry, psychology, anesthesiology, dentistry, otolaryngology, and oral and maxillofacial surgery. The book should be an excellent resource for trainees in sleep medicine. Their mentors also will find the cases useful as departure points for group discussion or as illustrations to accompany more formal lectures. If this book has any underlying emphasis, beyond its topical focus on sleep and health, readers will find that it highlights the importance of a good medical history and clinical judgment, rather than test results, as the primary foundation for good patient care.

This book also differs from many others in the field in that it is completely case-based. Whereas some books use short cases to enliven didactic textbook material, this edition of the Pitfalls series focuses on more detailed cases worth thinking about, from sleep clinicians seasoned "in the trenches," supplemented with didactic review targeted specifically to the problems at hand. The chapters do not provide focused coverage of a complete sleep nosology, with facts to memorize for each diagnostic category. Rather, case discussions are built around potential pitfalls, real-world challenges, and frequent problems from clinical practice, with underlying pearls that in many instances might not otherwise become apparent to a practitioner except through years of trial and error. This book addresses some areas of controversy and others that still lack evidence-based guidelines. It seeks to impart perspectives of individual authors, but to clarify where practice is supported by published data or the best judgment of the writer.

The authors themselves are another defining feature of this volume. Each is a current or past faculty or trainee at the University of Michigan in Ann Arbor, where Michael S. Aldrich established one of the earliest sleep disorders centers in 1985. Today, the University of Michigan Center for Sleep Science ranks among the largest and most widely respected academic sleep programs in the United States. With 48 faculty members, from 14 departments and 5 different schools on a single campus, it represents a unique critical mass of investigators who have, over the years, advanced understanding of sleepiness, sleep-disordered breathing, narcolepsy, insomnia, parasomnias, sleep laboratory techniques, and research tools. They have published new insights on sleep in the context of epilepsy, stroke, multiple sclerosis, neurodegenerative disorders, headache, attention-deficit/hyperactivity disorder, craniofacial disorders, pregnancy, infancy, childhood, older age, depression, asthma, arrhythmia, pain, hospitalization, the perioperative setting, and many other conditions or circumstances. Much of this research has been nurtured by the robust clinical and educational programs at the University of Michigan Sleep Disorders Center, directed by Ronald D. Chervin since 2000. More than two-dozen highly multidisciplinary clinicians involved with the Center each year provide about 5000 patient visits, perform 7000 sleep studies, train 7 new sleep physicians, and mentor new sleep researchers. Many individuals who learned sleep medicine or sleep science at the University of Michigan now have highly successful academic careers themselves, hold key responsibilities in their professional societies, and play leading roles in education. This unique book now offers some of the collective wisdom culled from many current and past members of a large, diverse, and storied sleep program that has long held education in sleep medicine as one of its highest priorities.

Acknowledgements

I would like to thank my many exceptional colleagues who brought enthusiasm and energy, amidst busy schedules, to describe their experiences for this volume. I am grateful to them, as well as my own mentors in sleep medicine, including Drs. Christian Guilleminault, Michael Aldrich, Alex Clerk, and Charles Pollak, for the considerable effort they each made to share with me their own fascination with sleep, sleep disorders, and the impact they have on human health. I extend sincere thanks to Nicholas Dunton and Jane Seakins, at Cambridge University Press, and to Alice Nelson, whose expertise, support, and copy-editing skills made this book feasible. Here at the University of Michigan Sleep Disorders Center, many thanks must go to Ms. Sarina Davis, whose exceptional skills in organization, communication, coordination, and computer software have been invaluable. Finally, I am grateful to my wife, Dr. Stephanie Chervin, Abby, and Nathan, for their patience during the time I spent to complete this project.

Introduction: the complexity, challenges, and rewards of effective sleep medicine

Ronald D. Chervin

Patients with sleep disorders often present with difficulty sleeping at night, or with daytime sleepiness and related complaints during the day. Frequently, the two issues are intertwined. In a diagnostic evaluation, to understand a patient's sleepiness the clinician should ask the patient directly to what extent he or she feels sleepy, perceives a problem with sleepiness, has had motor vehicle crashes or near-misses, or has experienced sleepiness in other sedentary circumstances. Obtaining a sleep history from a family member is also important and sometimes yields different perspectives. However, the history can be supplemented by standardized subjective or objective tests. Such tests can help the clinician to arrive at a correct diagnosis, judge the impact of a sleep disorder, or assess responses to intervention over time. Standardized tests help to compare results between patients, or in the same patients across time. Results should not be interpreted in isolation from the history, and they do not by themselves often dictate clinical decision-making. The following case describes a patient with complex sleep-related issues, and illustrates in part how subjective and objective assessments may be useful, but also discrepant or – if interpreted in isolation – misleading. More broadly, this patient's history and outcome show that effective amelioration of a patient's sleep complaints, to the point that he or she experiences fully restored healthy sleep, can require a systematically broad approach, trial and error, continued care over some time, and persistence in addressing what often turns out to be multiple underlying causes of inadequate sleep and daytime consequences.

Case

A 46-year-old woman who worked as a dental assistant presented with the chief complaints of non-restorative sleep and nocturnal awakenings for the previous 10 years. She sometimes had difficulty with sleep maintenance, but even after nights when she had slept soundly, she did not feel that her sleep had been refreshing. Her difficulties with sleep seem to have coincided with having had children, spaced 2 years apart, and associated weight gain of about 20 pounds (9 kg) that she was not able to lose thereafter. She endorsed feeling "tired" more than "sleepy" or "fatigued." She reported occasional snoring and frequent mouth breathing, but no witnessed apneas. Her Epworth Sleepiness Scale showed a total score of 6 points on a scale that ranges from 0 to 24. She would typically turn out the lights at 10:00 PM, fall asleep in 30 minutes or less, and wake up at 7:00 AM. She would wake up often, up to every hour. She felt as if she "does not get into deep sleep." The time to fall back asleep after each awakening would be variable. She did not feel refreshed in the morning. During the night, when she could not sleep, she would sometimes have ruminating thoughts and concerns. When she woke up, she would often look at her alarm clock to see what time it was. She watched television and read in bed. On occasion she would have the sensation after getting into bed in the evening that she would have to move her legs. This sensation would be relieved by getting up and walking around. She endorsed a history of depression, anxiety, and irritable bowel syndrome. Her examination showed a weight of 137 pounds (62 kg), and a height of 5 feet (152 cm) with a neck circumference of 13.5 inches (34 cm). Her oral examination showed a crowded oropharynx with Mallampati Class IV, minimal overjet, and a normal hard palate. She had mild septal deviation to the left and normal turbinates, with no collapse of the external nasal valves on inhalation. A recent thyroid-stimulating hormone level and free thyroxine (T4) were normal.

What diagnostic considerations and tests could be considered for this patient?

Several diagnostic considerations are raised by this history. She appears to qualify for restless leg syndrome, a clinical diagnosis defined by four main features: a sensation of the need to move the legs; circadian worsening at night; worsening at rest; and improvement with movement. She may also have psychophysiologic insomnia, an extremely common condition in which chronic insomnia arises from excessive concern about sleep itself. Psychophysiologic insomnia is suggested, for example, by her tendency to watch the clock during the night. However, she also snores, has mouth breathing, and complains of tiredness if not sleepiness per se. Moreover, her exam also suggests a crowded oropharynx that is predisposed to repeated collapse during sleep, as occurs in obstructive sleep apnea. In practice, evaluation for obstructive sleep apnea often takes precedence over investigation for other causes of insomnia, mainly because sleep apnea raises the likelihood of long-range risk for serious medical consequences, including cardiovascular morbidity and mortality.

This patient was scheduled for polysomnography in a sleep laboratory. The test showed normal results however, with an apnea/hypopnea index (AHI, events per hour of sleep) of only 1.3, where concern for an adult would begin at values closer to 5. The minimum oxygen saturation was also normal at 91%.

What should be evaluated or treated next?

False negative results can occur, though not frequently, with gold standard nocturnal polysomnography performed to assess for obstructive sleep apnea. One option, especially for patients with high pretest suspicion, would be to repeat the testing. In this case, the pretest suspicion was not considered to have been sufficiently high, and this patient also had other possibilities to consider as causes for her complaints. The patient's serum ferritin level was 29 µg and lower than the thresholds (50–75 µg) usually used to indicate that supplemental iron for restless leg syndrome may be helpful. She was treated with supplemental iron and with ropinirole as needed for symptoms of restless legs. However, her symptoms were only occasional and were not thought to be primarily responsible for her complaints. She was therefore referred to a psychologist who specializes in sleep medicine and is certified to provide cognitive behavioral therapy for insomnia (CBT-I).

Data from well-designed clinical trials suggest that cognitive behavioral therapy for chronic, psychophysiologic insomnia is highly effective, and in comparison to hypnotics more likely to retain long-term effectiveness.[1,2] The CBT-I was administered over six sessions, one approximately every 2 weeks. She made considerable progress, and 10 months later on follow-up, she continued to report that her nighttime sleep was still quite good. She had minimal difficulties initiating and maintaining sleep, with only occasional exceptions when she was particularly anxious. Although she was clearly grateful for this improvement – she estimated that her insomnia was about 75% better – she still complained that she continued to experience tiredness, a lack of energy, and also excessive sleepiness during the daytime. She still endorsed occasional snoring, and mouth breathing. She noted that she had gained about 10 pounds (5 kg) since her last sleep study. Her Epworth Sleepiness Scale showed a total score of 9, where abnormal subjective sleepiness is often considered to be reflected by scores of 10 or higher. She provided a 1-week sleep diary that showed an average bedtime at 10:30 PM and rise time at 6:30 AM, with average wake after sleep onset of only

25 minutes, and a 12-minute sleep latency. Sleep efficiency (time asleep divided by time in bed) was at 87%, which was 12% higher than before CBT-I, and she was indicating a 30-minute gain in total sleep time each night.

Just give up?

The sleep psychologist, realizing that CBT-I had achieved its aims, yet the patient still complained of daytime tiredness, wisely decided to refer this patient back to a sleep medicine physician. Restless legs symptoms were still present, but relatively infrequent. Continued snoring and weight gain led to recommendations for another laboratory-based polysomnogram. As the patient was not quite obese, with a body mass index even after the weight gain of 29 kg/m^2, and moreover had received one negative polysomnogram already, esophageal pressure monitoring was added to the polysomnogram. Esophageal pressure monitoring provides a gold standard measure of the work of breathing and assessment of upper airway resistance. This assessment can be especially useful in thinner or younger individuals, and women in particular, who present with symptoms that suggest obstructive sleep apnea, but show few frank apneas or hypopneas on polysomnography. Some of these individuals have a narrowed upper airway during sleep, and exert considerable effort to breathe despite having few discrete periods of diminished breathing that can be detected by standard sleep laboratory methods. Research has shown that some patients who exert continual, steady effort to breathe during sleep can be sleepy during the day as a result, and respond to treatment with continuous positive airway pressure.[3] In fact, some research over the past 10 years suggests that snoring patients with labored breathing may activate the cerebral cortex on a breath-to-breath basis throughout the night, possibly causing excessive daytime sleepiness in this subtle but recurrent manner above and beyond the impact of frankly observable, longer arousals or awakenings.[4]

The repeat polysomnogram showed 16 apneas or hypopneas per hour of sleep and a minimum oxygen saturation of 92%. Esophageal pressures reached an excessive maximum negative value of –19 cm of water during inhalation, whereas in normal circumstances this nadir should be closer to –10 cm of water. A Multiple Sleep Latency Test (MSLT) was also performed the day after the polysomnography. This is a gold standard objective measure of daytime sleepiness, and can also be used to assist in the diagnosis of narcolepsy. The main outcomes are the mean sleep latency, across five nap attempts, scheduled every two hours during the daytime, as well as the number of nap attempts on which rapid eye movement (REM) sleep was recorded. Abnormal daytime sleepiness is supported by the finding of a mean sleep latency of < 8 minutes, and narcolepsy as suggested if this finding is accompanied by REM sleep on two or more of the nap attempts. This patient in fact showed a mean sleep latency of 3.5 minutes, consistent with severe daytime sleepiness. No sleep-onset REM periods were recorded during the naps.

Given the evidence for obstructive sleep apnea on the polysomnogram, the patient subsequently returned to the sleep laboratory for a continuous positive airway pressure (CPAP) titration study. Settings from 4 to 10 cm of water were applied, and subsequent review of the study suggested that 9 cm of water effectively treated this patient's obstructive sleep apnea. She obtained a CPAP machine for home use 2 weeks ago, at the time of this writing. She reported success at using the machine each night, for the entire night, with the exception of 2 nights. When using the machine, she no longer snored. Her bed partner reported that her sleep appears to be "much more peaceful, as if she has simply passed out for the entire night." She no longer kicked her legs during the night. She felt as if most of her insomnia had been treated by the CBT-I, and that now her sleep was completely sound when using CPAP. She no longer experienced the restless legs symptoms that used to warrant occasional use of ropinirole.

However, despite this progress, this patient continued to complain that she felt no more refreshed on awakening than she had before having CBT-I or using CPAP. She still complained of a "general fatigue" that could limit her daytime activities, and also a degree of sleepiness that could limit her ability to read or work at a computer for extended durations. She did endorse feeling as if her mind was "a little more clear" but was still somewhat disappointed that despite all the improvement in her sleep, which she very much appreciated, she still did not feel more refreshed on awakening or less fatigued during the day.

Discussion

The large majority, but not all patients with sleep disorders, after appropriate assessment and treatment, can experience complete or nearly complete resolution of their original complaints. Although this patient was much improved, her original complaints of non-restorative sleep and daytime fatigue did not respond, even after treatment for three sleep disorders: psycho-physiologic insomnia; restless legs syndrome; and obstructive sleep apnea. We do not know whether her MSLT, which originally showed prominent sleepiness, would now show improved results. One possible explanation for the lack of subjective improvement at her last visit is that she had not yet used the CPAP for an adequate period of time to judge its effects on her fatigue. Up to 2 or 3 months of consistent CPAP use may be necessary in some cases to fully assess the impact on daytime symptoms. The patient believed that in recent years her depression and anxiety were well controlled, with bupropion and citalopram. However, if she was mistaken, then depression could certainly contribute to daytime fatigue that might not respond to treatment of sleep disorders. That said, sleepiness caused by depression is generally less likely than primary sleep disorders to cause abnormal MSLT results.

Finally, this case history illustrates another interesting point that surfaces frequently in sleep medicine, as well as other sections of this book. Whereas her Epworth Sleepiness Scale, the most commonly used standardized assessment of subjective daytime sleepiness, reached only 9 points – below the threshold (10) often taken for initial concern about daytime sleepiness – her MSLT showed objective evidence of severe daytime sleepiness. The 1-page Epworth costs only pennies, and it takes only minutes for a patient to rate his or her own tendency to doze, under eight variably soporific circumstances. The questionnaire was initially validated by evidence that Epworth scores showed some correlation with MSLT results.[5] However, that correlation was not strong, and subsequent studies have often showed little or no correlation between the Epworth and the MSLT.[6] Discrepancies such as this, between subjective and objective measures, are common in sleep medicine, and may indicate that such measures assess somewhat different constructs. Our measures – either subjective or objective – are not always as definitive in clinical practice as many clinicians would like to believe. For this patient, in retrospect, her clinicians would have been misled had they interpreted her normal Epworth score, in isolation, as an indication that her complaints should be ignored, and that further investigation after CBT-I, for possible obstructive sleep apnea, was unnecessary. In this case, persistent effort to understand this patient's complaint led to a clear diagnosis of obstructive sleep apnea, despite the older normal study, and demonstration on an MSLT of objective evidence for excessive daytime sleepiness that was quite significant.

In practice, an MSLT is usually obtained (and sometimes covered by medical insurance) only when narcolepsy is a diagnostic consideration, or when an objective assessment of sleepiness can be argued to be vital. This may be the case when fatigue and sleepiness seem difficult to separate on history, risk exists for driving and especially public transport accidents, or sleepiness and related symptoms appear to have complicated etiologies or inadequate response to treatment, as in this case. In contrast, a simple subjective measure such as the Epworth Sleepiness Scale may be best suited for routine use during clinical evaluations, in a manner that can make such evaluations comparable between clinicians or across time and treatments. Both subjective and objective assessments of sleepiness may have separate appropriate uses, but they must always be interpreted within the context of a thorough clinical history. They cannot be assumed to provide concordant results or redundant information.

Lastly, they should rarely if ever be expected, in isolation, to guide clinical decision-making.

Main points

Complaints such as non-restorative sleep and daytime sleepiness or fatigue raise the possibility of underlying sleep disorders, which can be multifactorial. Assessment of sleepiness can be performed by standardized subjective methods, laboratory-based objective testing, or both, but such results must be evaluated in the context of the clinical history to best serve each individual patient. Sleep medicine is a complex field, with multidisciplinary roots, that offers substantial opportunity to improve the health and quality of life for many patients. Nonetheless, not all patients experience complete resolution of their symptoms, and considerable more research will be necessary before this field achieves its full potential to eliminate many intersecting problems with nocturnal sleep and daytime function.

REFERENCES

1. Edinger JD, Wohlgemuth WK, Radtke RA, Marsh GR, Quillian RE. Cognitive behavioral therapy for treatment of chronic primary insomnia: a randomized controlled trial. *JAMA* 2001;**285**:1856–64.
2. Morin CM, Vallieres A, Guay B, et al. Cognitive behavioral therapy, singly and combined with medication, for persistent insomnia: a randomized controlled trial. *JAMA* 2009;**301**:2005–15.
3. Guilleminault C, Stoohs R, Kim Y, et al. Upper airway sleep-disordered breathing in women. *Ann Intern Med* 1995;**122**:493–501.
4. Chervin RD, Burns JW, Ruzicka DL. Electroencephalographic changes during respiratory cycles predict sleepiness in sleep apnea. *Am J Respir Crit Care Med* 2005;**171**:652–8.
5. Johns MW. A new method for measuring daytime sleepiness: the Epworth Sleepiness Scale. *Sleep* 1991;**14**:540–5.
6. Chervin RD, Aldrich MS. The Epworth Sleepiness Scale may not reflect objective measures of sleepiness or sleep apnea. *Neurology* 1999;**52**:125–31.

Sleepiness versus fatigue, tiredness, and lack of energy

In the field of sleep medicine, few issues are more critical than daytime sleepiness. Hypersomnolence represents the borderland between sleep and full alertness, and is important to recognize as one of the most common indications that nocturnal sleep has not been fully restorative. Sleep, which is critical to life, in essence tries to impose itself into wakefulness. Unfortunately, recognition of sleepiness is not always as simple as it sounds. As it usually develops insidiously, patients often are unaware that they are affected, or that everyone else does not feel the same. Moreover, patients choose many different words other than sleepiness – words often less clearly associated with sleep disorders, in the minds of their physicians – to describe their main complaints. This means that early in the process of obtaining a history, physicians can be misled into pursuing investigations and possible etiologies that deviate considerably from the true source of the problem.

This first section of the book, therefore, presents several cases that highlight a too-often non descript basket of terms, including sleepiness, fatigue, tiredness, and lack of energy, that often remain insufficiently understood or clarified by the clinicians who try to help the innumerable patients presenting with one or more of these issues as their chief complaint. The authors of these cases, each a neurologist whose clinical practice or research focuses on sleep, help to clarify how clinicians can distinguish between different sleepiness-related symptoms, as well as what can or cannot be assumed to underlie these symptoms. Some sleep disorders may be more likely than others to produce a complaint of sleepiness, as opposed to related constructs. Finally, some neurologic and other conditions may produce sleepiness and the other symptoms simultaneously. Fortunately, in some cases, standardized or objective testing, as discussed in the second section of this book, can provide some clarification. A thorough history and appropriate interpretation of any testing obtained are important because, in most cases, sleepiness, fatigue, tiredness, and lack of energy can all be improved by appropriate diagnosis and treatment for an underlying sleep disorder.

2

How to distinguish between sleepiness, fatigue, tiredness, and lack of energy

Anita Valanju Shelgikar

Case

A 40-year-old woman presented to the sleep clinic for evaluation of "daytime fatigue." This symptom began insidiously 4 years ago, but has been worsening over the past 18 months. Her main concern was that her "sluggish fatigue and unrefreshing sleep make me unmotivated to get my work done."

She reported that until 18 months prior to presentation, she felt her sleep quality was "reasonable" but since that time has "not been as deep" with approximately three awakenings for nocturia each night. She reported a bedtime of midnight, sleep latency of < 15 minutes, ability to resume sleep quickly after each nocturnal awakening, and wake time between 7:30 and 9:30 AM. She denied feeling refreshed upon awakening, and experienced persistent tiredness throughout the day.

Her Epworth Sleepiness Scale score was 3 out of 24; she reported a chance of dozing only while watching television or lying down in the afternoon. She previously tried multiple over-the-counter sleep aids, including melatonin and valerian root. She endorsed caffeine intake of one beverage daily, and started dextroamphetamine/amphetamine 20–30 mg daily for a diagnosis of possible attention-deficit/hyperactivity disorder. She continued to take bupropion, started 12 years ago, and attended counseling for management of a mood disorder.

Since onset of her fatigue 4 years ago, she had gained 30 pounds (14 kg), which she attributed to "eating to help stay awake." She reported rare snoring, witnessed apneas, and a sore throat upon awakening. She endorsed nasal congestion 2–4 nights per week and reported that her legs felt restless 3 times per month. This leg discomfort worsened in the evening, was associated with a strong urge to move, and transiently improved with walking. She reported occasional auditory hypnogogic hallucinations, described as a "loud bang that was not a real sound," along with occasional sleep paralysis, but denied hypnopompic hallucinations or cataplexy.

Past medical history included migraine headaches, depression, possible attention-deficit/hyperactivity disorder, and positive antinuclear antibody (ANA) without clinical manifestations of rheumatic disease. She continued to be followed by a rheumatologist. Medications included magnesium oxide, onabotulinumtoxinA injections for migraine headache, dextroamphetamine/amphetamine, bupropion, vitamin D3, folic acid, glucosamine, oral contraceptive, multivitamin, and valacyclovir.

Physical examination was notable for a body mass index (BMI) of 30.4 kg/m^2, a crowded oral airway, and a high-arched palate.

What evaluation was done and what was the diagnosis?

Limited serologic evaluation to assess for endocrinologic etiologies included a thyroid-stimulating hormone

Table 2.1 Key historical features of case

- Daytime fatigue for 4 years, worsening over 18 months
- Non-restorative sleep
- Use of stimulant medication
- Eating to stay awake, with subsequent 30-pound (14-kg) weight gain
- Decreased motivation
- Rare snoring and witnessed apneas
- Comorbid migraine headache and depression

(TSH) level of 1.96 mIU/l and a vitamin D level of 75 ng/ml, both of which were within normal limits. The patient was also advised to maintain follow-up with her psychiatrist for continued management of her mood disorder.

Table 2.1 highlights the key historical points raised by this patient. The clinical history suggested some features of sleep-disordered breathing, such as snoring, frequent nocturnal awakenings, and non-restorative sleep. Her oropharyngeal anatomy may have also increased the likelihood of sleep-disordered breathing in this patient. A baseline polysomnogram was obtained, with esophageal pressure (Pes) monitoring to quantitatively assess upper airway resistance. This study showed a total sleep time of 151 minutes, sleep latency of 29.5 minutes, and sleep efficiency of 42.9%. The apnea/hypopnea index (AHI, events per hour of sleep) measured 0.3 per hour of sleep, the respiratory effort-related arousal (RERA) index measured 0 per hour, and minimum oxygen saturation was 91%. The Pes signal was only reliable during one period of sustained non-REM sleep, during which esophageal pressures ranged from –8 to –17 cm of water as shown in Figure 2.1. Her periodic limb movement index was 15.9 per hour. The final study interpretation noted these findings to be suggestive of increased upper airway resistance, although the findings did not meet criteria for obstructive sleep apnea.

Discussion

Fatigue is reported in myriad medical and psychiatric conditions. Patients with depression, multiple sclerosis, congestive heart failure, fibromyalgia, cirrhosis (just to name a few) may endorse fatigue. This symptom is often attributed to a number of potential etiologies, such as a medication side effect, reduced exercise tolerance, or changes in dietary intake. Fatigue can profoundly impact a patient's quality of life through its effects on mood, job performance, and independence with activities of daily living. Patients with fatigue often undergo basic metabolic and endocrinology evaluations; if these are unrevealing, it is not uncommon for these patients to be referred for sleep medicine consultation.

Excessive daytime sleepiness, also a feature of many disparate conditions, can likewise have a negative impact on a patient's mood, job performance, and interpersonal relationships. As a result of motor vehicle crashes and other disasters that occur with loss of consciousness, daytime sleepiness also poses a significant public health risk. Given similarities in functional consequences of fatigue and sleepiness, discrimination between the two can be challenging. Traditional teaching distinguishes fatigue as a physical tiredness or lack of energy and sleepiness as propensity to doze or fall asleep.[1] Sleepiness is generally caused by an alteration or imbalance in sleep–wake mechanisms; fatigue may arise from the same factors, but can be caused by others as well.[2] Providers often ask a number of questions to categorize the patient's symptoms as either fatigue or sleepiness. However, consideration of these entities as mutually exclusive may hinder formulation of an accurate differential diagnosis and management plan.

Simple questions about when symptoms are worst – for example, after 2 hours of shopping, or 1 hour of sedentary reading – may help to distinguish fatigue from sleepiness. Some patients, though, are not detailed historians. Lack of collaborative history can further confound determination of the patient's primary symptom. Significant research has focused on fatigue, sleepiness, and even the interplay between the two. However, substantial variability remains in definitions of these two entities. Some studies define fatigue and daytime sleepiness as distinct entities, while others use the terms interchangeably. Formal study of these symptoms has been facilitated only to

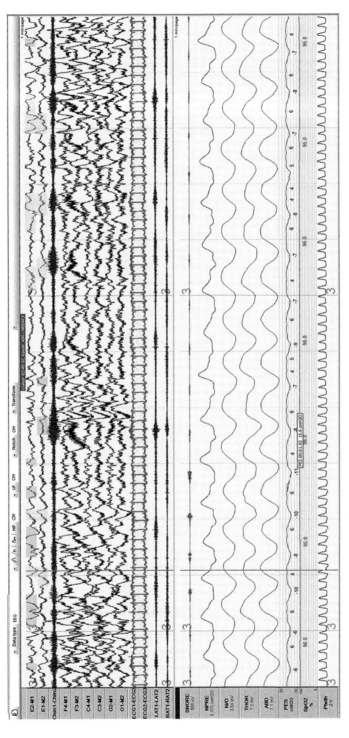

Figure 2.1 Baseline polysomnogram with esophageal pressure (Pes) monitoring. The Pes values suggest increased resistance of the upper airway, with pressure swings up to 15 cm of water shown. Pressure swings greater than about 10 cm of water often raise concern. The recording montage includes the following leads: central (C3-M2, C4-M1), frontal (F3-M2, F4-M1), and occipital (O1-M2, O2-M1) electroencephalograms; left and right eye electrooculograms (E1-M2, E2-M1); mental/submental electromyogram (Chin1-Chin2); electrocardiogram (ECG1-ECG2, ECG2-ECG3); left and right eye electromyograms (LAT1-LAT2, RAT1-RAT2); snore volume (SNORE); nasal pressure transducer (NPRE); nasal/oral airflow (N/O); thoracic (THOR) and abdominal (ABD) effort; esophageal pressure (PES); arterial oxyhemoglobin saturation (SpO2); and plethysmography (Pleth). See plate section for color version.

a limited extent by objective measures. The Multiple Sleep Latency Test (MSLT) is a validated objective measure of the ability or tendency to fall asleep, and is often used in the assessment of daytime sleepiness. While the MSLT is considered the gold standard for objective measurement of sleepiness, there remains no systematically collected data on normative values for mean sleep latency.[3] A validated, measurable biomarker of fatigue has yet to be determined, which leaves much room for variability in the definition and identification of fatigue.

Subjective questionnaires are often used in the clinical assessment of daytime sleepiness, and are used less often in the evaluation of fatigue. Of the multiple validated questionnaires available for subjective assessment of daytime sleepiness, the Epworth Sleepiness Scale[4] is the most widely used. This tool provides the respondent with a four-point Likert scale to assess the likelihood of dozing in eight distinct sedentary situations in recent times. The total score varies between 0 and 24, with scores of 10 or more raising concern (progressively) for subjective daytime sleepiness. Although concordance between Epworth scores and objective measurements of sleepiness is not strong, the Epworth can be a useful, cost-efficient tool for longitudinal use in a given individual.

The Fatigue Severity Scale[5] was initially used for multiple sclerosis and systemic lupus erythematosus patients. This questionnaire employs a seven-point Likert scale, ranging from "Strongly Disagree" to "Strongly Agree" for the ratings of statements about the effect of fatigue on mood and physical function. The Fatigue Severity Scale is a validated tool that differentiates between healthy controls and individuals with fatigue. Like the Epworth Sleepiness Scale, the Fatigue Severity Scale can be used in the clinical setting to track changes in a patient's score over time. Although the Epworth Sleepiness Scale is more commonly used in sleep medicine clinics, there may be a role for use of the Fatigue Severity Scale, particularly in certain patient populations. Table 2.2 summarizes some of the subjective and objective assessment tools that can be considered in the evaluation of sleepiness and fatigue.

Table 2.2 Subjective and objective assessment instruments that are often used in the evaluation of patients who complain of daytime sleepiness or fatigue

- Epworth Sleepiness Scale
- Fatigue Severity Scale
- Nocturnal polysomnography
- Multiple Sleep Latency Test

This patient reports "fatigue" as her chief complaint, and describes multiple medical and social factors that contribute to this symptom. While she does endorse physical tiredness, she also reports poor sleep quality and non-restorative sleep. She does not explicitly complain of daytime sleepiness, and her Epworth Sleepiness Scale score is low. However, she makes reference to inability to stay awake without medication or non-pharmacologic intervention (e.g. eating). In fact, her use of a pharmacologic stimulant (i.e. dextroamphetamine/amphetamine) and caffeine may mask some of her daytime symptoms, including sleepiness. Categorization of the patient's daytime symptoms is further confounded by her comorbid mood disorder, which is commonly associated with sleep disturbance. Her frequent nocturnal awakenings and non-restorative sleep, in the setting of her physical findings of obesity and a crowded oral airway, suggest that there may be undiagnosed sleep-disordered breathing as well. In this patient, symptoms of fatigue and sleepiness may, in fact, coexist. It is difficult to ascertain clearly distinct etiologies for each symptom, and some of her comorbidities may contribute to both symptoms. These considerations should be taken into account in medical decision-making and in formulation of a multifaceted treatment plan.

Main points

Fatigue and sleepiness are sometimes clues to different underlying conditions. However, these symptoms can also coexist and have additive effects on a patient's daytime functioning. Historical information, and particularly discussion of the contexts in which symptoms occur, may help elucidate the underlying etiology. The clinician should realize that patients may use these terms inter-changeably, and a broad differential diagnosis should be entertained during the diagnostic evaluation.

REFERENCES

1. Ancoli-Israel S, Savard J. Sleep and fatigue in cancer patients. In Kryger M, Roth T, Dement W, eds. *Principles and Practice of Sleep Medicine*, Fifth Edition. St Louis, MO: Elsevier;2010, pp. 1416–21.

2. Shen J, Barbera J, Shapiro CM. Distinguishing sleepiness and fatigue: focus on definition and measurement. *Sleep Med Rev* 2006;**10**:63–76.

3. Littner MR, Kushida C, Wise M, et al. Practice parameters for clinical use of the Multiple Sleep Latency Test and the Maintenance of Wakefulness Test. *Sleep* 2005;**28**:113–21.

4. Johns MW. A new method for measuring daytime sleepiness: the Epworth Sleepiness Scale. *Sleep* 1991;**14**:540–5.

5. Krupp LB, LaRocca NG, Muir-Nash J, Steinberg AD. The fatigue severity scale. Application to patients with multiple sclerosis and systemic lupus erythematosus. *Arch Neurol* 1989;**46**:1121–3.

3

A patient with prominent fatigue, tiredness, or lack of energy rather than sleepiness may still have a sleep disorder

Sarah Nath Zallek

Case

A 79-year-old man presented with "tiredness" and "decreased stamina" for the past 5 months. He had gained about 20 pounds (9 kg) over the preceding year. He reported a regular sleep schedule of about 7.5 hours a night. His wife heard him snore most nights, often loudly, but had not noticed him to stop breathing in his sleep. He had no difficulty initiating or maintaining sleep. Sleeping did not relieve his symptoms.

He denied feeling sleepy during his waking hours, and reported napping only rarely. His Epworth Sleepiness Scale score was 4 out of a possible 24 points. His Fatigue Severity Scale score was a 47 out of a possible 63 points. When asked to rate his sleepiness on a typical day, he reported a 2 on a scale of 0–10. He rated his fatigue on a typical day at 9 on a scale of 0–10.

He stated his mood was good, he was happily married, and he was enjoying retirement. He admitted to drinking one to two cups of coffee each day and one alcoholic beverage most evenings.

Past medical history included hypertension, tonsillectomy, colon cancer (in remission), and hyperlipidemia. Medications included terazosin, hydrochlorothiazide, atorvastatin, and topical testosterone.

On examination, he was mildly overweight, with a body mass index of 27 kg/m^2. His neck circumference was 17 inches (43 cm). He had a Class 1 dental occlusion (normal, without retrognathia or prognathia), a large uvula, and a long soft palate. The remainder of the general examination and the neurologic examination were unremarkable.

What is the differential diagnosis for his presenting symptoms of "tiredness" and "decreased stamina"?

These symptoms have many causes, including hematologic, metabolic, psychosocial, inflammatory, neoplastic, iatrogenic, and nutritional abnormalities. An exhaustive work up could be very inefficient and costly. As with any presenting symptom, a focused approach, guided by the details of the history and examination, is appropriate. His history of colon cancer raises a question of anemia. Complete blood count, electrolytes, hepatic and renal function prior to the sleep evaluation were normal. Depression can be associated with fatigue, but this patient's history does not suggest it. Hypothyroidism is common and can cause fatigue as a primary symptom. Thyroid-stimulating hormone was normal. His recent weight gain and onset of snoring raise a question of obstructive sleep apnea.

A polysomnogram recorded severe obstructive sleep apnea with an apnea/hypopnea index of 52 apneas or hypopneas per hour of sleep. A continuous positive airway pressure (CPAP) titration study was performed, after which he used CPAP at home on 100% of nights, for 7 hours per night on average according to data downloaded from his machine after the first 2 months.

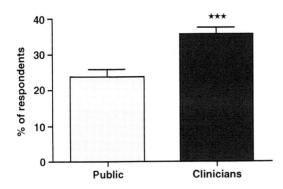

Figure 3.1 Percentage of respondents who chose drowsy when asked: "When you feel sleepy you feel _____?" *** indicates $P < 0.0001$; INI Sleep Center, unpublished data.

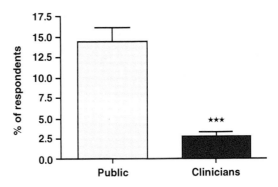

Figure 3.2 Percentage of respondents who answered "sleepiness" when asked: "Fatigue is best defined as _____?" *** indicates $P < 0.0001$; INI Sleep Center, unpublished data.

His "tiredness" and "decreased stamina" persisted, however. A CPAP mask leak was noted on the downloaded data, and once corrected, his symptoms resolved. His Epworth Sleepiness Scale score remained minimal and unchanged at 4, and his self-rated sleepiness on a typical day was unchanged at 2 (his response to a single question asking him to rate his sleepiness, on a typical day, on a scale of 0–10). However, his Fatigue Severity Scale score was reduced to 28. He rated his fatigue on a typical day at 1 on a scale of 0–10.

Discussion

Defining the symptom in any patient presentation is important. The use of language and the description of the symptom itself are both helpful to consider when one aims to determine exactly what the patient is experiencing.

Patients and clinicians use and hear the words sleepy, tired, fatigue, lack of energy, and other terms in quite variable ways. Each of these has some unique connotations, but their use may overlap and a complaint of one symptom may reflect an issue that the clinician does not suspect. Sometimes these terms are used very differently by patients to describe discreet symptoms that are specific to the way they feel. Distinguishing between them is possible through careful history and clarification of their intended meaning.

In a survey of 1073 people, 692 of whom were clinicians (physicians, advanced practice nurses, and nurses) and 381 of whom were lay persons (236 general public and 145 sleep center patients), significant differences were found in the ways each group defined various terms that refer to sleepiness or fatigue. For example, clinicians were more apt than the public (35% vs. 23%) to finish the statement, "When you feel sleepy you feel ____" with the word "drowsy" when choosing from a list of words (Figure 3.1). The public were more likely than clinicians (14% vs. 3%) to choose the word sleepiness to complete the statement, "Fatigue is best defined as ___" (Figure 3.2).

When this patient reported feeling tired, he might have meant a lack of physical or mental energy, or he could have meant he was sleepy. Making the distinction can be helpful in guiding the work up. In this patient's case, he specifically denied feeling sleepy or napping during the day. He also rated his fatigue much higher than sleepiness on two different types of rating scales.

Clarification could also have been made by asking the patient to further describe how he feels. For example, if he reports the symptom improving upon resting while awake, he is more likely to be referring to fatigue. If the symptom is temporarily alleviated by physical activity, he is more likely to be referring to sleepiness. Similarly, if he were to report a feeling of an urge to go to sleep, or relief of the symptom by sleeping, then he would be referring to sleepiness.

Features of the history that would raise a question of obstructive sleep apnea include snoring, particularly if frequent or loud, and witnessed apnea. Absence of either does not exclude the possibility of apnea, but their presence in the history is supportive.

Snoring may either be absent or go unnoticed. Bed partners sometimes do not notice snoring if they themselves are "sound sleepers," if the snoring is soft, or if they have hearing limitations. The history should also include whether the bed partner sleeps at the same times as the patient. People who work opposite shifts but share a bed might not actually be in bed at the same time often enough to observe the other's sleep. The apparent "bed partner" sometimes doesn't sleep in the same bed or bedroom as the patient. Patients who have no bed partner may report "no snoring" only because they are not aware of it themselves. So, a lack of snoring does not preclude a diagnosis of sleep apnea. Similarly, while witnessed apnea can be fairly specific for obstructive sleep apnea, it is not very sensitive. Cessation of breathing may be subtle and is quite easily missed by an observer.

Another clue to obstructive sleep apnea in the patient with fatigue is weight gain that preceded or coincided with the development of fatigue. Weight gain can narrow the upper airway and lead to sleep apnea, even if the weight gain is modest. Asking carefully about the timing of weight gain can help determine whether it was likely to have provoked sleep apnea and development of fatigue.

This patient's use of caffeine may have masked the symptom of sleepiness. He may have had an underlying increased drive to sleep that he did not perceive because of the underlying effects of caffeine. In any case, fatigue was his primary symptom.

Once the clinician understands the symptom, in whatever words the patient uses, he or she should clarify that symptom with the patient and use language the patient can relate to. For example, this patient complains of tiredness and decreased stamina, and he denies any urge to sleep or relief from symptoms after sleeping. He clearly describes a symptom other than sleepiness. With recognition of the actual symptom – in this case fatigue, not sleepiness – the clinician can reflect this back to the patient, distinguish it from

other symptoms, and continue to use words familiar to the patient in order to address the problem at hand. In this case, the clinician and patient agree the symptom of tiredness and lack of stamina represent a form of fatigue, and that the patient's words will be used to mean that when they discuss his care.

This may seem like linguistic acrobatics just to identify something seemingly so straightforward as fatigue or sleepiness, but it is a worthy investment and becomes natural over time. Confusing one symptom for another by hearing a word a clinician thinks means one thing, but the patient thinks means another, can misdirect the subsequent evaluation. Then again, using words patients cannot relate to, or believe do not reflect their symptoms, may keep them from knowing they have been understood. If the patient says he or she is tired, and the clinician determines this to mean sleepy, then he or she can call the symptom tiredness, agree on what it means, and aim to treat it.

Fatigue may be the most common symptom presenting in primary care, with a prevalence of 7–45%.[1] As the differential diagnosis is so broad, a careful history as described above is required to narrow the differential and carry out a prudent and efficient evaluation. In this case, obstructive sleep apnea was suggested by the history and was diagnosed with polysomnography.

The presence of greater fatigue than sleepiness can be helpful in discerning the cause. In a study of 462 adults, 121 with narcolepsy and 341 with obstructive sleep apnea, subjects with more fatigue than sleepiness were much more likely to have obstructive sleep apnea than narcolepsy. Those who rated sleepiness higher had an increased risk of narcolepsy. In other words, presenting with fatigue more than sleepiness makes a diagnosis obstructive sleep apnea much more likely than narcolepsy.[2]

Sleep disorders other than obstructive sleep apnea may also present with fatigue rather than sleepiness. Night or rotating shift work can lead to shift work-related sleep disorder, with circadian misalignment. Difficulty sleeping at desired times and excessive sleepiness during work hours are common. Fatigue can also occur, as shown in a study of nurses working 12-hour shifts.[3] Patients with insomnia often report significant daytime fatigue while being unable to sleep even if they lie down to nap.[4]

Quantifying fatigue can be challenging. The severity of fatigue and sleepiness can be described in words (such as mild or severe) by patients and followed over time. However, measuring those symptoms and quantifying change in a more standard manner can be especially helpful for a clinician. Ideally, the symptoms would be measured objectively. Objective measures for sleepiness do exist, but none has been developed to quantify fatigue.

Fortunately, a number of subjective rating scales are available to assess the degree of fatigue and sleepiness. The Multidimensional Fatigue Inventory (MFI-20) is a 5-point Likert scale questionnaire with subscales of general fatigue, physical fatigue, reduced activity, reduced motivation, and mental fatigue. The Chalder Fatigue Scale assesses mental and physical fatigue separately. The Fatigue Severity Scale asks nine questions to assess severity of fatigue.

Fatigue can improve with treatment of obstructive sleep apnea. In a study of 313 patients with obstructive sleep apnea, 183 used CPAP $\geq$ 5 hours per night, whereas 96 used it less or not at all; those who were adherent to CPAP reported less fatigue, tiredness, lack of energy, and sleepiness.[5] Cruz et al.[6] reported that the use of nasal automatic positive airway pressure controlled several symptoms of sleep-disordered breathing other than sleepiness, including fatigue. In another study of 164 patients with obstructive sleep apnea, fatigue improved with CPAP use, even among 89 subjects who were fatigued but not sleepy prior to treatment.[7] In the case presented in this chapter, the diagnosis of obstructive sleep apnea does not itself determine the cause of the symptoms. The relief of the patient's symptoms after effective treatment for the sleep apnea, however, makes a more convincing argument that the sleep disorder was the etiology.

Main points

Some sleep disorders can present with fatigue, tiredness, or lack of energy separate from sleepiness. Distinguishing between symptoms of sleepiness and other

symptoms may help to guide the diagnosis. For example, although many patients with obstructive sleep apnea do complain about sleepiness, at a sleep disorders center, patients with fatigue and not sleepiness are more likely to have obstructive sleep apnea than narcolepsy. Shift work-related sleep disorder and insomnia can also present with fatigue. The use of words to describe symptoms varies among patients and can differ between patients and clinicians, and a careful history is necessary to understand the symptom. Fatigue and other related symptoms besides sleepiness can improve with treatment of obstructive sleep apnea.

FURTHER READING

Malow, BA. Approach to the patient with disordered sleep. In Kryger M, Roth T, Dement W, eds. *Principles and Practice of Sleep Medicine*, Fifth Edition. St Louis, MO: Elsevier;2010, pp. 589–93.

REFERENCES

1. Shadid A, Shena J, Shapiro C. Measurements of sleepiness and fatigue. *J Psychosom Res* 2010;**69**:81–9.
2. Valerio TD, Fisk HL, Chervin RD, Zallek SN. Rating subjective fatigue greater than sleepiness predicts sleep apnea over narcolepsy; greater sleepiness is not predictive. *Sleep Abstract Supplement* 2005;**28**:A205.
3. Geiger-Brown J, Rogers VE, Trinkoff AM, et al. Sleep, sleepiness, fatigue, and performance of 12-hour-shift nurses. *Chronobiol Int* 2012;**29**:211–19.
4. Moul DE, Nofzinger EA, Pilkonis PA, et al. Symptom reports in severe chronic insomnia. *Sleep* 2002;**25**:548–58.
5. Chotinaiwattarakul W, O'Brien LM, Fan L, Chervin RD. Fatigue, tiredness, and lack of energy improve with treatment for OSA. *J Clin Sleep Med* 2009;**5**:222–7.
6. Cruz IA, Drummond M, Winck JC. Obstructive sleep apnea symptoms beyond sleepiness and snoring: effects of nasal APAP therapy. *Sleep Breath* 2012;**16**:361–6.
7. Zallek SN, Fisk HL, Chervin RD. Fatigue improves independently of sleepiness in treatment of sleep apnea. *Sleep Abstract Supplement* 2005;**28**:A201.

4

Fatigue, tiredness, and lack of energy, not just sleepiness, can improve considerably when a sleep disorder is treated

Wattanachai Chotinaiwattarakul

Sleep disorders are common in the general population and can contribute to impaired occupational performance, accidents at work or while driving, and disturbances of mood and social adjustment. A disturbance in sleep is frequently manifested as an intrusion of components of the sleep state into periods of wakefulness or vice versa and can result in a wide range of symptoms. Most patients referred to sleep centers present with one or a combination of three classic complaints: excessive daytime sleepiness; difficulty attaining or sustaining sleep; or snoring, abnormal movements, behaviors, or sensations during sleep or during nocturnal awakenings. These symptoms can be easily recognized as related to sleep and are not mutually exclusive. A given sleep disorder may be associated with more than one type of complaint. More subtle complaints, such as morning headache, difficulty concentrating, fatigue, tiredness, and lack of energy, may convey clues to the underlying pathology and sometimes indicate a potential sleep disorder.

Obstructive sleep apnea syndrome (OSAS) is found in up to 10% of the general population. Classic complaints in OSAS include excessive daytime sleepiness, loud snoring, gasping or choking at night, and witnessed apneas. Instead of self-reporting sleepiness, however, many OSAS patients may prefer other words to describe what affects them most prominently. Their chief complaints can be expressed as fatigue, tiredness, or lack of energy rather than sleepiness itself.

As in other fields of medicine, the foundation for the diagnosis of sleep disorders – especially OSAS – is the history of sleep complaints, risk factors, and medical comorbidities. A complete physical examination is required with special attention to body habitus and the upper airway. Fatigue, tiredness, and lack of energy can be caused by many different sleep disorders. Before possible OSAS is evaluated in patients with these chief complaints, several aspects such as sleep–wake history, circadian rhythm, and work load should be assessed. Finally, confirmation of a diagnosis of OSAS requires objective assessment of breathing during sleep.

Case

A 32-year-old architect sought medical attention mainly because of a 1-year history of fatigue that occurred almost every day. He felt physical and mental exhaustion that did not have any obvious trigger. He reported that his concentration and memory were not as good as they used to be. He was concerned that he lacked the energy to accomplish his work. He tried to exercise regularly in order to reduce fatigue, and he increased the amount of rest he obtained. He had a history of snoring for the past 10–15 years, and his wife had observed that his snoring disturbed her almost every night and seemed to increase in volume whenever he was in the supine position. She also reported he had a history of observed apneic episodes. On careful screening with structured sleep questionnaires and interviews, he reported having no history of

Common Pitfalls in Sleep Medicine, ed. Ronald D. Chervin. Published by Cambridge University Press. © Cambridge University Press 2014.

bruxism, sweating, coughing, gasping, choking, or excessive movements in bed. There was no history of cataplexy, autonomic behaviors, hypnagogic/hypno-pompic hallucinations, sleep paralysis, restless legs, periodic limb movement symptoms, frequent night-mares, night terrors, sleepwalking, or any unusual behaviors at night. The patient went to bed around 10:00 PM and fell asleep usually within 15 minutes without the use of hypnotics. He was aware of having on average one awakening at night after which he returned to sleep easily. He usually woke up at 7:00 AM every day. He favored sleeping on his side. He usually did not feel refreshed upon awakening and it took some time to feel fully awake. He took no daytime nap. His Epworth Sleepiness Scale score was borderline at 9 (on a scale of 0–24) but he reported several occasions of drowsiness while driving. He had no significant recent weight gain. He consumed three cups of coffee daily. No evidence of problems with alcohol or psychotropic medications was documented.

On physical examination, he was well-developed, slightly thin, and in no distress. His blood pressure was 152/86 mmHg, he weighed 168 pounds (76 kg), and was 5 feet, 6 inches (168 cm) tall (a body mass index of 26.5 kg/m^2). The patient's neck circumference was 16.5 inches (42 cm) and was supple with no thyromegaly or lymphadenopathy. Upper airway exam revealed a modified Mallampati Class IV classification. He had a narrow, high-arched hard palate. The tonsil grading score was 2+ bilat-erally. Neurologic examination was normal. The remainder of the physical examination was unremarkable.

What testing should be obtained and what is the diagnosis?

Fatigue is a common symptom and can also be associ-ated with a wide range of causes. About two-thirds of patients with fatigue will have an identifiable cause that can be elucidated with a careful history and appropriate laboratory tests. Endocrinologic, meta-bolic, and rheumatic disorders such as diabetes mellitus, cardiac failure, renal failure, liver failure, post organ transplantation, fibromyalgia, and psychiatric disease such as depression can be associated with fatigue without other significant complaints. Screening investigations to consider include full blood count and erythrocyte sedimentation rate, urea and electrolytes including calcium, blood sugar, liver function tests, thyroid function tests, and urinalysis. In addition, pri-mary sleep disorders must be considered, remember-ing that they are common. Factors to explore include time awake (sleep–wake history), time of day (circa-dian rhythm), and workload (time on task, task inten-sity, and task complexity). A sleep diary and structured interviews can be helpful.

The history of this patient provides several import-ant clues that point to a diagnosis of obstructive sleep apnea. First, the patient reports driving problems and unrefreshing sleep. Although his Epworth Sleepiness Scale is just within the normal range, significant day-time sleepiness may still be detected if the patient is asked directly whether sleepiness is a major problem or concern. Second, the patient and his wife began noticing problems of an increased volume of snoring, especially in the supine position, and witnessed apnea. Third, the upper airway is constricted, based on exam findings. Finally, all information or other possible causes is unrevealing.

Polysomnographic testing is a gold standard for diagnosis of sleep-related breathing disorders. It can reveal the type and severity, and guide appropriate treatment. Distinguishing sleepiness from fatigue can be difficult for clinicians. The Multiple Sleep Latency Test (MSLT) can be helpful to assess for objective evidence of daytime sleepiness. However, an MSLT is not indicated for routine evaluation of sleep-related breathing disorders. The MSLT is usually used as part of a clinical evaluation for patients with suspected narcolepsy.

This patient underwent polysomnography that showed 335 minutes of sleep time, with 198 minutes in the supine position. The study also showed a total of 182 apneic events, including 21 obstructive apneas, 159 obstructive hypopneas, and 2 central apneas. He had an overall apnea/hypopnea index (AHI, events per hour of sleep) of 32.6 apneic events per hour of sleep, consistent with severe OSAS. His supine AHI was 40.0 per hour. When on his side, the AHI was 21.9 per hour. His oxygen saturation fell from a baseline of 95% to a low of 79% during supine rapid eye movement (REM) sleep. In the lateral position, the lowest oxygen saturation was 91%. No MLST was performed.

What options should be considered for treatment?

Continuous positive airway pressure (CPAP) is usually the treatment of choice for OSAS, especially in moderate to severe cases. Home use of CPAP is also appropriate treatment for mild OSAS in symptomatic patients. The main limitations to CPAP use are the patient's acceptance and tolerance of treatment. The patient described above underwent in-laboratory CPAP titration to determine what level of pressure would provide the most effective control of his OSAS. During the titration study, the CPAP was titrated up from 4 cmH$_2$O pressure. At 12 cmH$_2$O pressure, even in REM sleep, CPAP prevented snoring and respiratory

events while supine, and maintained oxygen saturation at 90–95%.

When this patient was seen again 3 months later, after using the CPAP device on average for 5.5 hours each night, he noticed that his fatigue was markedly improved, and he regained a sense of sufficient energy. His Epworth Sleepiness Scale score was reduced to 4. No driving problem occurred. His well-being returned to normal in his view.

Discussion

Excessive daytime sleepiness, loud snoring, gasping or choking at night, and witnessed apneas are common complaints in OSAS. However, patients with polysomnographically confirmed OSAS may use other terms to express their chief complaints; fatigue, tiredness, or lack of energy are particularly common. In one study, the proportion of patients who preferred the term sleepiness to describe their chief complaints was about 22%, while about 40% preferred lack of energy, 18% preferred fatigue, and 20% preferred tiredness (Figure 4.1).[1]

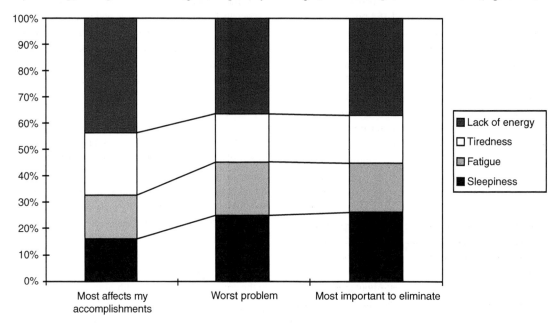

Figure 4.1 Frequency of terms as primary complaints among 190 patients with obstructive sleep apnea. Reproduced with permission from Chervin RD.[1]

Table 4.1 Reported symptom improvement (change from "*symptomatic*" to "*not symptomatic*") among positive airway pressure-adherent (PAP-adherent) and inadequately treated patients with obstructive sleep apnea

Complaints	No. of patients with complaint at baseline	Proportion of patients (%) with symptom improvement		
		PAP-adherent	Inadequately treated	P value (Chi-square test)
Sleepiness	107	48/72 (66.7%)	11/35 (31.4%)	0.001
Fatigue	127	45/80 (56.3%)	16/47 (34.0%)	0.03
Tiredness	148	56/96 (58.3%)	19/52 (36.5%)	0.02
Lack of energy	157	47/100 (47.0%)	21/57 (36.8%)	0.29

Reprinted with permission from Chotinaiwattarakul W, O'Brien LM, Fan L, Chervin RD.[3]

Women tended to report higher levels of fatigue, tiredness, or lack of energy than did men. The International Classification of Sleep Disorders (ICSD-2)[2] lists exhaustion among other complaints such as sleepiness and insomnia as part of the minimal criteria required to make a diagnosis of OSAS. The OSAS entry includes symptoms of loss of libido and morning headaches but does not mention the terms "fatigue," "tiredness," or "lack of energy" specifically. It is commonly taught in medical education that a complaint of excessive daytime sleepiness raises the possibility of a sleep disorder, while complaints of fatigue, tiredness, and lack of energy tend to suggest psychiatric and other medical diagnoses.

Nonetheless, many patients with OSAS may be aware of lack of energy and not perceive the degree of sleepiness, or confuse the symptom of fatigue with excessive daytime sleepiness. Patients may perceive no increased tendency to fall asleep during the day, but believe that a good night of sleep would improve lack of energy. Although frequently noted to occur in combination, fatigue is distinct from excessive daytime sleepiness. The complaint of fatigue is a complex symptom related to the perception of lack of energy. Objective measures of OSAS severity and measures of oxygen desaturation are not closely correlated with levels of subjective fatigue, tiredness, lack of energy, or sleepiness.

The most commonly used effective treatment for OSAS is CPAP, which generally eliminates apneas and hypopneas, and reduces oxygen desaturations during sleep. By either subjective or objective measures, sleepiness usually responds well to CPAP.

However, treatment effectiveness may be limited by variable adherence. Use of CPAP often averages between 3 and 5 hours per night in published series. A recent prospective follow-up survey shows that self-defined complaints of fatigue, tiredness, and lack of energy have potential for robust improvement, like sleepiness does, after adequate CPAP treatment (Table 4.1).[3] Greater positive airway pressure adherence may well result in better responses. Fatigue can improve substantially among patients without evidence of baseline sleepiness, and among those with only mild OSA. A randomized controlled trial showed an increase in energy as well as fatigue after 3 weeks of CPAP use.[4]

Main points

Fatigue, tiredness, and lack of energy, like excessive daytime sleepiness, may present as chief complaints in patients with OSAS. A careful relevant evaluation starts with a good history and physical examination, which often point toward a correct diagnosis. Use of CPAP can improve OSAS symptoms other than sleepiness.

REFERENCES

1. Chervin RD. Sleepiness, fatigue, tiredness, and lack of energy in obstructive sleep apnea. *Chest* 2000;**118**:372–9.
2. American Academy of Sleep Medicine. *International Classification of Sleep Disorders. Diagnostic and Coding*

Manual, Second Edition. Westchester, IL: American Academy of Sleep Medicine;2005.

3. Chotinaiwattarakul W, O'Brien LM, Fan L, Chervin RD. Fatigue, tiredness, and lack of energy improve with treatment for OSA. *J Clin Sleep Med* 2009;**5**:222-7.

4. Tomfohr LM, Ancoli-Israel S, Loredo JS, Dimsdale JE. Effects of continuous positive airway pressure on fatigue and sleepiness in patients with obstructive sleep apnea: data from a randomized controlled trial. *Sleep* 2011;**34**:121-6.

5

Patients with narcolepsy, in contrast to sleep apnea, more often choose to describe the problem as "sleepiness" rather than using other terms

Sarah Nath Zallek

Case

An 18-year-old woman presented with a chief complaint of feeling "sleepy during the day." She started noticing it at age 13 or 14 in her first year of high school. She would fall asleep in class. Her teachers said they thought she was bored, but she stated she was "literally unable to stay awake." She often dozed for about 5 minutes and felt refreshed. She admitted to nodding off at the wheel at times. She often fell asleep reading or watching television. She took an intentional nap every day and felt refreshed after about 30 minutes.

She admitted to dream-like experiences while awake, just before falling asleep, or after waking. She also frequently felt unable to move at those times. She described sudden weakness with laughter and other strong emotions.

She admitted to soft snoring on occasion but denied witnessed apnea. Her self-reported bedtime was about midnight, with a sleep latency of < 2 minutes. She slept until 9:00 AM most days and denied difficulty initiating or maintaining sleep. Although she was refreshed upon awakening, she would become quite sleepy by 10:00 AM.

When asked to rate her sleepiness on a typical day on a scale of 0–10, with 10 being the highest, she rated it a 10. She rated her fatigue on a typical day at 2 out of 10. Her Epworth Sleepiness Scale, which asks how likely one is to doze in each of 8 situations, was 22 out of a possible 24.[1] Her Fatigue Severity Scale score,

which is a 9 question subjective rating scale of fatigue, was 30 out of a possible 63.[2]

A polysomnogram recorded in a sleep laboratory showed a short sleep latency of 3 minutes and was otherwise unremarkable. A Multiple Sleep Latency Test (MSLT) demonstrated a short mean sleep latency of 0.5 minutes and sleep-onset rapid eye movement (REM) periods in each of 5 naps spread throughout the day (Figure 5.1).

What is the differential diagnosis of sleepiness in this patient?

This patient had adequate sleep opportunity for her age, good sleep continuity both subjectively and objectively, and appropriate circadian alignment. Her severe subjective and objective sleepiness is consistent with an increased drive to sleep.

The differential diagnosis from her history includes disorders of sleep regulation, such as idiopathic hypersomnia and narcolepsy. As she was sleepy on a daily basis, rather than for discreet periods of days to weeks, recurrent hypersomnia (e.g. Kleine–Levin syndrome) was not considered. While the sleepiness of idiopathic hypersomnia and narcolepsy can be difficult to distinguish from one another, her clear history of cataplexy makes narcolepsy with cataplexy nearly certain. The additional features of hypnagogic hallucinations and sleep paralysis, the refreshing nature of her short naps, and her symptom onset in the second decade are

Common Pitfalls in Sleep Medicine, ed. Ronald D. Chervin. Published by Cambridge University Press. © Cambridge University Press 2014.

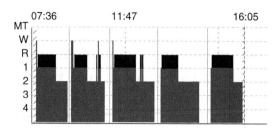

Figure 5.1 Hypnogram for this patient's Multiple Sleep Latency Test. A hypnogram is a plot of sleep stage against time for the duration of a sleep study. This hypnogram shows sleep onset almost immediately after lights out (vertical lines, which also represent elapsed wake time of about two hours between each nap). This study showed a mean sleep latency 0.5 minutes, and sleep-onset REM periods (black) occurred in each nap. Abbreviations used in figure: MT, movement time; W, wakefulness; R, REM sleep; 1 = non-REM stage 1 sleep; 2 = non-REM stage 2 sleep; 3 = non-REM stage 3 sleep; and 4 = non-REM stage 4 sleep. Currently the older designations of non-REM stage 3 sleep and non-REM stage 4 sleep are combined into stage N3 sleep.

highly supportive, though not as specific. Her combined clinical features, in conjunction with the short mean sleep latency and sleep-onset REM periods on the MSLT, were diagnostic of narcolepsy with cataplexy. On the MSLT, the patient has repeated daytime opportunities to fall asleep under conducive circumstances; a mean sleep latency < 8 minutes is considered consistent with excessive daytime sleepiness, and two or more sleep-onset REM periods support a diagnosis of narcolepsy, with or without cataplexy.

Discussion

Sleepiness is a propensity to fall asleep. Causes of excessive daytime sleepiness – sleepiness under inappropriate circumstances, severe enough to interfere with daily activities – can be grouped into four broad categories: insufficient sleep quantity, poor sleep quality, circadian rhythm disturbances, and an increased sleep drive. Insufficient sleep quantity is commonly due to insufficient sleep syndrome, in which typically sleep is curtailed on work or school days, with associated daytime sleepiness. Longer sleep on days off or vacations is refreshing.

At sleep disorders centers, obstructive sleep apnea is the most frequently diagnosed cause of poor sleep quality. Excessive daytime sleepiness results from discontinuous sleep, and possibly from intermittent hypoxemia as well. Sleep fragmentation can also arise from many other causes. Caffeine and other stimulants, environmental sleep disturbances, and pain may lead to poor sleep quality, for example.

Circadian rhythm disorders misalign sleep and wake from the desired schedule. Examples include advanced sleep-phase syndrome, delayed sleep-phase syndrome, and conditions as common as jet lag.

Disorders of increased sleep drive lead to sleepiness despite adequate quantity, quality, and timing of sleep. Narcolepsy and idiopathic hypersomnia fall into this category. In this group, the regulation of sleep and wakefulness is disturbed, and sleepiness presents itself at times intended for wakefulness, usually despite an adequate nighttime sleep opportunity.

Recognition and measurement of sleepiness are helpful if the symptom is a clue to a diagnosis. This patient clearly presented with sleepiness. She used the word "sleepy" in her chief complaint, which is not always the case with sleepy patients. She also rated sleepiness much more highly than fatigue on two different rating scales.

Clarifying the patient's symptoms is an important first step in diagnosis. This can be tricky. Not only can daytime symptoms be vague and overlap, but the words patients and clinicians choose to describe those symptoms vary widely. Listening to the patient's initial description is a start. The word "sleepy" is fairly specific, while "tired," "fatigued," and "exhausted" and other words are less so. As clinicians, we often assume we know what the patient means by the words they use. We all form expectations as the history is being provided, and sometimes we are at risk for hearing what we expect rather than what the patient is actually trying to convey.

Children and adults may present differently with sleepiness. While some adults may be able to articulate the symptom verbally, children may be less able to do so. A sleepy child may instead be labeled inattentive, unmotivated, or lazy.

In contrast to sleepiness, fatigue refers to difficulty with physical or mental exertion. In order to distinguish between sleepiness and fatigue, it may help to ask the patient if the symptom diminishes more with rest or physical activity. Sleepiness tends to diminish with physical activity, while fatigue typically lessens with rest.

In addition to being described by subjective verbal reports, sleepiness can be quantified. Several subjective scales of sleepiness are available, some of which have been validated. These include the Epworth Sleepiness Scale, the Stanford Sleepiness Scale, and several others.[3] Objective measures of sleepiness include the MSLT (the current gold standard) and the Maintenance of Wakefulness Test (MWT). Few normative data are available for the MWT, and it is not used as commonly as the MSLT in clinical practice.

The correlation between subjective and objective sleepiness measures varies. The Epworth Sleepiness Scale does not correlate well with MSLT mean sleep latency in narcolepsy or obstructive sleep apnea.[4,5] In the case of this patient, she subjectively described severe daytime sleepiness, and a very short mean sleep latency, typical of narcolepsy, was recorded on MSLT.

Sleep disorders present with a wide variety of symptoms. Nighttime symptoms include difficulty sleeping (insomnia) and unusual or unwanted behaviors (parasomnias). Daytime symptoms may be broader and sometimes vague, and can include sleepiness, fatigue, tiredness, inattention, irritability, emotional lability, cognitive dysfunction, and accidents. Recognition of any of these symptoms as the possible result of a sleep disorder is an essential first step in making the correct diagnosis. If the symptom is sleepiness, the differential diagnosis is broad, and includes narcolepsy.

Narcolepsy is a disorder of sleepiness and is classified in two forms: narcolepsy with cataplexy and narcolepsy without cataplexy.[6] Narcolepsy with cataplexy consists of a clinical tetrad of symptoms: excessive daytime sleepiness, often with periods of irresistible sleep (sleep attacks); sleep paralysis; hypnagogic hallucinations; and cataplexy. Cataplexy is sudden loss of muscle tone triggered by emotion. Laughter and anger are the most common triggers. Sleep fragmentation, with frequent brief awakenings, and automatic behavior, which is thought to be due to "microsleeps," are also common in narcolepsy. Daily excessive daytime sleepiness for at least 3 months, plus a clear history of cataplexy, is diagnostic. The diagnosis should be confirmed, whenever possible, by polysomnography followed by an MSLT. The findings should include a mean sleep latency of 8 minutes or less, and two or more sleep-onset REM periods.

Narcolepsy without cataplexy consists of daily excessive sleepiness for at least 3 months and must be confirmed by polysomnography followed by an MSLT with the findings as described above for narcolepsy with cataplexy. Sleep paralysis and hypnagogic hallucinations can be seen in either form of narcolepsy and are not required for the diagnosis of either one. In either form, there should be no alternative explanation, such as sleep apnea or medication effect, for the sleepiness.

Most patients who have narcolepsy with cataplexy have a deficiency of hypocretin (orexin), a neuropeptide produced in dorsolateral hypothalamus neurons with many projections to areas of the brain that affect sleep, including the locus coeruleus, suprachiasmatic nucleus, and the ventrolateral preoptic area.[7] Narcolepsy without cataplexy is usually not associated with hypocretin deficiency, but involves sleepiness just the same.

In order to diagnose narcolepsy, sleepiness must be recognized. Surprisingly, therein lies one potential pitfall for this condition. While sleepiness may be quite evident in adults by clear verbal description in the history, it can be trickier to identify in children. Adults are more likely to be able to articulate a feeling of sleepiness, if not as a chief complaint, then as an endorsed symptom. They may also be more apt to recognize the feeling than children. When an adult is sleepy, he or she may have the urge to lie down and sleep. In contrast, sleepy children may become more emotional, irritable, distractible, or "hyperactive" rather than showing a desire to lie down and sleep. It may be recognized either by the patient or an observer, but in children it is easily misconstrued as laziness or inattention.

Narcolepsy is typically symptomatic by the second or third decade of life but may be overlooked for many years before it is diagnosed. A child may not be able to articulate the symptom of sleepiness very well verbally. Observation of the child may identify sleepiness if naps or inadvertent sleep occur, but these are not always evident. Poor school or work performance may be the presenting sign of sleepiness in adolescents or adults, and may unfortunately be attributed by observers to low effort or interest, even if the patient feels excessively sleepy. Excessive sleepiness, largely due to insufficient sleep syndrome, is so common it may be thought to be normal or at least culturally acceptable among teens and young adults. This is unfortunate because, once medical attention is sought, a careful history can identify sleepiness that may have masqueraded for years as other signs. Diagnosis can then lead to excellent treatment and allow for good school and work performance.

Once chronic sleepiness is identified, narcolepsy should be considered in the differential diagnosis. Discerning the cause(s) of sleepiness requires a careful history. Consideration of all causes of sleepiness must be made, as broadly outlined above. Many causes will be easily eliminated by the history, which should routinely include sleep timing, continuity and perceived quality, duration, and daytime function. A "walk around the clock" approach is an organized way of asking about the details of sleep, wakefulness, and physical and mental activity through the 24-hour period. Starting at bedtime, continuing through the sleep period until wake time, and then through the day and evening, is an efficient tactic to address a sleep history systematically.

Comorbid conditions that also cause sleepiness may coexist in patients with narcolepsy. Insufficient sleep syndrome is a common reason for excessive sleepiness at all ages, including in children and adolescents. Obstructive sleep apnea can present at any age, as well. Diagnosis of underlying sleep disorders before making the diagnosis of narcolepsy is essential. Once identified, other causes of sleepiness should be treated effectively before a diagnosis of narcolepsy is made.

The type of sleepiness can sometimes help guide the diagnosis, but only to a point. Of course, sleepiness itself is not specific to narcolepsy, but sometimes features can give clues to the cause. Narcoleptic patients tend to feel refreshed on waking after a night of sleep. They also typically find short naps to be refreshing and may take several in a day. In idiopathic hypersomnia, patients awaken in the morning feeling unrefreshed and naps tend to be longer and not refreshing.

Daytime symptoms other than sleepiness, such as fatigue or tiredness, may feature more prominently in some other sleep disorders. If those are more significant than sleepiness, narcolepsy is not likely to be the primary diagnosis. In one study subjects who rated subjective fatigue greater than sleepiness were more likely to have sleep apnea than narcolepsy, but ratings of sleepiness more than fatigue were not helpful in predicting one of those diagnoses over the other.[8] Patients with narcolepsy are sleepy, which can be revealed in a careful sleep history.

Main points

Patients with narcolepsy are sleepy. Patients who present mainly with fatigue, tiredness, or other daytime symptoms are not likely to have narcolepsy. The symptom of sleepiness must be established with a careful history, especially in children and teenagers, as patients may not offer the words "sleepy" or "sleepiness" in their initial complaints.

FURTHER READING

Ahmed I, Thorpy M. Clinical features, diagnosis, and treatment of narcolepsy. *Clinical Chest Medicine* 2010;**31**:371–81.

Kryger M, Roth T, Dement W, eds. *Principles and Practice of Sleep Medicine*, Fifth Edition. St Louis, MO: Elsevier;2010.

Shadid A, Wilkingson K, Marcu S, Shapiro CM. *One Hundred Sleep Related Scales*. New York, NY: Springer;2010.

REFERENCES

1. Johns MW. A new method for measuring daytime sleepiness: the Epworth Sleepiness Scale. *Sleep* 1991;**14**:540–5.
2. Krupp LB, LaRocca NG, Muir-Nash J, Steinberg AD. The fatigue severity scale. Application to patients with multiple

sclerosis and systemic lupus erythematosus. *Arch Neurol* 1989;**46**:1121–3.

3. Shadid A, Shen J, Shapiro C. Measurements of sleepiness and fatigue. *J Psychosom Res* 2010;**69**:81–9.

4. Olson LG, Cole MF, Ambrogetti A. Correlations among Epworth Sleepiness Scale scores, Multiple Sleep Latency Tests and psychological symptoms. *J Sleep Res* 1998;**7**:248–53.

5. Chervin RD. The Epworth Sleepiness Scale may not reflect objective measures of sleepiness or sleep apnea. *Neurology*; 1999;**52**:125–33.

6. American Academy of Sleep Medicine. *International Classification of Sleep Disorders. Diagnostic and Coding Manual*, Second Edition. Westchester, IL: American Academy of Sleep Medicine;2005.

7. Taheri S, Ward H, Ghatei M, Bloom S. Role of orexins in sleep and arousal mechanisms. *Lancet* 2000;**355**:847.

8. Valerio TD, Fisk HL, Chervin RD, Zallek SN. Rating subjective fatigue greater than sleepiness predicts sleep apnea over narcolepsy; greater sleepiness is not predictive. *Sleep* 2005;**28** (Suppl):A205.

6

Patients with fatigue and sleepiness: multiple sclerosis

Tiffany J. Braley

Case

A 30-year-old man with a 2-year history of relapsing-remitting multiple sclerosis (MS) presented to his neurologist's office with a chief complaint of feeling "tired all the time." He described a constant sense of low energy that worsened throughout the course of his work day, particularly in the afternoon. He reported marginal relief with quiet periods of rest, but also admitted to an increased propensity to sleep in sedentary situations such as watching television, reading, or driving. He reported a bedtime of 9:30 PM, but denied feeling refreshed in the morning. He also endorsed frequent nocturnal arousals (waking up three to four times per night for no specific reason) and periodic snoring. When questioned about additional symptoms, he described significant lower extremity discomfort that was present at rest, worse at night, and relieved by walking. He denied any changes in his mood, or symptoms of anhedonia.

General examination was notable for a body mass index (BMI) of 26.7 kg/m^2 and a Mallampati Classification score of II. Neurologic exam was notable for a slightly diminished gag reflex and lower extremity hyperreflexia. Brain magnetic resonance imaging (MRI) was notable for multifocal hyperintense lesions in a periventricular pattern (consistent with known demyelinating disease), and an additional lesion at the cervico-medullary junction. Spinal cord MRI was notable for multiple demyelinating lesions throughout the cervical and thoracic spine. The patient's Epworth Sleepiness Scale score was 22 on a range of 0–24, where scores ≥ 10 are consistent with subjective daytime sleepiness. His Fatigue Severity Scale score was 6.9 on a scale of 0–7, where scores ≥ 4 suggest excessive fatigue.

Polysomnography showed an apnea/hypopnea index of 15.5 apneas or hypopneas per hour of sleep and a minimum oxygen saturation of 89%, diagnostic of moderate obstructive sleep apnea (OSA). A continuous positive airway pressure (CPAP) titration study revealed that a setting of 6 cm of water effectively treated his apnea. The patient was also diagnosed with restless legs syndrome (RLS) and was prescribed a dopamine agonist before bedtime.

At a follow-up appointment, the patient reported a "50% improvement" in his energy level and a sense of feeling more refreshed in the morning, which he attributed to CPAP use and improvement of his RLS symptoms. His Epworth Sleepiness Scale improved to 8/24. Despite this improvement, he was still somewhat dissatisfied with his energy level in the afternoon hours and scored 4.4/7 on the Fatigue Severity Scale. He was prescribed amantadine with little improvement in his symptoms. He was subsequently prescribed modafinil, which substantially improved his energy level.

Discussion

Fatigue is a highly individualized symptom with many overlapping descriptors. Although common synonyms

Common Pitfalls in Sleep Medicine, ed. Ronald D. Chervin. Published by Cambridge University Press. © Cambridge University Press 2014.

include tiredness, lack of energy, lassitude, decreased motivation, weariness, and asthenia, fatigue can also overlap with sleepiness – a more commonly recognized consequence of disordered sleep.

Fatigue and sleepiness have the potential to co-exist in many medical conditions, though more commonly in chronic disease states with a high prevalence of sleep disorders. Of these, one of the most extensively studied is MS. Multiple sclerosis is an autoimmune disease of the central nervous system that causes myelin destruction and axonal damage in the brain and spinal cord. This condition is the leading cause of non-traumatic neurologic disability among young adults and is associated with a variety of debilitating symptoms, including fatigue, which is experienced by at least 75% of MS patients.[1,2] Whereas fatigue may arise from MS-related cytokine dysregulation and neuronal dysfunction, several treatable comorbidities, including sleep disorders, also can contribute to fatigue and cause concomitant sleepiness. In particular, recent studies suggest that patients with MS are particularly vulnerable to OSA and RLS. Though reasons for these associations are not well-understood, MS-related central nervous system damage may contribute to an increased vulnerability to both sleep disorders.[3-6] Furthermore, sleepiness correlates with fatigue and tiredness in MS patients with OSA and disrupted sleep.[7] Given the overlap among these descriptions, the use of a systematic approach to disentangle fatigue from sleepiness can facilitate successful management of such symptoms.

The presented case provides a classic illustration of how fatigue and sleepiness can present within the same individual. As outlined above, our patient's history of MS puts him at risk for both primary fatigue (related to his underlying neurologic disease) and disordered sleep, which can contribute to both fatigue and sleepiness. At first glance, a complaint of feeling "tired all the time" in an MS patient may not trigger a detailed survey of symptoms, particularly in a young, non-obese man, as it is often assumed that all MS patients are tired by virtue of their neuroimmunologic condition. Additional questioning, however, reveals that this patient is experiencing both fatigue and sleepiness, and identifies several underlying causes for his symptoms.

A suggested approach to a patient who is at risk for both fatigue and sleepiness (Figure 6.1) is to start with an open-ended question, followed by a series of more focused questions depending on the patient's response. One useful strategy is to start by asking the patient about his or her level of energy. Often patients will endorse terms such as "low energy," "fatigue," or "tiredness"; but they should be allowed to provide their own descriptions to avoid any misconceptions. These open-ended questions should then be followed by a request for the patient to explain what is meant by their descriptor of choice. For example, if a man endorses "exhaustion," he should be asked to describe what "exhaustion" means to him, in his own words.

More specific queries regarding associated symptoms, as well as aggravating and alleviating factors, should then be employed. Certainly, reports of snoring should alert the examiner to the possibility of sleep apnea and consequential sleepiness. However, other elements of this patient's case also provide useful insight into his symptoms. In the case of our patient, sedentary situations were an aggravating factor for his symptoms. If the problem is reported to be worse during sedentary, monotonous activities than during extended physical activity, or if the patient endorses a propensity to doze off during sedentary activities, excessive sleepiness is more likely than fatigue. The use of sleep or napping as a recovery mechanism for symptoms, or reports of feeling unrefreshed after an adequate night of sleep (as in our patient's case) also suggest sleepiness secondary to an underlying sleep disorder, though patients may use other terms to explain what is meant by "unrefreshed." As patients with sleep disorders often prefer terms other than sleepiness to describe their symptoms, it is possible that the term "sleepiness" might not be endorsed by the patient, even with close-ended questioning. Given this subjectivity, the more germane question for the clinician may not be whether the patient is experiencing sleepiness versus fatigue, but whether the symptom described is likely to be related to an underlying sleep disorder or another cause.

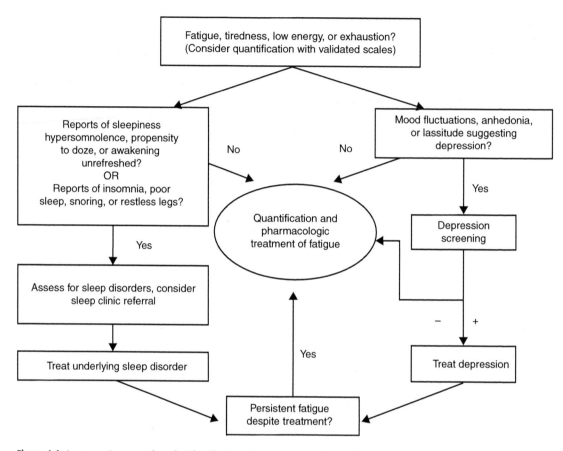

Figure 6.1 A systematic approach to the identification of common reversible causes of fatigue and sleepiness in patients with multiple sclerosis.

Another helpful approach is to ask the patient about his or her ability to initiate and sustain daily tasks. As previously mentioned, patients may suffer from fatigue related to chronic medical conditions or other comorbidities, as opposed to an underlying sleep disorder. Though no unified definition for fatigue exists, it is generally assumed to worsen with time or sustained mental or physical activity. If the patient feels energized at the start of their day or at the beginning of a specific activity, but develops a sense of diminishing physical or mental energy over time, fatigue is the more appropriate descriptor. Though our patient reported a constant feeling of low energy, he also developed worsening symptoms in the afternoon hours, which is consistent with MS-related fatigue.

Diagnostic testing for underlying causes and targeted treatment should be initiated only after symptoms have been clearly defined. Reversible causes of fatigue and sleepiness, such as a sleep disorder or depression, should be addressed before initiating symptomatic therapies. Patient and family education regarding proper sleep hygiene is another important initial step. If an underlying sleep disorder is suspected, referral to a sleep specialist should be considered.

In the case of our patient, successful treatment of OSA and RLS led to a significant improvement in excessive daytime sleepiness, but only a partial improvement in fatigue level, highlighting the need for additional pharmacologic therapy. A variety of pharmacologic agents are available to increase wakefulness and vigilance. Until recently, central nervous system (CNS) stimulants (such as methylphenidate) were the mainstays of treatment, but these have largely been replaced by newer agents such as modafinil, armodafinil, and, among patients with fatigue related to neurologic disorders, amantadine. Amantadine is approved by the US Food and Drug Administration (FDA) for treatment of influenza and Parkinson's disease. Though heterogeneity of clinical trial outcomes has precluded FDA approval of this medication for MS-related fatigue,[8,9] many clinicians advocate its use as a first-line agent for fatigue related to primary neurologic disorders. Amantadine is fairly well-tolerated with a mild side-effect profile, although caution should be used in patients with cardiovascular disease, cardiac arrhythmia, or seizure disorder. Modafinil, and its racemic analog armodafinil, are wake-promoting agents approved by the FDA for narcolepsy, shift-work sleep disorder, and OSA with residual excessive sleepiness despite optimal use of CPAP. In practice, modafinil is also commonly used in a variety of other conditions, including MS-related fatigue. Studies have demonstrated favorable results in regard to improved fatigue, focused attention, dexterity, and enhanced motor cortex excitability in MS patients with modafanil.[10,11] Nonetheless, modafinil is not FDA approved for MS-related fatigue, in part due to conflicting results from other studies. Modafinil and armodafinil are generally well-tolerated, but potential side effects include headache, psychiatric disturbance, gastrointestinal irritation, and decreased effectiveness of contraception.

Although use of a fatigue rating scale is not always necessary, a formal scale may be useful to evaluate treatment response. If a fatigue scale is desired, the clinician's level of comfort, time requirements, reliability, reproducibility, and applicability to patient's medical condition should also be considered when selecting the appropriate instrument. Taking these factors into consideration, the Fatigue Severity Scale is a reasonable option for most patients. Initially designed to identify common features of fatigue in both MS and lupus patients,[12] the Fatigue Severity

Scale assesses the impact of fatigue on multiple outcomes, with a physical focus. Each of nine responses is provided on a seven-point Likert scale. Prior studies have shown acceptable internal consistency and stability over time, and sensitivity to change afforded by clinical improvement.

Main points

Clinicians caring for patients with chronic medical conditions should be aware of the potential for concomitant fatigue and sleepiness. A detailed and systematic diagnostic approach that enhances understanding of patients' symptomatology and accounts for common underlying etiologies offers the best chance of successfully treating these complex patients.

ACKNOWLEDGEMENTS

This work was supported in part by a Bridge to K Research Award from the American Sleep Medicine Foundation.

FURTHER READING

Braley TJ, Chervin RD, Segal BM. Fatigue, tiredness, lack of energy, and sleepiness in multiple sclerosis patients referred for clinical polysomnography. *Mult Scler Int* 2012;**2012**:673936.

Braley TJ, Segal BM, Chervin RD. Sleep-disordered breathing in multiple sclerosis. *Neurology* 2012;**79**:929–36.

Krupp LB, LaRocca NG, Muir-Nash J, et al. The fatigue severity scale. Application to patients with multiple sclerosis and systemic lupus erythematosus. *Arch Neurol* 1989;**46**:1121–3.

Lange R, Volkmer M, Heesen C, Liepert J. Modafinil effects in multiple sclerosis patients with fatigue. *J Neurol* 2009;**256**:645–50.

Manconi M, Fabbrini M, Bonanni E, et al. High prevalence of restless legs syndrome in multiple sclerosis. *Eur J Neurol* 2007;**14**:534–9.

REFERENCES

1. Krupp L. Fatigue is intrinsic to multiple sclerosis (MS) and is the most commonly reported symptom of the disease. *Mult Scler* 2006;**12**:367–8.
2. Lerdal A, Celius EG, Krupp L, et al. A prospective study of patterns of fatigue in multiple sclerosis. *Eur J Neurol* 2007;**14**:1338–43.
3. Kaminska M, Kimoff R, Benedetti A, et al. Obstructive sleep apnea is associated with fatigue in multiple sclerosis. *Mult Scler* 2012;**18**:1159–69.
4. Braley TJ, Segal BM, Chervin RD. Sleep-disordered breathing in multiple sclerosis. *Neurology* 2012;**79**:929–36.
5. Manconi M, Fabbrini M, Bonanni E, et al. High prevalence of restless legs syndrome in multiple sclerosis. *Eur J Neurol* 2007;**14**:534–9.
6. Manconi M, Rocca MA, Ferini-Strambi L, et al. Restless legs syndrome is a common finding in multiple sclerosis and correlates with cervical cord damage. *Mult Scler* 2008;**14**:86–93.
7. Braley TJ, Chervin RD, Segal BM. Fatigue, tiredness, lack of energy, and sleepiness in multiple sclerosis patients referred for clinical polysomnography. *Mult Scler Int* 2012;**2012**:673936.
8. Cohen RA, Fisher M. Amantadine treatment of fatigue associated with multiple sclerosis. *Arch Neurol* 1989;**46**:676–80.
9. Taus C, Giuliani G, Pucci E, et al. Amantadine for fatigue in multiple sclerosis. *Cochrane Database Syst Rev* 2003: CD002818.
10. Rammohan KW, Rosenberg JH, Lynn DJ, et al. Efficacy and safety of modafinil (Provigil) for the treatment of fatigue in multiple sclerosis: a two centre phase 2 study. *J Neurol Neurosurg Psychiatry* 2002;**72**:179–83.
11. Lange R, Volkmer M, Heesen C, et al. Modafinil effects in multiple sclerosis patients with fatigue. *J Neurol* 2009;**256**:645–50.
12. Krupp LB, LaRocca NG, Muir-Nash J, et al. The fatigue severity scale. Application to patients with multiple sclerosis and systemic lupus erythematosus. *Arch Neurol* 1989;**46**:1121–3.

Assessment of daytime sleepiness

Daytime sleepiness is one of the most common complaints that patients bring to their physicians, and one of the main symptoms that prompt referral to sleep disorders centers. At those centers, multiple well-validated subjective and objective assessment options can supplement the clinical history that a sleep physician evaluates in an effort to find underlying causes. These tests do not always make the job of the clinician easier, and in fact offer many potential pitfalls that can obscure rather than clarify a helpful understanding of the patient's problem. The following cases illustrate such pitfalls. Although each case is different, they highlight some common mistakes in clinical practice and show, with hindsight, how care may be improved for other patients. Among the underlying themes, one important conclusion is that any test results must be considered in conjunction with other clinical data. Results from a history, subjective questionnaire, or objective sleep laboratory test alone often do not predict results of the other two types of assessments as closely as physicians – even sleep specialists at times – are prone to expect. The validated utility of each measure should be understood, but familiarity with the limitations of each assessment can be at least as important to good patient care, when it comes to understanding, diagnosing, and treating patients with complaints of daytime sleepiness.

7

Patient complaints, subjective questionnaires, and objective measures of sleepiness may not coincide

Michael E. Yurcheshen

Introduction

Three types of patients present to a sleep disorders center: those who are excessively sleepy, those who can't sleep, and those who do something unusual or unexpected when they sleep.

Characterization of sleepiness is an important task for the clinician. At a minimum, sleepiness can rob a patient of productivity and focus; at worst, it can be dangerous. New mothers, office workers, college students, and commercial drivers all benefit from an alert mind, but the consequences of sleepiness are different for each of them. It is critical for a clinician to identify and treat these patients quickly. On the other hand, many conditions can impair performance, but are not considered to be primary sleep disorders. Skill in separating sleepiness from other issues allows a clinician to devise a diagnostic and therapeutic path that will be of most benefit.

Sleepiness seems easy enough to identify, but clinicians can fall prey to formulaic thinking: Do you fall asleep during the day when reading or watching television? – turn to page 18. Can you endure an hour-long phone conversation with your mother-in-law without drifting off? – turn to page 34. But what happens when those pages are blank, or there's something on that next page that is unexpected? This is a conundrum in sleep medicine. What happens when objective and subjective sleepiness measures do not coincide? A disciplined approach to these cases while maintaining flexible thinking often serves best.

The following two cases illustrate what can happen when there is a disconnect between subjective and objective sleepiness.

Case 1: "Doc. ... it's hard to sleep at night"

A 37-year-old man presented complaining of difficulty falling and staying asleep. His sleep latency would last several hours, and he would wake countless times during the night. Eventually, he became dependent on prescription zolpidem to help him achieve and maintain sleep. Although insomnia was his primary complaint, the patient also complained of unrefreshing sleep. He woke feeling fatigued, and this continued throughout the day. Subjectively, he had minimal sleepiness. He could stay awake while watching televison or reading. His driving was seemingly unaffected. His Epworth Sleepiness Scale score was 4 (scale range of 0–24). When pressed, however, he did admit to daily napping, sometimes for several hours. Occasionally, he would even dream during these naps. The patient had a host of psychiatric and medical illnesses, including depression and anxiety, and had been out of work for many years due to disability.

On examination, the patient was obese with a body mass index of 33 kg/m^2. His neck circumference was 17 inches (43 cm). He had a crowded naso/oro-pharynx with a long, dependent palate, 1+ tonsil size, and a high riding tongue.

Primarily on the basis of snoring and his physical examination, a diagnostic nocturnal polysomnogram (NPSG) was performed. The patient had decreased sleep efficiency of 76%, primarily due to prolonged sleep latency of 76 minutes. The study demonstrated moderate obstructive sleep apnea (apnea/hypopnea index of 20.4 events per hour of sleep, minimum oxygen saturation 80%, with 3.9% of the night spent with an oxygen saturation of < 90%). The study also demonstrated frequent periodic leg movements (periodic limb movement index of 71).

The patient was scheduled for a continuous positive airway pressure (CPAP) titration, and clinic follow-up was planned thereafter.

Discussion

This is a case of obstructive sleep apnea and possible periodic limb movement disorder, although insomnia was the chief complaint. Conventional wisdom would say that obstructive sleep apnea rarely presents with sleep initiation insomnia. However, this patient may have had a component of concurrent sleep mis-perception syndrome. More important for the current discussion, however, is that this patient presented with an atypical history of sleepiness.

The Epworth Sleepiness Scale is a metric that has been in common use for well over a decade. It is often used by practitioners, researchers, and healthcare plans to assess subjective sleepiness. The scale aims to assess the likelihood of dozing under a number of sedentary situations, including while driving. The eight question-items, though, cannot account for many circumstances: What if a patient doesn't drive? There is no line item for feeling sleepy while working on the computer, certainly a common, present-day "at risk" time for daytime sleepiness. Daily napping that lasts for hours may only result in a normal score of 3 or 4, if the patient does not endorse sleepiness at other times (as in the present case). This said, most physicians would agree that napping at this patient's frequency and duration is highly suggestive of daytime sleepiness.

In this instance, the patient's Epworth score was misleading. Values of 10 or higher suggest sleepiness, and this patient's score was far below this threshold. This simple number does not always capture the degree to which sleepiness is *bothersome* to the patient, or whether the patient experiences unrefreshing sleep.

Attentive history taking, in conjunction with a detailed physical examination, were the most useful tools in unraveling this patient's case. As a result, the patient's sleep disorders were identified, and proper management was initiated. In this instance, as in others, an over-reliance on a low Epworth score might have led to myopic focus on insomnia, and a failure to recognize concurrent sleep-disordered breathing.

Case 2: "Doc. … I can't stay awake"

A 33-year-old gentleman presented with a complaint of: "I have narcolepsy and a circadian rhythm disorder and I'm undermedicated." The patient stated that for 15 years he had difficulty staying awake. He believed the sleepiness affected his college performance, forcing him to take 10 years to complete his degree. His current level of sleepiness was so debilitating to him that he could not hold a job, and could not even do artwork, which was his passion and avocation. His Epworth score was 18.

He had seen a sleep specialist in an outlying county, as well as a psychiatrist in a neighboring state. He was diagnosed with attention deficit disorder. Because of his ongoing complaints, he was treated with a host of wakefulness promoting agents including modafinil, methylphenidate, dextroamphetamine, and amphetamine salts. Even at high or maximum doses, the patient complained of ongoing sleepiness. He did not respond to a trial of γ-hydroxybutyrate.

The patient underwent an NPSG, followed by a Multiple Sleep Latency Test (MSLT) at an outside sleep disorders center. An MSLT is a daytime sleep study in which a patient is given the opportunity to fall asleep during five nap opportunities, though in the past this test was sometimes performed with only four naps. The nap opportunities are offered at 2-hour intervals.

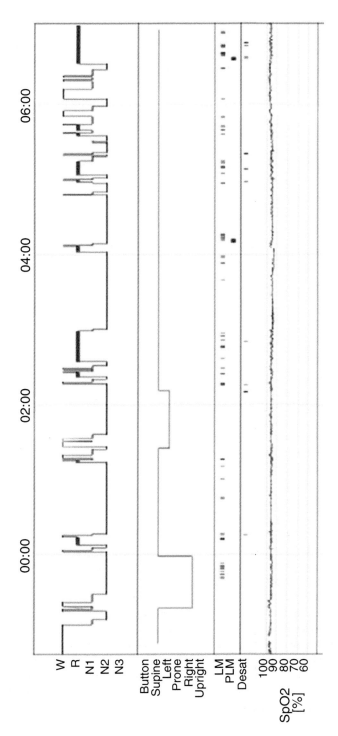

Figure 7.1 Hypnogram for overnight polysomnogram of patient in Case 2. The top bar signifies sleep staging from the beginning of the night to the end. The patient did demonstrate significant sleep fragmentation, including during rapid eye movement (REM) sleep. Although the patient had many awakenings, this can be common during sleep testing in an unfamiliar environment. Below the first bar are body position, limb movements, and oxygen desaturation. Abbreviations used in figure: Desat, desaturation; LM, limb movement; PLM, periodic limb movement; SpO2, oxygen saturation; R, REM sleep; W, wake.

	9:00 AM	11:03 AM	1:02 PM	3:02 PM
Lights off clock time:	9:00 AM	11:03 AM	1:02 PM	3:02 PM
Lights on clock time:	9:36 AM	11:25 AM	1:25 PM	3:24 PM
Total record time:	36.0	22.5	23.0	22.5
Total sleep time:	23.5	0.5	0.0	0.0
Sleep efficiency:	65.3	2.2	0.0	0.0
Latency to sleep:	11.0	20.0	20.0	20.0
Latency to N1:	11.0	20.0	20.0	20.0
Latency to N2:	28.0	–	20.0	20.0
Latency to N3:	–	–	40.0	40.0
Latency to R (from lights out):	–	–	20.0	20.0
Latency to R (from sleep onset):	–	–	20.0	20.0
Minutes of REM:	–	–	–	–

Figure 7.2 Results recorded as minutes of a Multiple Sleep Latency Test for the patient in Case 2. The patient did not fall asleep during the last three 20-minute nap opportunities, and by convention, 20 minutes was entered for each of these sleep latencies. No rapid eye movement (R) sleep was recorded during any nap. The mean sleep latency was 18 minutes. For adults, a mean sleep latency less than 5 minutes generally suggests severe excessive daytime sleepiness, 5–8 minutes reflects less severe excessive sleepiness that is still common in patients with sleep disorders, 8–10 minutes represents a gray zone, and 10+ minutes suggests little or no objective evidence for excessive daytime sleepiness.

Sleep latencies and stages are recorded, and a mean sleep latency across all naps of eight minutes or less is generally considered to provide objective evidence of daytime sleepiness. A mean sleep latency < 5 minutes is highly suggestive of severe excessive daytime sleepiness. In addition, the presence of more than one nap with rapid eye movement (REM) sleep is unusual in patients without sleep disorders.

During this NPSG, the patient slept for a total of 283 minutes, and had an overall sleep efficiency of 56%. He had 16% stage N1 sleep and 25% rapid eye movement (REM) sleep. His apnea/hypopnea index was 1. During the MSLT, the patient fell asleep during some of the five nap opportunities (number of naps not specified). He had an average sleep latency of 8.5 minutes, and achieved REM sleep on two nap opportunities.

He was diagnosed with narcolepsy, and referred to our sleep disorders center for further workup and management.

Sleep testing was repeated at our center, and the patient was requested to remain off modafinil for three days leading up to the study. He was not taking antidepressants in the days prior to the study. The hypnogram is reproduced in Figure 7.1. The patient had a prolonged rather than short REM sleep latency of 90.4 minutes. He did demonstrate fragmented sleep, and increased N1 sleep (15.5%). His REM sleep periods were truncated. During the MSLT (Figure 7.2), the patient fell asleep during one of four nap opportunities. He did not achieve REM sleep on any nap. He had an average sleep latency of 18 minutes.

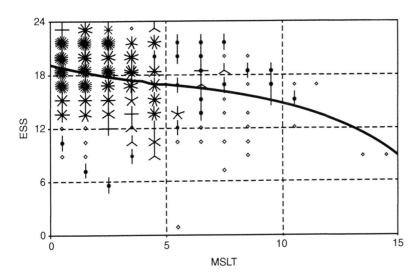

Figure 7.3 Regression fit estimation between Epworth Sleepiness Scale (ESS) and Multiple Sleep Latency Test (MSLT) scores in 522 patients with narcolepsy using best fit curvilinear line. The subjective Epworth scores did not appear to reflect closely the objective sleepiness as measured on the MSLT. Reproduced from Sangal RB, Mitler MM, Sangal JM,[1] with permission from Elsevier.

The patient was seen in follow-up to review the results of the sleep studies. He was informed that the test results did not provide objective evidence for hypersomnolence. Cerebrospinal fluid testing for hypocretin was discussed, but not pursued given the absence of sleepiness on the MSLT.

Discussion

In this case, the patient had a complicated history of psychiatric disease, and multiple medical evaluations. His sleep history was highly consistent with hypersomnolence, and sleep testing was certainly indicated.

This case brings attention to a common issue within the sleep community, namely the relationship between sleepiness and fatigue. These two symptoms can certainly coexist, although they also can be independent. In this case, two pieces of evidence suggest that the patient may suffer from fatigue more than hypersomnolence.

First, the patient's MSLT results are not consistent with hypersomnolence. The American Academy of

Sleep Medicine published guidelines for performing and interpreting MSLT results in 2005. The MSLT should always be performed in immediate conjunction with an NPSG. It should be performed after a minimum two-week washout of stimulants or REM suppressant medications. A toxicology screen can be performed before these tests (although it was not obtained in this case). The patient is not permitted to nap between nap periods on the MSLT, and should not take any sedating medications or stimulants during the study. Also, the results are only considered to be valid if the patient achieved six or more hours of sleep on the preceding NPSG. Although the results of this patient's initial MSLT initially appeared to raise the possibility of narcolepsy, the data should have been disregarded because he achieved only 283 minutes of sleep during his NPSG. During his repeat NPSG, the patient slept for over six hours prior to his repeat MSLT, which can then provide more interpretable information about his chronic level of daytime sleepiness (Figure 7.3[1]). Although prior-night sleep for six hours cannot precisely, in a physiologic manner, separate valid and invalid MSLT studies, this cut-point typically serves as a useful threshold in clinical practice.

Second, the patient did not respond to a half-dozen therapies, including ampakines, stimulants, and γ-hydroxybutyrate. Although non-response to medications is not a definitive diagnostic tool, his non-response to these therapies, in conjunction with an MSLT result that did not demonstrate sleepiness, suggests that this patient's presentation is more consistent with fatigue or another condition than true sleepiness.

This said, there are certainly cases in which an MSLT may yield a false negative result, suggesting little sleepiness when, in fact, sleepiness is present. The use of stimulants, and anxiety about the test or sleeping in a foreign environment, are two of the more common reasons.

This case also brings up the consideration of drawing cerebrospinal fluid (CSF) for hypocretin levels. Greater than 90% of patients who have narcolepsy with cataplexy have undetectable hypocretin levels, while virtually no individuals without the condition have levels < 110 pg. In this case, given non-sleepiness on his MSLT, and his non-response to stimulants, a CSF hypocretin level was not pursued, although this decision could certainly be debated.

FURTHER READING

Anonymous. A randomized, double blind, placebo-controlled multicenter trial comparing the effects of three doses of orally administered sodium oxybate with placebo for the treatment of narcolepsy. *Sleep* 2002;**25**:42–9.

Baumann C, Bassetti C, Scammell T. *Narcolepsy: Pathophysiology, Diagnosis, and Treatment.* New York, NY: Springer, 2011.

Buysse DJ, Reynolds III CF, Monk TH, et al. The Pittsburgh sleep quality index: a new instrument for psychiatric practice and research. *Psychiatry Res* 1989;**28**:193–213.

Littner M, Kushida C, Wise M, et al. Practice parameters for clinical use of the Multiple Sleep Latency Test and the Maintenance of Wakefulness Test. *Sleep* 2005;**28**:113–21.

Mignot E, Lammers GJ, Ripley B, et al. The role of cerebrospinal fluid hypocretin measurement in the diagnosis of narcolepsy and other hypersomnias. *Arch Neurol* 2002;**59**:1553–62.

Takei Y, Komada Y, Namba K. Differences in findings of nocturnal polysomnography and Multiple Sleep Latency Test between narcolepsy and idiopathic hypersomnia. *Clin Neurophys* 2012;**123**:137–41.

US Modafinil in Narcolepsy Multicenter Study Group. Randomized trial of modafinil as a treatment for the excessive daytime somnolence of narcolepsy. *Neurology* 2000;**54**:1166–75.

REFERENCE

1. Sangal RB, Mitler MM, Sangal JM. Subjective sleepiness ratings (Epworth Sleepiness Scale) do not reflect the same parameter of sleepiness as objective sleepiness (Maintenance of Wakefulness Test) in patients with narcolepsy. *Clin Neurophys* 1999;**110**:2131–5.

8

Daytime sleepiness and obstructive sleep apnea severity: where symptoms and metrics do not converge

Douglas Kirsch

Case 1

A 39-year-old commercial truck driver presented to the sleep clinic after a request for an evaluation from his Department of Transportation examiner. He denies knowledge of snoring or gasping during sleep, and had not been told of any witnessed apneas, though he does not have a current bed partner. He denies any daytime sleepiness, motor vehicle accidents, or near-miss accidents. He works long hours, often driving for 12 hours or more per day, but states that he is able to obtain 6.5–7.0 hours of sleep per night.

Past medical history:

Hypertension

Obesity

Physical examination:

Body mass index: 40 kg/m^2

Blood pressure: 130/87 mmHg

Neck circumference: 20 inches (51 cm)

Mallampati Class IV

His Epworth Sleepiness Scale score is 0.

He undergoes home sleep testing (HST) for apnea following the recommended guidelines for commercial drivers. A sample two-minute epoch from the HST is shown in Figure 8.1.

Polysomnographic data:

Apnea/hypopnea index: 75 events per hour of recording time

Minimum oxygen saturation: 62%

Case 2

A 48-year-old woman presented to the sleep clinic with significant daytime sleepiness. She has difficulty staying awake after lunch while at work and while commuting home from work by car. She has had these symptoms for 2–3 years, though they have worsened in the last several months. She obtains 8 hours of sleep at night, sleeping from 10:00 PM to 6:00 AM. She reports snoring and her husband has occasionally told her that she has pauses in her breathing during the night.

Past medical history:

Mildly overweight

Intermittent migraines

Depression

Physical examination:

Body mass index: 32 kg/m^2

Blood pressure: 134/75

Neck circumference: 16 inches (41 cm)

Mallampati Class IV

Her Epworth score is 14 out of 24.

She undergoes an HST.

A sample two-minute epoch from her HST is shown in Figure 8.2.

Polysomnographic data:

Apnea/hypopnea index: three events per hour of recording time.

Minimum oxygen saturation 89%

Common Pitfalls in Sleep Medicine, ed. Ronald D. Chervin. Published by Cambridge University Press. © Cambridge University Press 2014.

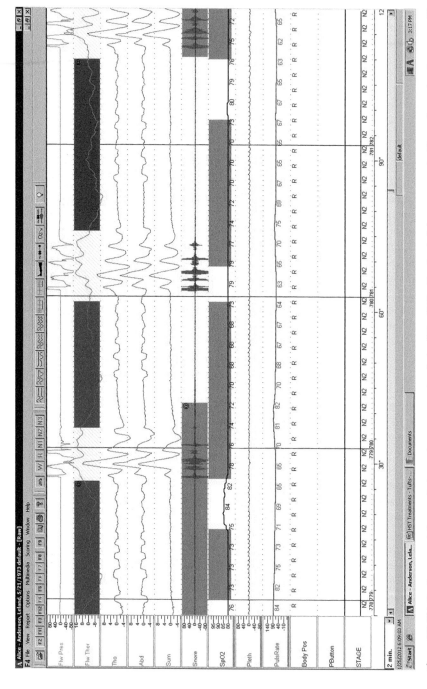

Figure 8.1 This 2-minute epoch from an in-home sleep apnea testing device (PDx, Philips Respironics) demonstrates significant obstructive sleep apnea. Three scored apneas are indicated by the shaded orange and gray boxes; note absent airflow, accompanied by continued respiratory effort for the majority of these events. The top two channels are nasal pressure and nasal–oral thermistor, followed by thoracic and abdominal effort bands with a combined sum effort channel. Below is a snore channel, oximetry, plethysmography, pulse rate, body position, patient event button, and "scored" sleep stage. See plate section for color version.

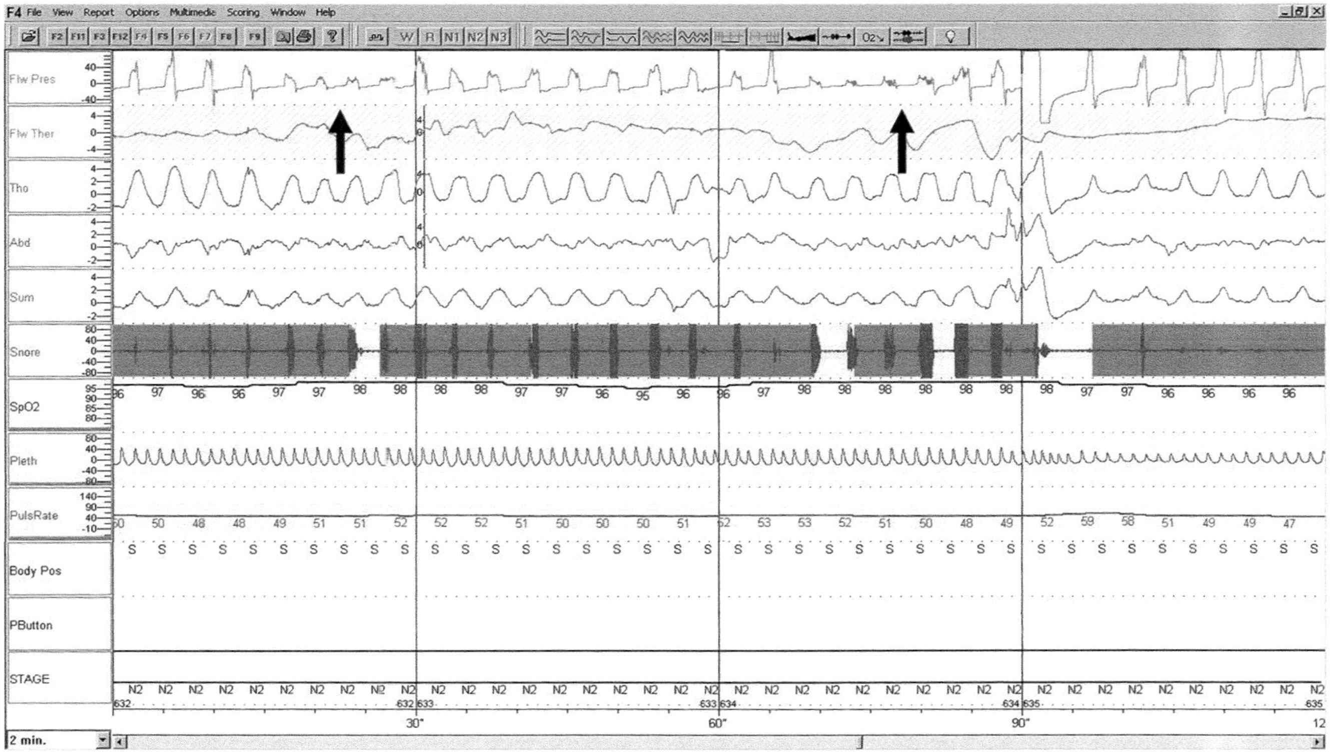

Figure 8.2 This 2-minute epoch from an in-home sleep apnea testing device (PDx, Philips Respironics) demonstrates two subtle, but unscored periods of decreased airflow (arrows). The top two channels are nasal pressure and nasal–oral thermistor, followed by thoracic and abdominal effort bands with a combined sum effort channel. Below is a snore channel, oximetry, plethysmography, pulse rate, body position, patient event button, and "scored" sleep stage.

Testing for obstructive sleep apnea and excessive daytime sleepiness

Obstructive sleep apnea (OSA) is a common sleep disorder, occurring in 2–4% of the population. The disorder is caused by repetitive collapse of the upper airway during sleep, leading to sleep fragmentation and intermittent hypoxia. Symptomatically, OSA can be associated with excessive daytime sleepiness (EDS), impaired cognition, mood disorders, or insomnia as well as increased risk for hypertension, ischemic heart disease, and stroke. The severity of OSA is commonly summarized by the apnea/hypopnea index (AHI). The AHI is defined as the number of apneas and hypopneas per hour of polysomnographic study. The most commonly used categorization of OSA severity is listed in Table 8.1.[1]

Excessive daytime sleepiness, or hypersomnia, is a core symptom of OSA. It is defined as "the inability to stay awake and alert during the major waking episodes of the day, resulting in unintended lapses into drowsiness or sleep."[2] Many patients are not aware of EDS; it may be brought to their attention by coworkers or family members who notice them nodding off. When sleepiness occurs while the patient is operating a motor vehicle or during other jobs requiring alertness, the safety of the patient and the general public may be at risk.

Many methods exist to assess for daytime sleepiness. Subjective methods tend to be easier and cheaper, but are prone to error due to poor patient insight or patient misrepresentation. Objective testing for daytime sleepiness may be more accurate and reproducible, though these evaluations are expensive and may not represent the patient's experience in real-world situations.

Table 8.1 Obstructive sleep apnea (OSA) severity by apnea/hypopnea index (AHI)

OSA severity	AHI (events/hour)
Normal	0.0–4.9
Mild	5.0–14.9
Moderate	15.0–29.9
Severe	30 or more

Adapted from Epstein LJ, Kristo D, Strollo P, et al.[1]

The most widely used questionnaire specific for daytime sleepiness is the Epworth Sleepiness Scale (ESS). The ESS was developed in Australia by Murray Johns in 1991 and has been demonstrated to be consistent when testing and retesting individuals over time. The ESS contains eight-question items that evaluate a patient's self-assessment of sleepiness in different sedentary situations "in recent times." The Likert response scale ranges from 0 ("would never doze") to 3 ("high chance of dozing"). The sum of the eight-item responses then quantifies subjective sleep propensity. Initial studies demonstrated that patients with narcolepsy, idiopathic hypersomnolence, or moderate-to-severe OSA often had high ESS scores (> 15). Scores of 10 or higher raise concern for excessive sleepiness, whereas lower scores are considered normal. The ESS has been studied frequently. However, the instrument does not predict objective measures of daytime sleepiness or sleep apnea strongly, if at all, and few data have emerged to support the ability of the ESS score to predict likelihood of motor vehicle accidents. Longitudinal tracking of ESS scores on an individual level appears useful in assessing change or treatment response over weeks to months. Medicare adopted the ESS in 2008 as a standard in the evaluation of all patients with suspected sleep apnea as a requirement for some forms of treatment.

An alternate method of assessment is the Stanford Sleepiness Scale (SSS), which measures instantaneous levels of subjective sleepiness. The SSS is a single question, about instantaneous subjective sleepiness, that is answered with a seven-point Likert scale. In contrast to the ESS, the SSS is most appropriately used by the same individual several times in a single day. Another questionnaire is the Functional Outcomes of Sleep Questionnaire (FOSQ), which assesses the impact of daytime sleepiness on activities of daily living. The FOSQ is designed to take 15 minutes to complete. The instrument assesses six domains as well as daily endeavors potentially affected by daytime sleepiness. A modified short form of the FOSQ, the FOSQ-10, has also been validated and may be easier for clinical use in following patients over time.

The Multiple Sleep Latency Test (MSLT) is the gold standard for objective evaluation of EDS. This test measures the physiologic tendency of a patient to fall asleep in a dim and quiet laboratory environment. The January 2005 practice parameters published by the American Academy of Sleep Medicine describe the testing protocol in detail.[3] This test is primarily validated for the diagnosis of narcolepsy; it has been applied by many practitioners as a tool for the assessment of sleepiness of all causes. The test results in two major data points: the mean sleep latency (MSL), which is the arithmetic average of how quickly the patient had an epoch scored as sleep in each nap, and the number of sleep-onset rapid eye movement (REM) periods (SOREMPs), the number of naps in which the patient had at least one epoch scored as REM sleep. Based on the International Classification of Sleep Disorders (ICSD-2)[2] a diagnosis of narcolepsy requires a mean sleep latency of < 8 minutes and 2 SOREMPs. However, physicians should recognize that other sleep disorders (including OSA, behaviorally induced insufficient sleep, and circadian rhythm disturbances, for example) may cause similar findings, so assessment of the results from an MSLT should always be performed within a clinical context.

The Maintenance of Wakefulness Test (MWT) is effectively the inverse of the MSLT. Though similar in that the patient is tested four times over the course of a day for 40 minutes per "nap" opportunity in a dim room while reclining, the subtle, but important, difference in the instructions for the MWT is that the patient should attempt to "remain awake as long as possible." The MWT has been used by the Federal Aviation Administration to test pilots who have been diagnosed with OSA and treated, assessing whether they are alert enough to return to work safely. While this test evaluates the ability of patients to stay awake in a circumscribed set of conditions, it has not been clearly predictive of motor vehicle accidents or other activities where reduced alertness may impact safety. The MWT can also be somewhat difficult to interpret, for example when the test does not demonstrate either "no sleep/clearly alert" or "clearly abnormally sleepy." The meaning of SOREMPs on an MWT is also unclear.

Discussion

Case 1 demonstrates a situation in which the patient's severe OSA is not reflected by an abnormal ESS score. There are multiple potential reasons for this finding. The patient may not be sleepy in any scenario, he may not perceive a propensity to sleep though he may be sleepy when in certain situations, or he may be falsifying answers on the subjective test. With regards to the last scenario, Tregear et al.[4] note that the ESS "... depends upon driver honesty in answering questions and upon driver awareness of sleepiness. Drivers may misrepresent sleepiness levels to prevent license revocation and those aware of sleepiness may develop compensatory strategies."

Case 2, on the other hand, is a patient who is quite sleepy, though her AHI is quite low. This finding may be reflected by an underdiagnosis of OSA severity by home sleep apnea testing (which would be less likely with an in-laboratory test), possible respiratory-related arousals causing sleepiness even in the absence of an OSA diagnosis from in-laboratory polysomnography, or sleepiness caused by an alternate sleep disorder.

While these cases represent the outside extremes, they are representative of the difficulty in assessing the relationship between OSA and EDS. In each of the cases, the following questions arise: (i) Is there a predictable relationship between OSA severity and EDS; and (ii) What are the potential causes for sleepiness in OSA?

Relationship between OSA and EDS

The relationship between OSA severity and EDS is unpredictable and to some extent dependent on the methods used to determine OSA severity and level of EDS. In particular, research studies have been inconsistent with regards to the relationship between sleep study data (particularly AHI) and ESS results. A significant proportion of OSA patients do not report subjective daytime sleepiness on this test, though it remains unclear whether these patients have an objectively measureable functional effect from OSA.

Table 8.2 The respiratory disturbance index (RDI) versus the Epworth Sleepiness Scale (ESS) score for the Sleep Heart Health Study

RDI	$RDI < 5$	$5 \leq RDI < 15$	$15 \leq RDI < 30$	$RDI \geq 30$
Mean ESS (standard deviation)	7.2 (4.3)	7.8 (4.4)	8.3 (4.6)	9.3 (4.9)

Adapted from Gottlieb DJ, Whitney CW, Bonekat WH, et al.[5]

Gottlieb et al.[5] used data from the Sleep Heart Health Study to review the relationship between the respiratory disturbance index (RDI, similar to AHI) on an unattended full polysomnogram and the ESS. The 1824 patients were broken into four categories based on RDI, as shown in Table 8.2.

The limited differences between groups were statistically significant, which suggested that excessive sleepiness was related to RDI in a small, but statistically significant manner. Adjusting for common confounders, such as age, sex, body mass index, and sleep times did not change this relationship. If EDS is defined by an ESS score > 10, patients with moderate to severe elevations of RDI were 67% more likely to have EDS than patients with a normal RDI. However, even in the highest RDI classification, the mean ESS score was in the normal range, suggesting that a reasonable portion of patients with significant sleep-disordered breathing either did not subjectively recognize sleepiness or did not have EDS. In a more recent study, a trend (which was not statistically significant) existed for patients with a high AHI to have an ESS score ≥ 13, compared to an ESS score ≤ 6, suggesting that AHI may play only a minor role in predicting EDS.

In 2006, Pack et al.[6] examined a group of more than 400 truck drivers, some of whom were at high risk for OSA and some of whom were at low risk for OSA. This study revealed that ESS scores did not correlate with sleep apnea in this population, again demonstrating the limitations of self-reported ESS scores in identification of patients with OSA. However, the study also established that an AHI ≥ 20 events per hour was a risk factor for EDS as measured by the MSLT. Only a very small proportion (4%) of subjects with severe OSA (AHI ≥ 30 events per hour) had completely normal mean sleep latencies of 10 minutes or more.

Fewer data have been obtained on the relationship between OSA and the MWT. Sleep apnea has been linked to shorter sleep latencies on the MWT in some studies, though a minority of OSA patients still have normal sleep latencies on the test. Attempts to understand the factors that influence MWT results have not resulted in a clear picture; though, in one study, age, previous sleep history, and the number of greater than 4% oxygen saturation dips explained a minority of the variance.[7] Motivation has also been demonstrated to affect the results of the MWT.

Understanding excessive sleepiness in OSA

The pathogenesis of EDS in OSA is unclear. Thus, it is difficult to design a measure to optimally link severity of OSA with daytime sleepiness. Early research on 100 patients with OSA (AHI > 10) at Stanford University distinguished between patients who were sleepy (MSL ≤ 5 min), mildly sleepy (5 min $<$ MSL < 8 min), and not sleepy (MSL ≥ 8 min).[8] The respiratory disturbance index, oxygen saturation indices, body mass index, and total nocturnal sleep time did not significantly correlate with daytime sleepiness, as measured by the MSLT. Other early research suggested that EDS was potentially related to nocturnal hypoxemia or sleep fragmentation.

A more recent study[9] of 40 subjects with at least moderate OSA (AHI > 20 per hour) evaluated polysomnographic characteristics of those subjects who were sleepy (as defined by an ESS score > 10 and an MSL score < 5 min) and compared them to those who were not sleepy (an ESS score < 10 and an MSL score > 10 min). The sleepy subjects exhibited a longer duration of apnea than did those without EDS. This finding may be related to intrinsic differences in their threshold for arousal or may represent the effect of increased sleep pressure. As the AHIs in the two groups were similar, the frequency of respiratory events did not explain the mechanisms of EDS in this study. Another potential cause of EDS is the increased sleep-related hypoxemia in that group; the effect of low oxygen levels could damage wake-promoting neural structures. Although the mechanisms linking intermittent hypoxemia and EDS in humans are not clearly established, mouse studies demonstrate that sleep-specific intermittent hypoxemia damages neurons in wake-promoting brain regions ultimately leading to the manifestation of sleepiness. Evidence also exists from human studies that the cognitive deficits in OSA patients may be secondary to repetitive nocturnal intermittent hypoxemia.

Though nocturnal oxygen saturation is one element likely to affect EDS, additional variables also need to be considered. Closer examination of respiratory-related arousals and comparison to other arousals has been performed, demonstrating positive correlation with daytime sleepiness. Patients with OSA may also have other individual variables that contribute to vulnerability to daytime sleepiness, including genetic factors, acute or chronic sleep deprivation, other medical conditions, and duration of OSA.

Main points

Excessive daytime sleepiness is a common symptom among patients with OSA. However, common metrics of OSA severity, including the AHI, do not always predict the severity of daytime sleepiness.

FURTHER READING

Bedard MA, Montplaisir J, Richer F, Malo J. Nocturnal hypoxemia as a determinant of vigilance impairment in sleep apnea syndrome. *Chest* 1991;**100**:367–70.

Chervin RD, Aldrich MS. The Epworth Sleepiness Scale may not reflect objective measures of sleepiness or sleep apnea. *Neurology* 1999;**52**:125–31.

Jacobsen JH, Shi L, Mokhlesi B. Factors associated with excessive daytime sleepiness in patients with severe obstructive sleep apnea. *Sleep Breath* 2013;**17**:629–35.

REFERENCES

1. Epstein LJ, Kristo D, Strollo P, et al. Clinical guideline for evaluation, management, and long-term care of obstructive sleep apnea in adults. *J Clin Sleep Med* 2009;**5**:263–76.
2. American Academy of Sleep Medicine. *International Classification of Sleep Disorders. Diagnostic and Coding Manual*, Second Edition. Westchester, IL: American Academy of Sleep Medicine;2005.
3. Littner MR, Kushida C, Wise M, et al. Practice parameters for clinical use of the Multiple Sleep Latency Test and the Maintenance of Wakefulness Test. *Sleep* 2005;**28**:113–21.
4. Tregear S, Reston J, Schoelles K, et al. Obstructive sleep apnea and risk of motor vehicle crash: systematic review and meta-analysis. *J Clin Sleep Med* 2009;**5**:573–81.
5. Gottlieb DJ, Whitney CW, Bonekat WH, et al. Relation of sleepiness to respiratory disturbance index: the Sleep Heart Health Study. *Am J Respir Crit Care Med* 1999;**159**:502–7.
6. Pack AI, Maislin G, Staley B, et al. Impaired performance in commercial drivers: role of sleep apnea and short sleep duration. *Am J Respir Crit Care Med* 2006;**174**:446–54.
7. Banks S, Barnes M, Tarquinio N, et al. Factors associated with maintenance of wakefulness test mean sleep latency in patients with mild to moderate obstructive sleep apnoea and normal subjects. *J Sleep Res* 2004;**13**:71–8.
8. Guilleminault C, Partinen M, Quera-Salva MA, et al. Determinants of daytime sleepiness in obstructive sleep apnea. *Chest* 1988;**94**:32–7.
9. Mediano O, Barcelo A, de la Pena M. Daytime sleepiness and polysomnographic variables in sleep apnoea patients. *Eur Respir J* 2007;**30**:110–13.

9

Neither subjective nor objective measures allow confident prediction of future risk for motor vehicle crashes due to sleepiness

Anita Valanju Shelgikar

Case

A 31-year-old woman initially presented with excessive daytime sleepiness and symptoms of restless legs syndrome for 5 years. At the time of presentation, she was enrolled in college for the summer semester. Her courses required long periods of prolonged sitting and reading, during which she often fell asleep. She had difficulty with attentiveness without taking a nap between classes. A classmate once observed that she had a "blank stare" during class, but the patient had no recollection of this behavior. She remarked, "I feel like I'm spacing out or that my mind is foggy," and then she loses track of time; this can last for minutes to an hour if she is by herself. There is no associated extremity movement with these episodes. She denies any associated oral trauma or fecal or urinary incontinence. She has no history of head injury, central nervous system infections, or febrile convulsions, and no family history of seizures.

Her grades did suffer because she often slept through class. Her restless legs symptoms were extremely bothersome at the time, and this was presumed to be the etiology of her daytime sleepiness. She was started on pramipexole, with significant improvement in her leg symptoms, but persistent daytime sleepiness. Soon thereafter she started work at 4:30 AM, and began to attribute her daytime sleepiness to her shift work and self-induced sleep deprivation, which she combated with coffee. When she transitioned to a desk job, she was fired after a few weeks "because I had trouble getting there on time at 8:00 AM and I wasn't alert enough."

The patient has often felt uncomfortable driving due to her daytime sleepiness. She never sustained a motor vehicle collision, but has swerved off the road and drifted out of her lane fairly often. As a result, she has limited her driving. She asks her husband to drive if she feels that she is unable to drive.

The patient reported that she was usually in bed by midnight and could fall asleep easily. Some nights she would wake after 3–4 hours and remains awake for 1.5 hours, largely due to restless legs symptoms. She would often wake spontaneously at 6:00–6:30 AM. Her husband has heard her snoring. She reported that "my arms tingle and go limp if I'm laughing really hard." One time she was carrying a box while her brother was making jokes, and she found it hard to hold on to the box "because they [her arms] started to go limp while I was laughing." She has never had sleep paralysis. She rarely had hypnagogic hallucinations but reported frequent visual hypnopompic hallucinations.

Past medical history included migraine headaches, depression, papillary microcarcinoma treated with right thyroid lobectomy, and hypothyroidism (postsurgical). Medications included vitamin D3, norgestimate-ethinyl estradiol (oral contraceptive), levothyroxine, and venlafaxine. Her venlafaxine was initially prescribed for treatment of depression. In the past, she had also tried duloxetine, lamictal, lithium, and venlafaxine hydrochloride, extended release for treatment of her mood disorder and found venlafaxine to work best.

Physical examination was notable for a body mass index of 23.4 kg/m^2, patent oral airway, and normal, non-focal neurologic exam.

What test was done and what was the diagnosis?

A baseline polysomnogram showed a total sleep time of 492 minutes, apnea/hypopnea index of 5.2 apneas or hypopneas per hour of sleep, and a minimum oxygen saturation of 90%. The rapid eye movement (REM) sleep latency on that study was 20.5 minutes and no snoring was noted. Her periodic limb movement index was four movements per hour of sleep. This study was followed by a 4-nap Multiple Sleep Latency Test (MSLT) that showed a mean sleep latency of 2.3 minutes with sleep-onset REM periods (SOREMPs) in all naps. She had discontinued use of venlafaxine for at least 2 weeks prior to her studies. Interpretation of the baseline polysomnogram indicated that there was no clear evidence of sleep-disordered breathing. The MSLT was found to support a diagnosis of narcolepsy. Given the patient's history of bilateral arm weakness with laughter, she was given a diagnosis of narcolepsy with cataplexy.

The patient noted significant symptomatic improvement after treatment of her narcolepsy with cataplexy, and with continued use of pramipexole for her restless legs syndrome. Her cataplexy resolved and her daytime sleepiness decreased with nightly use of sodium oxybate. She remained on venlafaxine for treatment of her comorbid depression. Her Epworth Sleepiness Scale score with treatment was 7 (normal) out of 24. She noted that staying awake in the afternoon was still, at times, a "struggle" that prompted her to nap for 1 hour. She reported overall improvement in her alertness while driving, though she continued to avoid driving in the early morning hours due to her concern that she may have slight residual sleepiness at that time.

Discussion

No evidence-based, consensus guideline on assessment of a sleepy individual's fitness to drive currently exists. The issue of drowsy driving has garnered particular interest in occupational medicine, with focus on commercial drivers and shift workers, but is pertinent to all drivers. A random digit-dialed telephone survey of non-institutionalized adults aged above18 years of age showed that 4.2% of the 147 076 respondents reported having fallen asleep while driving at least once during the previous 30 days. Reports of falling asleep while driving were more common in those respondents who reported usually sleeping ≤ 6 hours per day, snoring, or unintentionally falling asleep during the day.[1] Due to the public health implications of drowsy driving, this topic has been the source of extensive study. Research to date includes evaluation of various subjective or objective assessment tools, or a combination of testing modalities, to use in clinical settings to predict risk of motor vehicle crashes and fitness to drive. Table 9.1 lists evaluation modalities that may be considered in the clinical assessment of driving safety.

The Epworth Sleepiness Scale is commonly used for subjective assessment of excessive daytime sleepiness in recent times. This instrument asks the respondent to rate the likelihood of dozing during eight different sedentary situations. The summed result can provide a standardized measure of self-assessed sleepiness across different time points or treatment conditions. However, validity studies have reported only weak to moderate[2] or absent[3] associations between Epworth scores and objective assessments of sleepiness. A recent survey of over 35 000 highway drivers did suggest an association between the Epworth score

Table 9.1 Tools that may be utilized in the clinical evaluation of sleepiness and safety to drive

Essential:
- Detailed clinical history
May be considered:
- Epworth Sleepiness Scale
- Karolinska Sleepiness Scale
- Multiple Sleep Latency Test
- Maintenance of Wakefulness Test
- Psychomotor Vigilance Task
- Driving simulator

and the risk of sleepy driving accidents. In this study, respondents with an Epworth score of 11 or above, in comparison to those with lower scores, had a higher odds ratio for having had a sleepy driving accident.[4] Despite retrospective data such as these, however, available literature does not yet make clear whether the Epworth in fact predicts driving risk going forward.

Even if a low Epworth score does provide some reassurance of lower crash risk, it cannot guarantee that any elevated risk is eliminated. The patient described has an Epworth score of 7 out of 24 with treatment, but still "struggles" to stay awake in the afternoon. Driving at that time of day, when she is most susceptible to dozing, may still confer a risk of a crash. The Epworth score must be interpreted in the clinical context if it is to inform the clinician and patient about driving safety and risk of crash due to sleepiness.

Objective sleep testing, specifically the MSLT and Maintenance of Wakefulness Test (MWT), has been studied to determine whether either assessment may predict risk for sleepy driving crashes. A study of 618 subjects selected from the general population demonstrated that shorter mean sleep latencies on MSLTs (consistent with increased sleepiness) were associated with likelihood of documented automobile collisions during the previous 10 years.[5] Another study of 38 untreated sleep apnea patients and 14 healthy control subjects compared mean sleep latencies on four 40-minute MWT trials, Epworth scores, and Karolinska Sleepiness Scale scores to an important outcome: the number of inappropriate line crossings during 90-minute real-life driving sessions.[6] The Karolinska Sleepiness Scale seeks to assess how sleepy the respondent is at a particular moment. In this study, the number of inappropriate line crossings correlated with MWT scores, Karolinska Sleepiness Scale scores measured at halfway in total driving distance, and Epworth scores. For example, participants with MWT mean sleep latencies of 33 minutes or less, in comparison to remaining subjects, had more inappropriate line crossings, as shown in Figure 9.1.[6] Again, however,

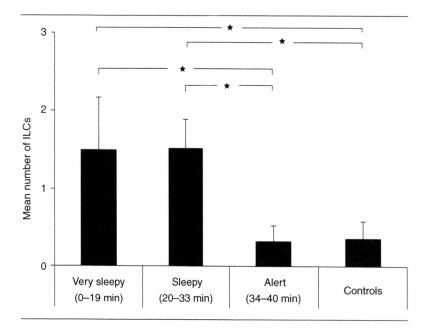

Figure 9.1 Mean number of inappropriate line crossings (ILCs, mean and standard error) during real driving in 14 control subjects and 38 untreated sleep apnea patients, grouped according to mean sleep latency on the Maintenance of Wakefulness Test. *$P < 0.05$. Reproduced with permission from Philip P, Sagaspe P, Taillard J, et al.[6]

as with subjective assessments, data have not yet been generated to make a convincing case that objective assessments of daytime sleepiness have predictive value for future motor vehicle crashes.

A robust body of literature examines the utility of driving simulators in assessment of sleepiness, driving performance, and crash risk, with many studies to suggest that simulated driving performance may be predictive of real driving performance.[7] While use of driving simulators has shown much promise in research settings, logistic difficulties currently preclude these devices to be incorporated into routine clinical evaluation. As technology continues to evolve, driving simulators may become more readily obtainable in clinical determination of driving safety. The Psycho-motor Vigilance Task (PVT)[8] is commonly used in research on sleep deprivation and performance. The PVT measures reaction time in response to a visual stimulus, and studies have shown that various degrees of sleep deprivation yield increased reaction times. However, performance on the PVT has not been shown to indicate poor performance on a driving simulator. Thus, the PVT should not be used as a stand-alone measure of fitness to drive in the setting of a known sleep disorder or sleepiness.[9]

In short, although published data certainly suggest a likely role for objective testing in evaluation of fitness to drive, more data are needed before an evidence-based guideline can be applied to clinical practice. From a practical standpoint, MSLTs and MWTs are not routinely pursued in the evaluation and management of all patients with excessive daytime sleepiness. For example, patients with obstructive sleep apnea are often sleepy, but their sleepiness is seldom assessed by objective means because treatment is indicated once the diagnosis is established, and in most cases thorough evaluation of sleepiness will not change treatment decisions. The same holds true for patients whose excessive daytime sleepiness is attributed to other factors, such as medication side effect, comorbid medical disorders, or behavioral influences such as chronic partial sleep deprivation. Furthermore, for this diverse group of individuals, all of whom may report daytime sleepiness, a well-validated and reliable method to predict future crash risk remains to be established.

Main points

Drowsy driving presents a major individual and public health risk. Currently no evidence-based guidelines, with use of either subjective or objective testing, are available to guide determination of an individual's fitness to drive, with respect to his or her daytime sleepiness. This assessment must be performed on a case-by-case basis, with consideration of all factors that pertain to the etiology and timing of a patient's daytime sleepiness and driving habits. An experienced clinician cannot use any current combination of approaches or testing to determine confidently that a patient will or will not have a crash because of daytime sleepiness. Some available subjective and objective assessments do have face validity and at least retrospective data to suggest that they may help in assessment for future driving risk. The clinician's most important roles are to identify and treat underlying contributors to daytime sleepiness, educate patients on risks of drowsy driving, and encourage patients to either forgo driving or to pull over if sleepiness develops while sitting behind the wheel.

REFERENCES

1. Centers for Disease Control and Prevention. Drowsy driving – 19 states and the District of Columbia, 2009–2010. *MMWR Morb Mortal Wkly Rep* 2013;**4**:1033–7.
2. Akerstedt T, Gillberg M. Subjective and objective sleepiness in the active individual. *Int J Neurosci* 1990;**52**:29–37.
3. Benbadis SR, Mascha E, Perry MC, et al. Association between the Epworth Sleepiness Scale and the Multiple Sleep Latency Test in a clinical population. *Ann Intern Med* 1999;**130**:289–92.
4. Philip P, Sagaspe P, Lagarde E, et al. Sleep disorders and accidental risk in a large group of regular registered highway drivers. *Sleep Med* 2010;**11**:973–9.
5. Drake C, Roehrs T, Breslau N, et al. The 10-year risk of verified motor vehicle crashes in relation to physiologic sleepiness. *Sleep* 2010;**33**:745–52.
6. Philip P, Sagaspe P, Taillard J, et al. Maintenance of Wakefulness Test, obstructive sleep apnea syndrome, and driving risk. *Ann Neurol* 2008;**64**:410–16.

7. de Winter JC. Predicting self-reported violations among novice license drivers using pre-license simulator measures. *Accid Anal Prev* 2013;**52**:71-9.

8. Dinges DF, Powell JW. Microcomputer analyses of performance on a portable, simple visual RT task during sustained operations. *Behav Res Meth Instr* 1985;**17**:652-5.

9. Baulk SD, Biggs SN, Reid KJ, van den Heuvel CJ, Dawson D. Chasing the silver bullet: measuring driver fatigue using simple and complex tasks. *Accident Anal Prev* 2008;**40**: 396-402.

10

A sleep apnea patient with excessive daytime sleepiness and subtle respiratory events may be misdiagnosed with narcolepsy or idiopathic hypersomnia

Alp Sinan Baran

Case

A 41-year-old otherwise healthy man presented with a long history of worsening daytime fatigue and sleepiness. Symptoms became more problematic recently after starting a new job that involved predominantly sedentary work at a computer workstation, as compared to his prior position, which required more physical activity. After finding him nodding off at his desk, his employer encouraged him to seek medical evaluation. The patient was then referred by his family physician to a local sleep laboratory, where he was tested with a polysomnogram (PSG) and Multiple Sleep Latency Test (MSLT). He was determined to have an apnea/hypopnea index (AHI) of 4.8 apneas or hypopneas per hour of sleep on the PSG. The MSLT yielded a mean sleep latency of 8.2 minutes with a sleep-onset rapid eye movement (REM) episode on the first nap (Table 10.1). As he did not formally qualify for a diagnosis of obstructive sleep apnea (OSA) or narcolepsy, he was given a diagnosis of idiopathic hypersomnia and was prescribed modafinil 200 mg once daily. With this regimen, he experienced improvement in daytime sleepiness, but had new onset of frequent headaches attributed to the medication, ultimately leading to discontinuation. His primary physician decided to obtain a second opinion from a sleep physician at a sleep disorders center before consideration of prescribing a stimulant medication.

During his reevaluation at the sleep disorders center, the patient denied a history of snoring but admitted to occasional awakenings with a snort. Physical examination was remarkable for normal body habitus (body mass index of 23 kg/m^2), unrestricted nares, mildly elongated soft palate, and retropositioned mandible with Class II malocclusion and 7 mm overjet of his incisors.

Should sleep testing be repeated?

Despite previously negative PSG results and the absence of snoring, the patient's clinical history of awakenings with a snort, combined with physical findings consistent with a retropositioned mandible, were suggestive of sleep-disordered breathing. Therefore, a repeat PSG was performed and analyzed with special attention to respiratory effort-related arousals (RERAs), which were not tabulated on the original study. Though the AHI was again borderline at 5.3, the respiratory disturbance index (RDI), which includes RERAs in addition to apneas and hypopneas, was 19.8. The respiratory events were subtle but nevertheless caused significant sleep disturbance. Snoring was mild and occurred more frequently during REM sleep, as did apneic events. The percent of the night spent in REM sleep was below the lower limit of normal, which is 20% (Table 10.2). When REM sleep is fragmented, in this case by obstructive respiratory events, the overall percentage may be lower than normal.

The patient was presented with treatment options, which included continuous positive airway pressure,

Common Pitfalls in Sleep Medicine, ed. Ronald D. Chervin. Published by Cambridge University Press. © Cambridge University Press 2014.

Table 10.1 Results of the patient's polysomnogram and Multiple Sleep Latency Test

Polysomnogram results

Sleep architecture		Respiratory parameters	
% Stage N1	18	AHI	4.8
% Stage N2	45		
% Stage N3	2		
% REM	17		

MSLT results

	Sleep latency (mins)	REM latency (mins)
Nap 1	7.0	10.6
Nap 2	8.5	N/A
Nap 3	8.1	N/A
Nap 4	9.2	N/A

AHI, apnea/hypopnea index; MSLT, Multiple Sleep Latency Test; REM, rapid eye movement.

Table 10.2 Results of patient's repeat polysomnogram with scoring of respiratory effort-related arousals

	Non-REM	REM
AHI ([apneas + hypopneas] / total sleep time)	4.5	8.8
RDI ([apneas + hypopneas + RERAs] / total sleep time)	17	33
% Total sleep time	82	18

AHI, apnea/hypopnea index; RDI, respiratory disturbance index; REM, rapid eye movement; RERAs, respiratory effort-related arousals.

oral appliances, and surgical considerations. Given his retropositioned mandible and the predominance of RERAs, he was thought to be a good candidate for an oral appliance to position his mandible more anteriorly. He was agreeable to the use of a mandibular advancement device during sleep, and another PSG was performed to optimize the appliance and confirm efficacy. The AHI and RDI were both within normal limits, and REM sleep percentage increased into the normal range of 20–25% (Table 10.3). The mandibular advancement device was prescribed for home use. When the patient returned for follow-up 3 weeks later,

Table 10.3 Results of patient's polysomnogram with mandibular advancement device

	Non-REM	REM
AHI ([apneas + hypopneas] / total sleep time)	1.5	2.4
RDI ([apneas + hypopneas + RERAs] / total sleep time)	2.7	3.8
% Total sleep time	78	22

AHI, apnea/hypopnea index; RDI, respiratory disturbance index; REM, rapid eye movement; RERAs, respiratory effort-related arousals.

he reported subjective improvements in sleep quality and daytime alertness. If he slept at least 7–8 hours per night, he no longer experienced excessive daytime sleepiness. At the time of follow-up 3 months later, he again reported excellent results and was tolerating the treatment well, with only mild transient temporomandibular joint discomfort during the first 1–2 hours after awakening. With the subjective resolution of excessive daytime sleepiness, a repeat MSLT was not deemed necessary.

Discussion

The diagnosis of OSA may not always be obvious, especially in a patient of normal or nearly normal weight and with no history of snoring. Though OSA is certainly not confined to patients who are obese and snore, this stereotype tends to influence many clinicians. Not all patients with OSA snore loudly and some may not snore noticeably at all, but they can still present with poor sleep quality and excessive daytime sleepiness as the main symptoms. To further complicate matters, such patients may not have obvious apneas or hypopneas on a PSG, resulting in an unremarkable apnea/hypopnea index, and a missed diagnosis or else misdiagnosis based on presence of EDS without apparent cause. Some of these patients may end up living with the short- and long-term consequences of untreated OSA until the condition progresses, with worsening of signs and symptoms to a degree that makes diagnosis more obvious. Others with more prominent excessive daytime sleepiness may be given a diagnosis of idiopathic hypersomnia or narcolepsy and treated with wakefulness promoting medications, resulting in symptomatic improvement in excessive daytime sleepiness without addressing the underlying condition. This was the situation in the case described. Had it not been for the intolerance of modafinil due to headaches, the patient may not have been reevaluated for definitive diagnosis of his condition.

Craniofacial features can predispose to OSA

Some patients have OSA as a consequence of various syndromes that involve craniofacial abnormalities, such as Crouzon syndrome and Pierre Robin syndrome. These patients are usually readily identifiable and many have OSA that is prominent enough to make diagnosis straightforward. However, more subtle craniofacial features can also predispose to sleep-disordered breathing, as in this case. A retropositioned mandible may not be obvious if it is not extreme, and can be missed unless examined carefully, especially in a male patient with a beard that may compensate for an appearance of a deficient chin. With mandibular retropositioning, the posterior airway space is narrowed, and even in the absence of excessive adipose tissue, OSA may result. During examination of mandibular position, some patients may have a tendency to close the mouth in an unnatural manner, bringing the tips of the incisors together. This disguises the retropositioning of the mandible, which can be better demonstrated by asking the patient to move the jaw in a chewing motion.

Though not present in this case, nasal obstruction can also cause or worsen sleep-disordered breathing, and is another feature to keep in mind during the evaluation of patients without other obvious abnormalities. A restricted nasal airway is thought to result in oropharyngeal collapse by at least two mechanisms. If nasal flow restriction is severe enough to cause mouth-breathing, upper airway collapsibility is increased by the open position of the mandible.[1] Additionally,

during supine sleep with the mouth open, the mandible and tongue are more likely to fall posteriorly. Even if obstruction is not to a degree that necessitates mouth breathing, increased resistance requires increased inspiratory effort, which can cause narrowing of the oropharynx. Skeletal nasal abnormalities, whether developmental of traumatic – e.g. nasal septal deviation and turbinate hypertrophy – can create increased nasal resistance. Soft tissue abnormalities – e.g. polyps and congestion secondary to rhinitis – can also cause a significant increase in upper airway resistance.

Respiratory effort-related arousals

A milder variant of OSA, as described in this case, was originally termed "upper airway resistance syndrome."[2] With the subsequent addition of RERAs to apneas and hypopneas as features of OSA, this diagnosis now encompasses upper airway resistance syndrome as well. A RERA is characterized by an electroencephalographic (EEG) arousal lasting at least 3 seconds, preceded by evidence of increased respiratory effort, with airflow reduction and oxygen desaturation that do not qualify for scoring an apnea or hypopnea. The increased respiratory effort associated with a RERA can be identified most definitively by esophageal pressure monitoring (with intrathoracic pressure swings to values of –10 cm H_2O or more negative). However, standard PSG using a nasal pressure transducer can also reveal RERAs. EEG arousals preceded by $\geq$ 10 second intervals of flattening of the inspiratory portion of the nasal pressure tracing can be used to identify episodes of flow limitation even when criteria for an apnea or hypopnea are not met.[3] Crescendo snoring or upper airway vibration – detected using nasal pressure or a piezoelectric snore sensor – often occurs during RERAs and also can help to identify these events, though they are not a required criterion.

AHI versus RDI

Terminology used to quantify breathing abnormalities on PSG reports can be confusing. In the past, the RDI and AHI were equivalent terms and were used interchangeably to indicate the mean number of apneas and hypopneas per hour of sleep. With formal definition of RERAs, the RDI can now include this respiratory event type, and some sleep laboratories have taken advantage of this option, though many still use the RDI as a synonym of the AHI. Only careful examination of the definitions used on a PSG report can clarify the variable use of this terminology.

Are RERAs important?

There remains a significant focus on oxygen desaturation as a key issue in OSA, but strong evidence suggests that the sympathetic nervous system activation with EEG arousals also plays an important role in the long-term health consequences of OSA, including hypertension and associated complications.[4] Of course, EEG arousals are also the cause of sleep fragmentation and are likely to contribute to EDS in patients with OSA. Despite the pathophysiologic importance of RERAs, the American Academy of Sleep Medicine has deemed the scoring of these events as optional, while the scoring of apneas and hypopneas is mandatory.[3] With this optional status, and the fact that some health insurance providers do not recognize RERAs as legitimate obstructive respiratory events qualifying patients for coverage of treatment, many sleep laboratories do not include the identification and reporting of RERAs

within their scoring protocols. This omission can lead to a missed diagnosis of mild OSA, as initially occurred in this case. Abundant data show that OSA classified as mild, based on the frequency of apneic events, can nonetheless have effects, for example on sleepiness, that are as severe as those produced by severe OSA. Physicians should keep the possibility of unidentified subtle obstructive respiratory events in mind when reviewing the results of a PSG, especially in patients whose clinical outcomes are unsatisfactory, or when a discrepancy arises between the clinical history and PSG results.

REFERENCES

1. Meurice J, Marc I, Carrier G, Series F. Effect of mouth opening on upper airway collapsibility in normal sleeping subjects. *Am J Respir Crit Care Med* 1996;**153**:255–9.
2. Guilleminault C, Stoohs R, Clerk A, Cetel M, Maistros P. A cause of excessive daytime sleepiness. The upper airway resistance syndrome. *Chest* 1993;**104**:781–7.
3. American Academy of Sleep Medicine. *The AASM Manual for the Scoring of Sleep and Associated Events: Rules, Terminology and Technical Specifications*. Westchester, IL: American Academy of Sleep Medicine;2007.
4. Shepard JW Jr. Hypertension, cardiac arrhythmias, myocardial infarction, and stroke in relation to obstructive sleep apnea. *Clin Chest Med.* 1992;**13**:437–58.

Diagnosis of narcolepsy

Narcolepsy affects about 0.03% of the population, but often patients remain undiagnosed for many years before their condition is recognized and treated. Much progress has been made in understanding the neurophysiologic basis for narcolepsy with cataplexy. This condition appears to be caused at least in part by near absence of a neurotransmitter, hypocretin-1 (also called orexin A), that is normally produced in the hypothalamus and distributed widely to many regions of the brain, where it plays a critical function in maintaining alertness. In practice, the diagnosis of narcolepsy with cataplexy is still accomplished in large part by a good clinical history and examination. Sleep laboratory testing for confirmation is also sought whenever possible, especially when the history of

cataplexy is ambiguous. Narcolepsy without cataplexy, in contrast, does not appear likely to have the same neurophysiologic basis, and its diagnosis requires sleep laboratory confirmation. The clinical cases in this section show that significant pitfalls exist for the clinician in the assessment of patients for suspected narcolepsy, of either type. The history alone can often reveal the diagnosis, but the history, like the Multiple Sleep Latency Test and other clues to the presence of narcolepsy, can also at times be deceiving. With the advantage of the hindsight provided in the cases that follow, the reader will appreciate that persistence and a combination of serial investigations may be necessary, for some patients, to firmly establish a diagnosis that leads to the most effective treatment plans.

11

Narcolepsy with cataplexy can occur in the absence of a positive Multiple Sleep Latency Test

Daniel I. Rifkin

Case

J. W. presented as a 20-year-old college student with a 3-year history of progressive daytime sleepiness. In high school, she started to fall asleep in both her morning and afternoon classes and took a nap when she returned home from school. Despite her frequent napping, she maintained good grades and graduated high school with honors. However, she was now performing poorly in college because she had trouble staying awake to study for tests or to complete papers. She "only wanted to sleep." She didn't want to go out with friends or even go to class for that matter. As she was having so much difficulty in college and seemed to "withdraw" from her usual activities, her primary care provider suspected clinical depression and placed her on paroxetine.

However, J. W. did not improve. She saw a sleep medicine specialist, Dr. P., but she did not report hypnogogic hallucinations or sleep paralysis. However, she did report a more recent "funny and weird" feeling with profound laughter. Interestingly, this feeling only occurred when she laughed with this one particular friend. She never fell to the ground or "felt weak" per se. She always "grabbed" her friend though, when she laughed, which seemed odd to her. Otherwise, J. W. was healthy, had a normal exam, and was no longer taking the paroxetine. With a suspicion of narcolepsy without cataplexy (as Dr. P. did not feel that her "funny feeling" represented cataplexy), Dr. P. pursued a polysomnogram (PSG) followed by a Multiple Sleep Latency Test (MSLT). A negative urine toxicology screen was obtained at the time of the sleep laboratory testing. On the PSG, J. W. fell asleep quickly with a sleep onset latency of 2.5 minutes. Latency to rapid eye movement (REM) sleep was 58 minutes, with 23% of total sleep spent in REM sleep. Sleep architecture appeared fragmented without a clear ultradian non-REM/REM pattern. The longest consolidated REM sleep period was 18 minutes. Neither sleep apnea, nor any other disorder that could explain non-restorative sleep was identified. The 5-nap MSLT on the following day revealed a mean sleep onset latency of 9.6 minutes (Nap 1: 8.5 min; Nap 2: 6.5 min; Nap 3: 5.5 min; Nap 4: 9.5 min; and Nap 5: 18.0 min). A single sleep-onset REM period (SOREMP) was noted in Nap 3 (Figure 11.1). However, the suggestion that REM sleep was imminent – appearance of a REM sleep-consistent electroencephalogram (EEG), with saw-tooth waves – was noted on two separate occasions in Nap 2. The technician notes were unremarkable except for "the patient looked anxious" and was "pacing back and forth" in the room after Nap 3. With these findings of a mean sleep onset latency of 9.6 minutes and 1 SOREMP, the test was interpreted as negative for narcolepsy, but more specifically was interpreted as negative for excessive daytime sleepiness. And because of the reported negative MSLT findings, and in spite of the PSG findings of a shortened sleep onset latency, slightly decreased REM-sleep latency, and prominent sleep fragmentation,

Common Pitfalls in Sleep Medicine, ed. Ronald D. Chervin. Published by Cambridge University Press. © Cambridge University Press 2014.

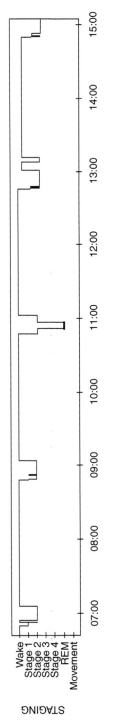

Figure 11.1 Hypnogram from this patient's initial Multiple Sleep Latency Test (MSLT). A hypnogram summarizes the sleep stages attained during a sleep study. In this case, only the third nap showed rapid eye movement (REM) sleep. Appearance of REM sleep within 15 minutes of sleep onset, during a 20-minute MSLT nap opportunity, qualifies the nap as a sleep-onset REM period (SOREMP). However, two or more SOREMPs on an MSLT are required to confirm a diagnosis of narcolepsy without cataplexy. (Note, this hypnogram shows an older convention in which non-REM sleep was scored as stage 1, 2, 3, and 4. Current standards divide non-REM sleep into stages N1, N2, and N3, which includes former stages 3 and 4.)

60

Dr. P. suspected generalized anxiety disorder and placed J. W. on alprazolam and buspirone. Her symptoms worsened and her mother insisted J. W. obtain a second opinion, which led her to Dr. E. about 1 year after originally seeing Dr. P.

Dr. E. obtained a similar history, but questioned J. W. further regarding her "funny feeling" with laughter. Not only did she feel "funny" but she described a feeling like her "face was melting" and that it was hard for her to form words when she was laughing so hard. Even though the feeling only lasted seconds, it occurred repetitively at times during the laughing spell. Dr. E. was convinced her symptoms represented cataplexy. Dr. E. thus diagnosed J. W. with narcolepsy with cataplexy, and although he didn't believe that repeat testing was absolutely required, he sought to confirm his suspicion with a repeat PSG followed by MSLT. This PSG revealed a shortened sleep onset latency with a REM-sleep latency of 26 minutes. The 4-nap MSLT uncovered a notably short mean sleep onset latency of 2.4 minutes, with 4 out of 4 SOREMPs. Narcolepsy with cataplexy was confirmed.

What went wrong?

For more than a year after initially presenting to a sleep medicine physician, J. W. remained misdiagnosed as a non-narcoleptic. Even her daytime sleepiness was questioned and labeled as depression and anxiety despite clinical evidence to the contrary. Unfortunately, the missed diagnosis of narcolepsy or the delay in diagnosis is common, with some authors reporting excessively long intervals from the time of initial symptom presentation to the time of ultimate diagnosis.[1] Often times, one lacks the confidence to make the diagnosis of narcolepsy, or the diagnosis of excessive sleepiness for that matter, based on clinical evidence alone, and instead one relies too heavily on laboratory data. In this particular case, the initial MSLT findings did not confirm the presence of narcolepsy without cataplexy (as originally considered by Dr. P.) based on International Classification of Sleep Disorders (ICSD-2)[2] criteria, so the diagnosis was erroneously abandoned.

Or was the initial MSLT incorrectly interpreted, especially in conjunction with the PSG the previous night, which revealed fragmented sleep with shortened sleep onset and REM-sleep latencies? What if Dr. P. eliminated the results of the last nap, due to concern about a "last nap effect" that can prevent sleep when younger patients are "anxious" for their imminent opportunity to finally leave the laboratory?

With Nap-5 eliminated, the mean sleep onset latency would have been 7.5 minutes, within the range of pathologic sleepiness (< 8 min) based on ICSD-2 criteria.[2] Even if one accounts for the "last nap effect" and the re-calculated mean sleep onset latency, how does one address the single SOREMP? One published study found 2 or more SOREMPs on the initial MSLT – a required criterion for the diagnosis of narcolepsy in the absence of cataplexy – in only 83.5% of narcoleptics with cataplexy.[2,3] In a later study, those findings were confirmed with only 74% of narcoleptics yielding 2 or more SOREMPs.[4] The MSLT results differ from one testing date to another, and the test–retest reliability for the number of SOREMPs on an MSLT can be poor. One study explored the diagnostic utility of repeat MSLTs in patients with clinical features of narcolepsy and normal PSG. Mean sleep latency data were gathered between 2004 and 2009 for 125 patients; of these, 10 patients with repeat MSLT data were identified for the study. The results showed that 2 patients among the 10 met narcolepsy criteria on the second MSLT, despite not having met these criteria during the first MSLT. Both patients showed no substantive difference between the two testing periods in terms of preceding night sleep quality. Additionally, only 50% of patients met sleepiness criteria during the first MSLT; with repeat MSLT the number rose to 90%. The authors note that the increase in narcolepsy diagnosis was based on a decrease in the average sleep latency in the second study, not necessarily an increase in SOREMPs.[5]

Further, in an abstract entitled, "The Multiple Sleep Latency Test is not infallible," Jahnke and Aldrich[6] reviewed sleep evaluations of 13 patients with non-diagnostic initial MSLTs that were significantly different from subsequent MSLT results. The authors described multiple cases in which insufficient sleep obscured narcolepsy. One patient, at the age of 15, developed excessive daytime sleepiness, along with sleep paralysis and hypnagogic hallucinations. At age 20, nocturnal REM sleep latency was 51.5 minutes, with an MSLT that showed a mean sleep latency of 4.6 minutes, and no SOREMPs. After a month of increased nocturnal sleep, the mean sleep latency on a repeat MSLT was still short at 5.1 minutes, and the test now showed 5 SOREMPs.[6]

Many narcoleptics have a negative MSLT initially, and since the sensitivity for identification of two or more SOREMPs in patients with narcolepsy is not 100%, the current standard of practice is to repeat an MSLT test if narcolepsy remains suspect.[7] Thus, one should not rely solely on a single MSLT to discount the diagnosis of narcolepsy if the clinical suspicion is high.

Additional clues

The nighttime PSG also can be a valuable tool in the diagnosis of narcolepsy, especially if the MSLT result is suspect. One study found that the positive predictive value for narcolepsy of a SOREMP at the onset of a nighttime PSG **exceeds** that of the occurrence of SOREMPs on an MSLT.[4] As much as sleep intrudes into wakefulness in narcoleptics, an altered and fragmented sleep pattern with wakefulness often intrudes into sleep. The mechanism of disrupted or fragmented sleep in narcolepsy may differ from one patient to the next, and may be due to REM-intrusion phenomena such as nightmares or even REM-sleep behavior disorder. Non-REM parasomnias such as sleepwalking and confusional arousals are also more prevalent in patients with narcolepsy. Although important, "fragmented sleep" as part of the narcolepsy diagnostic criteria is often overlooked and under-recognized.

Laboratory tests including HLA genotyping or hypocretin-1 (also known as orexin A) analysis from cerebrospinal fluid can also be utilized. The HLA-DQB1*06:02 allele is strongly associated with narcolepsy and has a clinical sensitivity of 85–95% depending on ethnicity. In Caucasians, > 99% of affected narcoleptics with cataplexy have the HLA-DQB1*06:02 allele; however, the specificity is low as

15–25% of unaffected Caucasians have the HLA-DQB1*06:02 allele. Similarly, low cerebrospinal fluid hypocretin-1 levels can be found in a number of neurologic conditions other than narcolepsy, and the finding has a relatively low specificity, but it is most predictive of narcolepsy with cataplexy when the HLA-DQB1*06:02 allele is also present. Bourgin et al.[8] reaffirm the notion that "determination of CSF hypocretin-1 concentration to diagnose narcolepsy might be most useful in ambulatory patients with cataplexy but with a normal MSLT result, or if the MSLT is not interpretable, conclusive, or feasible." As 98% of patients with hypocretin-1 deficiency are positive for HLA-DQB1*06:02 allele, they also suggest HLA typing before lumbar puncture is performed. Unfortunately, however, hypocretin testing is not yet commercially available in many areas, including the United States.

Lastly, the clinical history is perhaps the most important and valuable tool in the diagnosis of narcolepsy with cataplexy. J. W. fits the typical profile of a young, otherwise healthy patient with the onset of hypersomnolence in the second decade of life and the ultimate development of cataplexy. Although she did not feel "weak" with her episodes, nor buckle her knees and fall to the ground, she clearly manifested limited cataplectic attacks that involved the head, neck, and face. A study of 40 young cataplectic patients (age range 13–23 years) reported that sagging of the jaw, inclined head, drooping of the shoulders, and transient buckling of the knees were the most common presentations.[9] J. W. was never asked whether her "funny feelings" had resolved when she was taking paroxetine, a serotonin uptake inhibitor and known treatment for cataplexy.

Any symptom associated with laughter or strong emotion should be explored in great detail when narcolepsy is suspected. More extensive questioning by Dr. P. might have uncovered the facial weakness later identified by Dr. E. In essence, one can make the diagnosis of narcolepsy with cataplexy based on the clinical history, and not rely solely on the MSLT results. The interpretation of the MSLT, when performed, should be made in conjunction with the PSG and within the context of the patient history. With that in mind, narcolepsy with cataplexy can be diagnosed in the absence of a positive MSLT.

REFERENCES

1. Morrish E, King MA, Smith IE, Shneerson JM. Factors associated with a delay in the diagnosis of narcolepsy. *Sleep Med* 2004;**5**:37–41.
2. American Academy of Sleep Medicine. *International Classification of Sleep Disorders. Diagnostic and Coding Manual*, Second Edition. Westchester, IL: American Academy of Sleep Medicine;2005.
3. Guilleminault C, Mignot E, Partinen M. Controversies in the diagnosis of narcolepsy. *Sleep* 1994;**17**:S1–6.
4. Aldrich M, Chervin R, Malow B. Value of the Multiple Sleep Latency Test (MSLT) for the diagnosis of narcolepsy. *Sleep* 1997;**20**:620–9.
5. Coelho F, Hlynur G, Murray B. Benefit of repeat Multiple Sleep Latency Testing in confirming a possible narcolepsy diagnosis. *J Clin Neurophysiol* 2011;**28**:412–14.
6. Jahnke B, Aldrich M. The Multiple Sleep Latency Test is not infallible. *Sleep Res* 1990;**19**:240.
7. Littner MR, Kushida C, Wise M, et al. Standards of Practice Committee of the American Academy of Sleep Medicine. Practice parameters for clinical use of the Multiple Sleep Latency Test and the Maintenance of Wakefulness Test. *Sleep* 2005;**28**:113–21.
8. Bourgin P, Zeitzer J, Mignot E. CSF hypocretin-1 assessment in sleep and neurological disorders. *Lancet Neurol* 2008;**7**:649–62.
9. Guilleminault C, Arias V. Cataplexy. In Bassetti C, Mignot E, eds. *Narcolepsy and Hypersomnia*. New York, NY: Informa Healthcare;2007.

12

Narcolepsy is not the only cause of sleep-onset rapid eye movement periods

Shelley Hershner

Case

A 22-year-old college student, with a past medical history of attention-deficit disorder (ADD), presented with a 2-year history of sleepiness. The patient was falling asleep in class, especially during her 9:00 AM and 11:00 AM classes, and frequently fell asleep while studying. Her Epworth Sleepiness Scale score was 14 on a scale of 0–24. Despite taking 20 mg of methylphenidate daily for her ADD she still struggled with sleepiness throughout the day. Sleepiness was problematic even during her senior year in high school, but had gotten progressively worse during college. She denied hypnogogic hallucinations, sleep paralysis, and cataplexy.

What are the important clinical questions to ask about sleep duration when evaluating a young adult for excessive daytime sleepiness?

A detailed history of the patient's sleep pattern is vital in the evaluation of excessive daytime sleepiness. Detailed questions should include bedtime, how long it takes to fall asleep, the frequency of nighttime awakenings, and the final rise time, both during the week and weekends. Young adults often have insufficient sleep during the week with catch-up sleep on the weekends. This "catch-up" sleep may also be an indication of delayed sleep-phase disorder, as affected patients will sleep later on the days that they do not

have morning obligations such as class or work. Sleep patterns may also clarify the patient's baseline sleep requirements. To determine this sleep requirement, it is best to explore the sleep pattern and duration during a period of the time when the patient had no restrictions on adequate sleep. For many teenagers and young adults, this may be their sleep schedule during the summer or while on vacation.

In this case, the patient got in bed at 1:00 AM, took an hour to fall asleep, and woke up at 8:30 AM on Monday, Wednesday, and Friday as she had a 9:00 AM class. On Tuesday and Thursday, she slept until 10:30 AM as her class started at 11:00 AM. She did not have nighttime awakenings. During the summer and weekends, she went to sleep at 3:00 AM, fell asleep in < 10 minutes, and woke up at 12:00 PM. She felt less sleepy when she got 8–9 hours of sleep each night.

In this case, the patient may be relatively sleep deprived during the school year as she only has 6.5–9.0 hours of sleep per night.

A polysomnogram and a Multiple Sleep Latency Test (MSLT) are ordered for the evaluation of excessive daytime sleepiness.

How should an MSLT for evaluation of excessive daytime sleepiness be ordered and interpreted?

The MSLT is a validated objective measure of the propensity to fall asleep during the daytime, with the

Common Pitfalls in Sleep Medicine, ed. Ronald D. Chervin. Published by Cambridge University Press. © Cambridge University Press 2014.

Table 12.1 Recommendations for the Multiple Sleep Latency Test protocol

- Five-nap opportunities offered at 2-hour intervals
- Four-nap test may be performed but this is not reliable for the diagnosis of narcolepsy unless at least 2 sleep-onset rapid eye movement (REM) periods have occurred
- The first nap should occur 1.5–3.0 hours after the overnight polysomnogram
- The overnight polysomnogram should occur during the patient's major sleep period
- A minimum of 6 hours of total sleep time is recommended
- A Multiple Sleep Latency Test should not occur following a diagnostic and titration study (split-night)
- A nap session is stopped after 20 minutes if sleep does not occur. The latency for that nap is recorded as 20 minutes
- Sleep onset is defined as the first epoch with > 15 seconds of any stage of sleep
- In order to assess for REM sleep, a nap is continued for 15 minutes after the onset of sleep. This means an individual nap could be as long as 34 minutes in duration
- Prior to each nap the patient is instructed, "Please lie quietly, assume a comfortable position, keep your eyes closed and try to fall asleep."

Adapted from Littner MR, Kushida C, Wise M, et al.[1]

assumption that sleep latency is an accurate measure of sleepiness.[1] If possible, the preceding overnight polysomnogram must be performed during the usual major sleep period. The patient should complete at least 7 days of sleep logs, actigraphy, or both just prior to the sleep study. Drug screening, typically a urine toxicology test on the morning of the MSLT, can exclude the presence of medications or substances that may affect the sleep study. The MSLT is interpreted with an understanding of technical and standard protocols (Table 12.1[1]), and in the context of the clinical history; this should include current sleep patterns, sleep duration, medications, and the results of the preceding overnight polysomnogram.

In the case above, the polysomnogram did not show significant obstructive sleep apnea; the apnea/hypopnea index (AHI, events per hour of sleep) was 1.7 and the lowest oxygen saturation was 93%. The MSLT showed a mean sleep latency of 5.6 minutes with 2 sleep-onset rapid eye movement (REM) periods

(SOREMPs); these occurred on the first and second nap. The naps were conducted at 2-hour intervals starting at 8:00 AM after a rise time at 6:00 AM.

Discussion

Several important considerations are necessary when evaluating the results of an MSLT, as narcolepsy is not the only cause for SOREMPs. The American Academy of Sleep Medicine practice parameters defines a SOREMP as the first epoch of REM sleep at any time during the nap opportunity; or, in other words, REM sleep within 34 minutes of the time at which the patient is first instructed to try to fall asleep. Although an MSLT nap opportunity is 20 minutes, the protocol is to continue the nap for an additional 15 minutes after the first epoch of sleep (any stage) to determine whether REM sleep will appear. The presence of SOREMPs on 2 or more of the 5 nap attempts, spaced through the day, has a sensitivity of 0.78 and a specificity of 0.93 in the evaluation of narcolepsy. However, patients without narcolepsy may also have SOREMPs. In a community sample of adults without cataplexy, 13.1% of males and 5.6% of females had multiple SOREMPs.[2] Although no subject had cataplexy, many had other sleep disorders, including behaviorally induced insufficient sleep syndrome and shift work disorder, and some were taking REM and non-REM suppressing medications.

The presence of SOREMPs by itself is not diagnostic of narcolepsy, therefore, and requires evaluation in the clinical context as there are other causes. An early onset of REM sleep may be influenced by:

1. The patient's sleep schedule
2. Current medications
3. The presence of obstructive sleep apnea and other sleep disorders.

Standard protocol recommends that the preceding polysomnogram should be performed during the patient's normal sleep period. For many, this means a lights out at 10:00 PM and lights on at 6:00 AM, but this may not be appropriate in all patients. For patients with circadian rhythm sleep disorders, such as delayed sleep-phase disorder or shift work disorder, the timing of the naps should begin after normalization of their

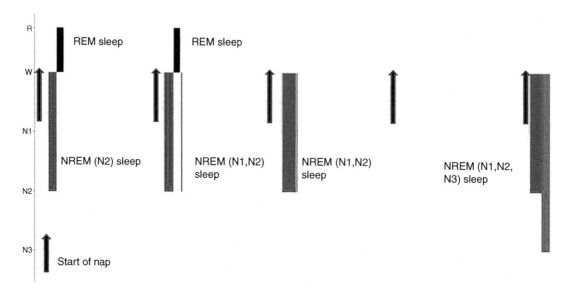

Figure 12.1 Multiple Sleep Latency Test (MSLT) hypnogram. This is the hynogram of the patient's MSLT with a mean sleep latency of 5.6 minutes and 2 sleep-onset REM (R) periods in the first 2 naps. The patient slept during 4 out of the 5 nap opportunities. The sleep-onset REM periods may be influenced by circadian factors as the patient often had a late rise time. Nap 1 (N1) started at 8:09 AM and Nap 2 (N2) at 10:07 AM.

sleep schedule or modification of the MSLT protocol with the naps starting 1.5 hours after the patient's normal rise time. In adults, the normal sleep consists of 4–5 major episodes of non-REM sleep which cycle to REM sleep approximately every 90–120 minutes. The REM sleep periods get progressively longer and much of the total REM sleep occurs in the early morning hours near the expected rise time.[3,4] If a patient is woken earlier than normal, this could result in what appears to be an inappropriately early REM sleep onset.

In the above example, the patient had a typical sleep time between 1:00 and 3:00 AM and a rise time between 9:00 and 12:00 PM. On the day of her MSLT, she was woken at 6:00 AM with her first and second nap scheduled at 8:00 AM and 10:00 AM respectively (Figure 12.1). It would be expected, based on her normal sleep schedule, that she would have substantial REM sleep during these sleep opportunities. Better options might have been to have shifted her MSLT to accommodate her rise time of 9:00 AM or later, with the first nap at 11:00 AM or later, or to try to entrain

her circadian rhythm to a more typical sleep schedule of 10:00 PM to 6:00 AM during the weeks that preceded the testing.

The abrupt discontinuation of a REM-sleep suppressant medication can cause a rebound in REM sleep that can create a false positive SOREMP on an MSLT. The American Academy of Sleep Medicine practice parameters recommend that REM-sleep suppressant medications be discontinued 14 days prior to the MSLT. How long REM sleep may be altered after medication discontinuation is not precisely known, but may relate to the half-life of the medication. For medications such as fluoxetine, which has a half-life of 42–72 hours, 14 days may not be adequate. Desipramine, a tricyclic antidepressant, had maximal REM sleep rebound on day 4 after discontinuation, and on day 27, REM sleep was still slightly increased from baseline.[5] In a sample size of 6 patients, REM sleep rebound was present 18 days after discontinuation of amitriptyline, but only for those patients whose depression had improved.[6] Discontinuation of REM-sleep suppressing medications may not be the

Table 12.2 The odds ratio for the presence of multiple sleep-onset REM periods in a Multiple Sleep Latency Test in male and female patients on non-REM-sleep- and REM-sleep-suppressing medications

	Non-REM-sleep-suppressing medications Odds ratio	REM-sleep-suppressing medications Odds ratio
Male	8.24 (1.50–45.24)	2.01 (0.55–7.36)
Female	11.19 (2.34–53.52)	0.30 (0.05–1.63)

Adapted from Mignot E, Lin L, Finn L, et al.[2]

Table 12.3 Rapid eye movement-sleep-suppressing medications

- Selective serotonin reuptake inhibitors
- Venlafaxine
- Irreversible monoamine oxidase inhibitors
- Tricyclic antidepressants
- Risperidone
- Quetiapine
- Trazadone
- Opioids
- Marijuana (tetrahydrocannabinol)
- Stimulants (amphetamine and methylphenidate)
- Beta-blockers (specifically propranolol, metoprolol, pindolol)
- Clonidine
- Corticosteroids
- Benzodiazepines and benzodiazepine receptor agonists (mild REM-sleep effect)
- Carbamazepine
- Phenobarbital
- Chloral hydrate

only medication effect. In a community sample of healthy, non-cataleptic adults, both REM and non-REM suppressing medications taken at the time of the MSLT were related to the presence of SOREMPs, with the non-REM suppressing medications having a stronger association (Table 12.2).[2]

In general, before an MSLT, REM-sleep-suppressing medications should be held for a minimum of 14 days or 5 half-lives of the specific medication (Table 12.3). A urine or serum toxicology screen the morning of the MSLT can help confirm the absence of confounding medications.

In this case, the patient had discontinued methylphenidate 14 days prior to her sleep study.

Chronic partial sleep deprivation also can affect the results of an MSLT. A minimum of 6 hours of sleep is suggested on the polysomnogram that directly precedes the MSLT. Chronic partial sleep deprivation during the days before a nocturnal polysomnogram and daytime MSLT can cause excessive daytime sleepiness and potentially result in alterations in REM sleep.

In experimental protocols, chronic partial sleep deprivation of 6 hours nightly for 4 consecutive nights resulted in a sleep latency of around 8 minutes, and total, acute sleep deprivation for 24 hours produced a sleep latency of around 2 minutes.[7] Total and partial sleep deprivation change the sleep cycle during recovery sleep; however, much of the available literature on recovery sleep focuses on acute, total sleep deprivation. Following chronic partial or acute total sleep

deprivation, slow-wave sleep will rebound first, followed by REM sleep rebound. The REM sleep rebound will occur either on the first or second night of recovery sleep and depends on how quickly there was a rebound of slow-wave sleep.[8] The first night of recovery sleep could show a prolonged REM sleep latency and decreased REM sleep due to the high percentage of slow-wave sleep. When slow-wave sleep normalizes, then REM sleep rebounds causing a shortened REM sleep latency and increased amount of REM sleep. This could occur on the second night of recovery sleep. Older patients may have an earlier REM sleep rebound than younger patients due to a lower amount of slow-wave sleep; 20% of geriatric subjects had a SOREMP on the first night of recovery sleep following total sleep deprivation.[9] When sleep duration is at least 4 hours, slow-wave sleep is conserved and theoretically recovery sleep may than consist of REM sleep rebound.[10] An auditory stimulus which fragmented sleep, but kept total sleep time intact, resulted in REM sleep rebound with a shortened REM sleep latency and an increase in the percentage

Table 12.4 Percentage of patients, evaluated for suspected obstructive sleep apnea and daytime sleepiness, who had specified numbers of sleep-onset rapid eye movement periods (SOREMPs) during a Multiple Sleep Latency Test

No. of SOREMPs	Percentage
4	0.0
3	0.9
2 or more	4.7
2	3.8
1	9.7
0	85.6

Adapted from Chervin RD, Aldrich MS.[12]

of REM sleep.[11] Currently no available literature indicates the frequency of SOREMPS following chronic partial sleep deprivation. The American Academy of Sleep Medicine practice parameters recommend that 7 days of sleep logs are available to the physician interpreting the polysomnogram and MSLT.

Sleep disorders other than narcolepsy can result in SOREMPs. In a large series of patients tested for possible obstructive sleep apnea and excessive daytime sleepiness, 4.7% were found to have 2 or more SOREMPs on an MSLT (Table 12.4).[12] Patients were not on psychoactive medications. Predictors of having two or more SOREMPs were: male gender; short mean sleep latency on the MSLT; a relatively short nocturnal REM sleep latency; and a low minimum oxygen saturation. Shift-work disorder in men is highly associated with the presence of SOREMPs (odds ratio 5.95 [2.35–15.20 $P = 0.0002$]).[2] The frequency with which other sleep disorders may result in SOREMPs is not well known.

Outcome

In this case, following evaluation in clinic, the patient was diagnosed with delayed sleep-phase disorder, with the intention of repeating the polysomnogram and MSLT once her sleep schedule was entrained to a less delayed schedule. Over the next several months,

through the use of bright light in the morning, melatonin in the evening, and improved sleep hygiene, she was able to fall asleep at 12:30 AM. She also changed her school schedule, which allowed her to sleep until 9:00 AM. She no longer overslept on the weekends.

In a repeat clinic visit 6 months after her polysomnogram and MSLT, the patient was no longer falling asleep in class or while studying. Her Epworth Sleepiness Scale score improved to 8 out of 24, from 14 out of 24. As her sleepiness had resolved with adequate sleep, further evaluation for excessive daytime sleepiness and possible narcolepsy was deferred.

Main points

The presence of two SOREMPs on an MSLT that follows adequate overnight sleep supports the diagnosis of narcolepsy, under appropriate clinical circumstances. Caution is required in the interpretation of MSLT results, as narcolepsy is not the only cause of SOREMPs. Careful consideration of other sleep disorders is required, as patients with untreated obstructive sleep apnea or shift-work disorder may meet the MSLT diagnostic criteria for narcolepsy. The presence or recent history of REM sleep-suppressing medications should be considered, as their abrupt discontinuation can cause REM sleep rebound. Consideration must be given to the patient's normal sleep times, as abrupt changes for the MSLT can result in SOREMPs that more accurately reflect the typical sleep schedule rather than the presence of narcolepsy. The risk of inappropriately diagnosed narcolepsy, as a result of a false positive MSLT or unsuspected confounders, could lead to many years of stimulant medication and a missed opportunity to treat the real underlying problem.

REFERENCES

1. Littner MR, Kushida C, Wise M, et al. Practice parameters for clinical use of the Multiple Sleep Latency Test and the Maintenance of Wakefulness Test. *Sleep* 2005;**28**:113–21.

2. Mignot E, Lin L, Finn L, et al. Correlates of sleep-onset REM periods during the Multiple Sleep Latency Test in community adults. *Brain* 2006;**129**:1609–23.

3. Carskadon MA, Dement WC. Normal human sleep: an overview. In Kryger MH, Roth T, Dement WC, eds. *Principles and Practice of Sleep Medicine*, Fourth Edition. St Louis, MO: Elsevier Saunders;2005, pp. 13–23.

4. Sasaki Y, Fukuda K, Takeuchi T, Inugami M, Miyasita A. Sleep-onset REM period appearance rate is affected by REM propensity in circadian rhythm in normal nocturnal sleep. *Clin Neurophysiol* 2000;**111**:428–33.

5. Oswald I. Drug research and human sleep. *Annu Rev Pharmacol* 1973;**13**:243–52.

6. Gillin JC, Wyatt, RC, Fram D, Snyder F. The relationship between changes in REM sleep and clinical improvement in depressed patients treated with Amitriptyline. *Psychopharmacology* 1978;**59**:267–72.

7. Roehrs T, Dement WC, Roth T. Daytime sleepiness and alertness. In Kryger MH, Roth T, Dement WC, eds. *Principles and Practice of Sleep Medicine*, Fourth Edition. St Louis, MO: Elsevier Saunders;2005, pp. 39–50.

8. Bonnet MH. Acute sleep deprivation. In Kryger MH, Roth T, Dement WC, eds. *Principles and Practice of Sleep Medicine*, Fourth Edition. St Louis, MO: Elsevier Saunders;2005, pp. 51–66.

9. Bonnet MH. Effect of 64 hours of sleep-deprivation upon sleep in geriatric normals and insomniacs. *Neurobiol Aging* 1986;**7**:89–96.

10. Dinges D., Banks, S. Sleep deprivation: cognitive performance. In Amlaner FP, ed. *Basics of Sleep Guide*. Westchester, IL: Sleep Research Society;2009: pp. 257–64.

11. Bonnet MH, Berry RB, Arand DL. Metabolism during normal, fragmented, and recovery sleep. *J Appl Physiol* 1991;**71**:1112–18.

12. Chervin RD, Aldrich MS. Sleep onset REM periods during Multiple Sleep Latency Tests in patients evaluated for sleep apnea. *Am J Resp Crit Care* 2000;**161**:426–31.

Diagnosis of obstructive sleep apnea

Obstructive sleep apnea affects several percent of the population. It is by far the most common problem evaluated and treated at sleep disorders centers. Consequences that stem from missed opportunities to diagnose, and then treat, affected individuals can be substantial. The cases in this section highlight some of the common challenges and pitfalls that clinicians encounter in evaluation of patients for possible obstructive sleep apnea. The authors describe their own perspectives, in the context of challenging patients and experiences that they have encountered. Recurring themes are that a clinical history and examination form the foundation of a diagnosis, which can then be confirmed or illuminated by objective testing. Despite the precision with which numbers are reported following sleep laboratory or home testing for sleep apnea, a good number of limitations exist and must be taken into account when test results are considered in the context that each patient's history has provided.

Cost-containment efforts increasingly motivate the use of home studies rather than sleep laboratory-based studies. Although the former may offer the important advantage of making sleep apnea diagnosis available to many more patients, at a cost society can more readily afford, home studies generally do not record sleep itself, and have specific limitations that must be taken into account before the studies are requested, and when they are interpreted. Many types of home studies exist, and data to support the effectiveness of each varies considerably.

Finally, data from home or laboratory studies can be affected by many variables that cannot be controlled, in addition to those that can be minimized by attention to good protocols and clinical care. Sleep medicine fellows usually spend the initial few months of their 1-year training program learning what sleep studies can do for patients. Many spend the majority of the year thereafter focusing more on understanding the limitations of these tests. This understanding often distinguishes highly effective sleep specialists from clinicians less well prepared to provide optimal care for sleep disorders.

13

A strict cut-off for the apnea/hypopnea index does more harm than good in clinical practice

Sheila C. Tsai

Over a century ago, physicians recognized irregular breathing patterns and pauses in breathing occurring during sleep, and associated this pattern with consequent daytime somnolence. This disorder was eventually labeled as obstructive sleep apnea syndrome (OSAS), and criteria were developed for its diagnosis. The diagnosis was made based on clinical history and observation, but an objective test performed during sleep, the polysomnogram (PSG), was developed to confirm the diagnosis. Effort has been made to standardize the procedure and optimize validity and reliability, but methodologic and biologic or night-to-night variability still can influence the test and interpretation of the results. Available laboratory data must still be reviewed and analyzed within the specific clinical context.

Case

A 45-year-old man presented for evaluation of excessive sleepiness. He noted fragmented sleep, unintentional dozing during the day, and loud snoring. His other medical conditions included hypertension and diabetes. Physical examination was notable for a morbidly obese man with a body mass index of 60.3 kg/m^2, a neck circumference of 21 inches (53 cm), and a modified Mallampati Class IV airway. His Epworth Sleepiness Scale score was 20 out of 24 (where scores of 10 or more often raise concern). A very high clinical suspicion for obstructive sleep apnea prompted an in-laboratory sleep study. This patient's information supported a high pretest probability of severe OSAS, and suggested that he would benefit from treatment. However, the apnea/hypopnea index (AHI, events per hour of sleep) on his sleep study was only 7.1 events per hour of sleep. This number is often considered the single most important polysomnographic result in the assessment for OSAS: 5–14 is often considered to reflect "mild" OSAS, 15–29 "moderate," and 30 or above "severe." For this patient, a continuous positive airway pressure (CPAP) titration study in the sleep laboratory was recommended, and during this follow-up study an effective therapeutic pressure was determined. Unfortunately, the patient had difficulty tolerating CPAP therapy. Given the "mild" degree of sleep apnea, the patient's primary care physician felt that further attempts at CPAP or other therapy were not warranted.

How is this interpretation of the patient's sleep study results flawed?

Unfortunately, this view of the patient's sleep apnea as "mild," based on the AHI alone, provided a disservice to the patient and the clinician. First, categorizing the obstructive sleep apnea severity as mild minimized the importance of its role in the patient's symptoms and overall health. Second, although the AHI provided helpful information, the wealth of other data provided in the study were ignored. In fact, investigating the study details further (Figure 13.1), the lowest oxygen

Common Pitfalls in Sleep Medicine, ed. Ronald D. Chervin. Published by Cambridge University Press. © Cambridge University Press 2014.

SLEEP SUMMARY

Lights out:	22:52:36
Lights on:	5:40:36
Total recording time:	408.0 mins
Total sleeptime:	176.5 mins
Sleep efficiency:	43.3 %
WASO:	223.0 mins
Sleep latency:	8.5 mins
Stage R latency:	79.5 mins

SLEEP STAGE SUMMARY	Duration (mins)	% TST
Stage N1	36.5	20.7
Stage N2	108.0	61.2
Stage N3	18.5	10.5
Stage R	13.5	7.6
Total NREM	163.0	92.4
Supine	153.5	87.0
Supine REM	0.0	0.0
Non-supine	23.0	13.0

AROUSAL SUMMARY	Count	Index
Respiratory	14	4.8
RERA	26	8.8
Spontaneous	134	45.6
PLM	0	0.0
TOTAL	**174**	**59.2**

RESPIRATORY DISTURBANCE SUMMARY

	Apnea			Hypop	Total	
	# Obst.	# Central	# Mixed	#	# (A+H)	Index
REM events	9	0	0	0	9	40.0
Supine	0	0	0	0	0	0.0
Non-supine	9	0	0	0	9	40.0
NREM events	1	0	0	11	12	4.4
Supine	0	0	0	11	11	4.3
Non-supine	1	0	0	0	1	6.3
TOTAL EVENTS	10	0	0	11	21	7.1
Supine	0	0	0	11	11	4.3
Non-supine	10	0	0	0	10	26.1
Overall indices	OAI	CAI	MAI	HI		**AHI**
	3.4	0.0	0.0	3.7		**7.1**

HEART RATE VALUES

	Sleep	All stages
Mean	59.9	60.4
Max	84	85
Min	50	50

LIMB MOVEMENT SUMMARY

	Count	Index
PLM	0	**0.0**

OXYGEN SUMMARY

Saturation	Mean	Max	Min
Sleep	90.2%	98.0%	**68.0%**
All stages	90.1%	98.0%	**64.0%**
Cumulative minutes w/sats </=88%:			**60.0**

Figure 13.1 Details from the case patient's sleep study. Abbreviations used in figure: NREM, non-rapid eye movment; PLM, periodic limb movment; REM, rapid eye movement; RERA, respiratory effort-related arousal index; WASO, wake after sleep onset.

desaturation was 64%, in association with an obstructive apnea. The patient's typical apneic events were prolonged, up to 143 seconds in duration (Figure 13.2). His events were more severe during rapid eye movement (REM) sleep, as seen in many obstructive sleep apnea patients, but only 13 minutes of REM sleep were recorded during the limited 176 minutes of sleep that were captured over the course of the entire night. In addition, no REM sleep was recorded in the supine position, which often gives rise to the most severe sleep apnea. It was clear from the additional measured variables and careful review of the data that the severity of the patient's sleep apnea was underestimated, at least in part because of the prolonged duration of the obstructive respiratory events, the significant oxygen desaturation, the limited amount of REM sleep, and

the lack of supine-REM sleep in the recording. These details provide more information than does interpretation of the PSG based on a strict AHI cut-off alone.

Discussion

In this case, there was over-reliance on an "objective" sleep study and the resultant AHI, despite a clinical history that strongly supported the diagnosis and the importance of treatment. The sleep history and physical examination are crucial to optimal patient care, although they too have variable predictive value when evaluated alone without further testing or objective data. Conversely, although the PSG provides a valuable diagnostic tool, the results cannot be interpreted

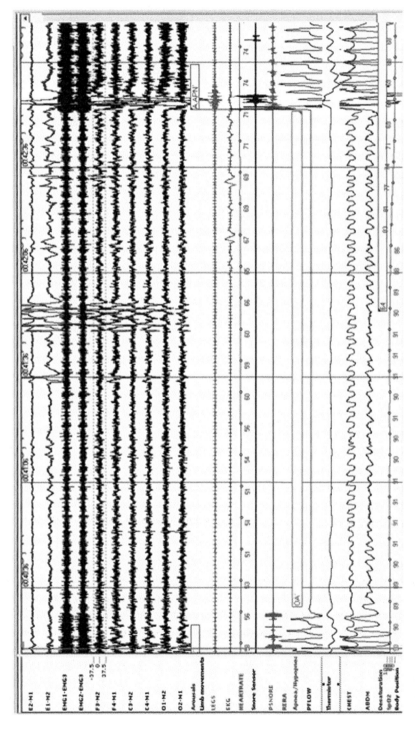

Figure 13.2 A prolonged apneic episode lasting 143 seconds in duration and occurring during REM sleep. (This frame represents a 3-minute epoch.) See plate section for color version.

75

without understanding clinical details, which are important in establishing the context for interpretation of PSG results.

The PSG has too often become the most heavily weighted factor when making the diagnosis. It has become the gold standard for the diagnosis of OSAS, and the interpretation of results is often over-simplified to one number, the AHI. If the threshold AHI is met, then the patient has sleep apnea. If it is not met, then the patient does not have sleep apnea. However, clinical care in reality is not so straightforward. Sleep-disordered breathing follows a continuum, and reliance on a strict cut-off AHI value brings inherent problems with under- or over-diagnosis of sleep apnea. Although it is important to review the AHI, it is also crucial to understand other details and limitations of the PSG. In addition to the amount of recorded total sleep, REM sleep, and supine sleep, many other considerations can also affect the outcome of a PSG. For example, a shifted sleep schedule could influence the sleep study results. If a patient with delayed sleep-phase syndrome undergoes a sleep study at conventional times, the sleep latency and REM sleep latency may be significantly prolonged, influencing the results and possibly leading to underestimation of the severity of concurrent obstructive sleep apnea.

Furthermore, it is important to understand how criteria and thresholds were determined for interpreting PSG data. Adequate outcomes-based data have yet to inform ideal criteria to use in the diagnosis of OSAS. The initial PSG criteria used to confirm sleep apnea were somewhat empiric, and changes to the recommended criteria for diagnosis have occurred over time. Investigators have demonstrated a correlation of sleepiness with the total apneas, hypopneas, and flow limitation events per hour of sleep. However, this number of events per hour of sleep – the respiratory disturbance index (RDI) – showed a low sensitivity and specificity.[1] Current standards recommend the somewhat more stringent measure of the AHI, which includes only apneas and hypopneas, and make additional consideration of respiratory effort-related arousals (based on flow limitation and other features of the recording) optional. Further complicating the diagnosis, the definition of a hypopnea, often the largest

component of the AHI or RDI, has been somewhat variable. The importance of oxygen desaturation as a contributor to the consequences associated with untreated sleep apnea was recognized, and therefore, this criterion was included in the definition of a hypopnea. Research studies and clinical practices varied, however, on the degree of oxygen desaturation that was considered significant. Some reports defined a hypopnea in part by the requirement of at least a 3% oxygen desaturation, whereas others required a 4% desaturation. In 1999, the American Academy of Sleep Medicine (AASM) released recommendations for the definition of OSAS and for sleep study measurement techniques in attempts to unify scoring in clinical research.[2] These criteria were often referred to as the "Chicago criteria" and were adopted by many in clinical practice. In the recommendations, a hypopnea was defined by a 10-second duration and a 50% decrease in baseline air flow, though air flow was, and continues to be, measured by non-quantitative signals. If there was a clear decrease in flow but not by 50% of baseline, then an associated oxygen desaturation of $\geq 3\%$ or a subsequent arousal was required to score a hypopnea. In 2007, the AASM released a manual for the scoring of sleep and related events.[3] In this version, the recommended scoring criteria for a hypopnea changed. An oxygen desaturation of $\geq 4\%$ in addition to $\geq 30\%$ decrease from baseline airflow was recommended in order to score this respiratory event. This recommendation had the advantage that it conformed with Medicare expectations in the United States, but it lacked strong literature support. Use of different criteria, including recognition that an arousal rather than a desaturation could help define a hypopnea, were listed as an alternative option. In 2012 the AASM updated the recommended scoring criteria for hypopneas again, this time with no alternative definition. A 30% decrement in baseline air flow is still required, the oxygen desaturation must be $\geq 3\%$, and in the absence of a desaturation, an arousal can also allow scoring of a hypopnea.[4] As before, expert consensus more than new, significant published evidence appears to have motivated the change. Thus, there have been inconsistencies in scoring respiratory events, which lead to inconsistencies in diagnosing sleep apnea. A standing committee now exists to review polysomnographic standards and definitions annually. Changes will be posted online.

With the recommended PSG scoring criteria for OSAS varying in different years, interpretation of sleep study results could be quite different. An individual may or may not meet criteria for the diagnosis of sleep apnea depending on the recommendations at the time. In addition, if they do meet criteria for sleep apnea, the severity likely varies with the recommended criteria adopted. This inconsistency in AHI outcome was noted with the change in hypopnea scoring criteria from 1999 to 2007. Indeed, in one study, over 5000 PSGs were evaluated using various definitions of apneas and hypopneas. When comparing the most liberal criteria for respiratory events to the most conservative criteria that required a $\geq$ 5% oxygen desaturation, the median RDI varied 10-fold, from a normal RDI to a moderately-to-severely-elevated RDI.[5]

Conclusion

The somewhat arbitrary definition of OSAS and the ever-changing scoring recommendations should further encourage the thoughtful clinician to exercise caution when reviewing the AHI. Over-emphasis on an absolute AHI cut-off minimizes the importance of the clinical history and findings even in a highly suspicious case. If a study does not meet AHI criteria for sleep apnea, the diagnosis may have been missed because of night-to-night variability in testing. In addition, categorizing the severity of sleep apnea based on AHI values can be problematic. Viewed alone, as in our case patient, the AHI may clearly underestimate the severity of sleep apnea. Although the PSG measures a number of variables, including arousal index and oxygen desaturations, in addition to the AHI, there has been an over-reliance on the AHI alone. Medical insurers have often required specific AHI levels as a prerequisite for reimbursement of treatment for OSAS. However, the conventional stratification of sleep apnea severity based on the AHI is arbitrary, and derived primarily from consensus. This stratification considers only the number of respiratory events while trivializing

the importance of the event durations and the degree of associated oxygen desaturation. If a patient has "mild" sleep apnea but these events lead to severe oxygen desaturation or significant cardiac consequences, then a clinician may incorrectly under-emphasize the importance of this medical, sleep-related issue. In addition, other factors should be considered when evaluating a person for OSAS because the AHI itself has been shown to correlate poorly with key outcomes as salient to OSAS as self-reported sleepiness.[6] These data suggest that additional polysomnographic and clinical factors are also important contributors to the symptoms and consequences of sleep apnea.

Main points

While the sleep study provides important diagnostic information when combined with the clinical history and physical examination, it is not a gold standard without limitations. Interpreting the results of the sleep study based on a strict AHI cut-off alone is a mistake. To diagnose OSAS, the astute clinician should understand the sleep study results in the context of the clinical history and physical examination findings, recognize the limitations of the PSG, and review the full data available from the study. If there is discordance between the clinical pretest suspicion and the test results, then the clinician should investigate further.

REFERENCES

1. Hosselet J, Ayappa I, Norman RG, Krieger AC. Classification of sleep-disordered breathing. *Am J Respir Crit Care Med* 2001;**163**:398–405.
2. American Academy of Sleep Medicine Task Force. Sleep-related breathing disorders in adults: recommendations for syndrome definition and measurement techniques in clinical research. *Sleep* 1999;**22**:667–89.
3. Iber C, Ancoli-Israel S, Chesson, Am Quan SF. *The AASM Manual for the Scoring of Sleep and Associated Events: Rules, Terminology, and Technical Specifications*, First

Edition. Westchester, IL: American Academy of Sleep Medicine;2007.

4. Berry RB, Brooks R, Gamaldo CE, et al. *The AASM Manual for the Scoring of Sleep and Associated Events: Rules, Terminology, and Technical Specifications, Version 2.0.* Westchester, IL: American Academy of Sleep Medicine;2012.

5. Redline S, Kapur VK, Sanders MH, et al. Effects of varying approaches for identifying respiratory disturbances on sleep apnea assessment. *Am J Respir Crit Care Med* 2000;**161**:369–74.

6. Weaver EM, Kapur V, Yueh B. Polysomnography vs. self-reported measures in patients with sleep apnea. *Arch Otolaryngol Head Neck Surg* 2004;**130**:453–8.

14

One night of polysomnography can occasionally miss obstructive sleep apnea

Raman K. Malhotra

Case

A 58-year-old woman presented to the clinic with complaints of excessive daytime sleepiness for the last 3 years. She also described fatigue and low energy levels during the day, despite adequate amounts of sleep at night. She felt her sleepiness affected her work as a sales manager owing to inattentiveness and poor concentration. She also had drowsiness during her commute home in the evening.

She reported occasional snoring during sleep. The snoring could only be heard inside the bedroom. On occasion, her husband noticed pauses in breathing during sleep, though she was unaware of this. She also complained of mouth breathing and acid reflux that awoke her from sleep. She denied morning headaches, night sweats, restless legs symptoms, cataplexy, sleep-related hallucinations, and sleep paralysis. She typically slept on her side and her back.

She went to bed at 10:30 PM every night, with a sleep latency of 5–10 minutes. She had one nightly awakening during sleep; she would go to the restroom to urinate and then return to bed. Wake after sleep onset was < 15 minutes. She woke by alarm in the morning at 6:30 AM on work days. On weekends, she slept until 8:00 AM.

She had a past medical history of borderline hypertension and gastroesophageal reflux disease. Physical examination was remarkable for obesity (body mass index of 38 kg/m^2), an enlarged neck circumference of 17 inches (43 cm), and a Mallampati score of Class III airway.

How do you make the diagnosis of obstructive sleep apnea?

A diagnosis of obstructive sleep apnea is strongly suspected, based on her history of snoring, witnessed apneas, daytime sleepiness, mouth breathing, nocturnal acid reflux, and nocturia. Her physical exam findings of obesity, enlarged neck circumference, and a crowded airway also increase her risk for obstructive sleep apnea. When a detailed history and physical exam are consistent with a high risk of obstructive sleep apnea, objective confirmation is required because the sensitivity and specificity of a clinical history and exam alone are considered to be insufficient. The gold standard for diagnosis is attended, in-laboratory polysomnography, though in specific circumstances, an unattended, home test can be considered.

An overnight, attended in-laboratory polysomnography was performed on this patient and was interpreted as not consistent with obstructive sleep apnea. The respiratory disturbance index was 4.2 and the minimum oxygen saturation was 90%. See Table 14.1 for the patient's polysomnography data and Figure 14.1 for the patient's hypnogram.

Common Pitfalls in Sleep Medicine, ed. Ronald D. Chervin. Published by Cambridge University Press. © Cambridge University Press 2014.

Table 14.1 Polysomnography data regarding sleep architecture and position

Time in bed	485 min
Total sleep time	228 min
Sleep latency	8 min
REM sleep latency	360 min
% Stage N1 sleep	28%
% Stage N2 sleep	38%
% Stage N3 sleep	25%
% Stage REM sleep	9%
% Supine sleep	23%

Is there any benefit to repeating the study?

A single night of polysomnography can occasionally miss obstructive sleep apnea. Further review of her polysomnographic data and hypnogram showed decreased sleep efficiency, with minimal recorded rapid eye movement (REM) sleep and supine sleep. As clinical suspicion remained high for obstructive sleep apnea, a repeat in-laboratory polysomnogram was performed. Increased REM sleep was observed on the repeat study. Also supine sleep was encouraged by the sleep technologist. Her repeat polysomnogram was interpreted as consistent with obstructive sleep apnea, with a respiratory disturbance index of 12.3 and a minimum oxygen saturation of 85%, which occurred during supine-REM sleep.

Discussion

Though attended, in-laboratory polysomnography is considered the gold standard for diagnosis of obstructive sleep apnea in adults, several studies have demonstrated that one night of polysomnography can miss up to 20% of patients with obstructive sleep apnea. The following discussion will focus on possible reasons why one night in the laboratory may not accurately characterize the severity of sleep-disordered breathing in a patient at high risk for obstructive sleep apnea.

The patient may not sleep well on the first night in the laboratory owing to discomfort with the recording equipment, unfamiliar environment, or anxiety. This "first-night effect," which has been reported in the literature, is associated with less total sleep time, lower sleep efficiency, more intermittent waking time, and longer REM sleep latency than would most likely be observed in a sleep laboratory during a second night of recording. This decreased total sleep and lack of consolidated sleep may decrease opportunities to observe an adequate number of respiratory events.

In addition, due to first-night effect or other reasons (e.g. unfamiliar environment, anxiety about the test, discomfort from sensors and wires), a decreased amount (or even absence) of REM sleep may occur on polysomnography. This can lead to underestimating the severity of obstructive sleep apnea and a lowering of the overall respiratory disturbance index, especially in patients who have REM-related obstructive respiratory events. In many patients, obstructive events are predominantly noted during REM sleep, primarily due to the muscle atonia that normally occurs during REM sleep, leading to a propensity for upper airway collapse during this stage.

Furthermore, one night of polysomnography may miss obstructive sleep apnea due to lack of sufficient recorded supine sleep. Obstructive sleep apnea is often more severe in the supine position in many patients, and the absence or decreased total amount of supine sleep may lead to a missed opportunity for diagnosis. Patients may sleep in different positions in the laboratory than at home owing to an altered sleeping environment and recording sensors which may limit mobility in bed. Neck position and elevation of the head of the bed may also significantly alter airway mechanics. A tilt of the neck may exacerbate or conversely, alleviate obstructive respiratory events during sleep.

Additionally, patients are often advised to bring medications used at home for the sleep study. Substances, such as alcohol, along with certain prescription medications, can cause upper airway muscle relaxation and worsen sleep-disordered breathing. If a patient normally drinks alcohol or uses medications at bedtime at home, but does not mimic the same circumstances in the sleep laboratory, the polysomnography may be falsely negative for obstructive sleep apnea.

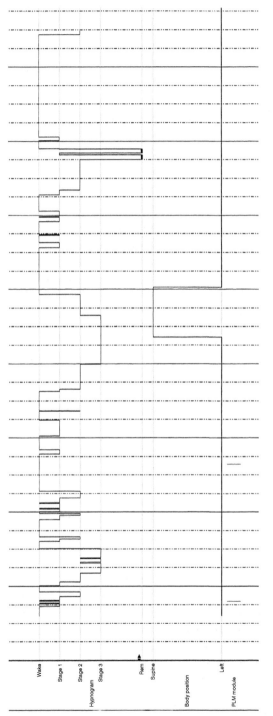

Figure 14.1 Hypnogram from the overnight sleep study demonstrating time at different stages of sleep and wake along with sleep position. Abbreviation used in figure: PLM, periodic limb movement.

Variability in the night-to-night degree of sleep-disordered breathing may also be noted in relation to comorbid medical conditions. Many medical conditions fluctuate and can lead to variability in the degree of sleep apnea noted on one night of polysomnography. Examples include chronic obstructive pulmonary disease (COPD), asthma, and myasthenia gravis. There are also reports of variability in apnea/hypopnea indices in patients on hemodialysis related to whether dialysis occurred that day or the previous day. Nasal congestion, due to either an upper respiratory infection or allergic rhinitis, can also have some effect on the presence of obstructive sleep apnea. Treatment of nasal congestion has been shown to lower apnea/hypopnea index in patients, especially in patients with mild-to-moderate obstructive sleep apnea.

It is also important to note what type of recording equipment and sensors were used for the attended in-laboratory polysomnography. The American Academy of Sleep Medicine (AASM) standards regarding technical specifications and appropriate sensors to measure sleep and respiration are not followed by all sleep centers in the United States, and may not be followed by many sleep centers around the world. Equipment needs to be well maintained and calibrated, and should meet the applicable technical standards. One example of an AASM standard that may affect results of the sleep study is the usage of both a nasal pressure transducer and a nasal–oral thermistor to monitor respiration during a sleep study. Omission of one of these sensors may lead to under- or over-estimation (respectively) of the severity of sleep-disordered breathing.

In addition, the assessment of mild obstructive sleep apnea may be improved by the use of esophageal pressure (Pes) monitoring during polysomnography. Pes monitoring provides quantitative data on negative intrathoracic pressures during the respiratory cycle. The results offer a gold-standard assessment of the work of breathing during sleep. Use of Pes monitoring in addition to the standard monitoring of respiration and sleep may help to detect mild obstructive sleep apnea or obstructed breathing that is otherwise missed. For example, some patients have continued increased respiratory effort, through a continuously narrowed airway, rather than discrete events that can be identified as apneas, hypopneas, or respiratory effort-related arousals. In these cases, standard scoring will not reflect a problem, whereas excessive negative Pes swings may do so. Pes monitoring is usually not routinely performed but can be requested at sleep disorders centers that have experience in the placement of the esophageal catheter and interpretation of the results. Studies suggest that the use of the catheter has a negligible adverse impact on the quality of sleep, so its use should be determined mainly by the anticipated medical benefit for the patient. Thin, young, or female patients whose history suggests sleep-disordered breathing may be the most likely to benefit from Pes monitoring.

Following adequate data collection, it is equally as important to score data correctly. For years, no agreed upon consensus existed as to what constituted a respiratory event during sleep for calculation of the apnea/hypopnea index or respiratory disturbance index. In fact, prior to 2012, two definitions existed for hypopnea in the AASM Scoring Manual. This has now been clarified and one definition of hypopnea – scored if a 10-second reduction in airflow is associated with either an oxygen desaturation of $\geq 3\%$ or a cortical arousal – is recommended. Some previous criteria for hypopneas required an oxygen desaturation of 4%, and dismissed "arousal-based" scoring. This narrow definition leads to lower apnea/hypopnea indices owing to a disregard of respiratory events associated with sleep fragmentation. Studies have shown that omission of arousal-based scoring of hypopneas can miss diagnosis of obstructive sleep apnea in a substantial portion of patients. In one study, up to 40% of lean patients with good pulmonary function were found to be misclassified as not having obstructive sleep apnea when arousal-based scoring for hypopneas was not used. Hypopnea definitions requiring a 4% oxygen desaturation and a lack of scoring of arousal-based events are still required by the Centers for Medicare and Medicaid Services (CMS) at the time of writing.

Main points

If a negative polysomnogram is noted in a patient considered to be at high risk for obstructive sleep apnea by clinical history and exam, a repeat study may be warranted to evaluate for obstructive sleep apnea that may have been missed on the one night of recording.

FURTHER READING

Ahmadi N, Shapiro GK, Chung SA, Shapiro CM. Clinical diagnosis of sleep apnea based on single night polysomnography vs. two nights of polysomnography. *Sleep Breath* 2009;**13**:221-6.

Chediak AD, Acevedo-Crespo JC, Seiden DJ, Kim HH, Kiel MH. Nightly variability in the indices of sleep-disordered breathing in men being evaluated for impotence with consecutive night polysomnograms. *Sleep* 1996;**19**:589-92.

Hutter DA, Holland BK, Ashtyani H. Occult sleep apnea: the dilemma of negative polysomnography in symptomatic patients. *Sleep Med* 2004;**5**:501-6.

Le Bon O, Hoffmann G, Tecco J, et al. Mild to moderate sleep respiratory events: one negative night may not be enough. *Chest* 2000;**118**:353-9.

Levendowski D, Zack N, Rao SM. Assessment of the test–retest reliability of laboratory polysomnography. *Sleep Breath* 2009;**13**:163-7.

15

Unattended, full polysomnography can be a good alternative to attended polysomnography, but technical limitations are common

Q. Afifa Shamim-Uzzaman

Introduction

Obstructive sleep apnea (OSA) is increasingly being recognized and confirmed primarily through attended, in-laboratory polysomnograms (PSGs). However, PSGs are expensive, labor-intensive studies that are not always readily accessible. Portable monitors with a wide range of complexity have emerged as alternatives to in-laboratory PSGs, primarily because they do not require the constant presence of a sleep technologist. However, limitations of portable monitors must be considered when choices are made among available diagnostic options.

Case

A 68-year-old former smoker had a history of bladder cancer (resected 8 years prior), hypertension, hyperlipidemia, and recently diagnosed diabetes complicated by neuropathy. He presented with a 30-year history of excessive daytime sleepiness. He is frustrated that he cannot sit down to rest without falling asleep, and he frequently dozes in and out of sleep unintentionally for 5–10 minutes at a time, missing portions of his favorite television shows. The sleepiness is even worse when he is reading, and he is no longer able to enjoy a good book. He was involved in a motor vehicle accident 20 years ago when he fell asleep at the wheel; since then, he has been more vigilant while driving, but still admits to falling asleep when stopped in traffic. He reports that he can stay awake if he keeps himself busy, but he falls asleep quickly during sedentary activities. His Epworth Sleepiness Scale score is 16 (on a scale that can range from 0 to 24, where 10 or higher often raises concern).

He is a restless sleeper who tosses and turns throughout the night, waking unrested in the mornings with his bed in "a mess." He has had no bed partner for the past 20 years, but his ex-wife and more recently his close friend have told him he snores loudly. In fact, he has woken himself up because of his snoring. He goes to bed at 10:00 PM, falls asleep within 30 minutes, but wakes up every 1–2 hours during the night to use the restroom. Rarely, he awakens gasping for air. He denies any witnessed apneas. His dentist has told him that he has damaged his teeth by clenching them so hard. He has occasional heartburn for which he takes famotidine. He also has chronic nasal congestion for which he uses a nasal spray.

The patient is a Vietnam veteran who worked at the Ford Motor Company when he returned from his tour of duty in 1967, then as a manager at a fast-food restaurant until he retired in February 2009. His symptoms have not improved in retirement, and he sometimes feels worse now than when he was working. His primary care physician sent him to a sleep disorders center 3 years ago, but the patient rescheduled his visit once because of transportation issues, and later cancelled his appointment because of bad weather (snow). He has not had a sleep evaluation until now.

Common Pitfalls in Sleep Medicine, ed. Ronald D. Chervin. Published by Cambridge University Press. © Cambridge University Press 2014.

On physical examination, he is an obese Hispanic male in no apparent distress. His body mass index is 38 kg/m^2 (increased from 34 kg/m^2 3 years ago), and his neck circumference is 17.5 inches (44 cm). He has mild retrognathia without micrognathia. He has a narrow, high-arched hard palate, long low-lying soft palate, and thickened uvula. His tongue is large and scalloped. He has 2+ tonsils and a Mallampati Class III oropharynx. Molar occlusion is Class II bilaterally, and anteriorly he has a few millimeters of overjet and overbite. Maxillary sinuses are tender without periauricular or cervical lymphadenopathy. Cardiorespiratory exam is normal. Neurologic exam is intact except for visual acuity (for which he wears glasses) and a stocking sensory deficit in bilateral lower extremities, where he was unable to differentiate between soft touch and pinprick.

The patient underwent a level II portable sleep study the following week. The study was unattended, performed on an outpatient basis in a room of a hospital that does not have a sleep laboratory. He was found to have severe sleep apnea, with an apnea/hypopnea index (AHI, apneas or hypopneas per hour of sleep) of 39 and a minimum oxygen saturation of 74%. He was treated with an automatically titrating continuous positive airway pressure unit (auto-PAP) set to deliver between 5 and 20 cm of water. Initial use and downloaded data from his machine suggested that 15 cm of water would be sufficient 95% of the time. The median delivered pressure had been 11.4 cm of water and the maximum delivered pressure had been 16 cm of water. A trial at home of CPAP fixed at 15 cm of water showed that he could not tolerate it. He was transitioned back to auto-PAP, set to range between 11 and 16 cm of water. After compliant use, he reported an 80% improvement in both daytime and nighttime symptoms.

Discussion

There is no simple blood test for OSA; diagnosis is based on history, physical examination, and the results of objective sleep testing. A full, attended in-laboratory PSG is the gold standard for diagnosis, but use of unattended portable monitors, in conjunction with a comprehensive sleep evaluation, can also provide good results under many circumstances.

In 1994, the American Academy of Sleep Medicine categorized sleep-monitoring devices into four levels, as outlined in Table 15.1.[1] Level I studies mandate the recording of electroencephalograms (EEGs), electrooculograms (EOGs), chin surface electromyograms (EMGs), airflow, respiratory effort, oxygen saturation, and electrocardiograms (ECGs) or heart rate; the additional recordings of body position and leg EMG channels are recommended. Video and a snoring microphone are also commonly used. Additional variables that may be recorded in level I studies include end-tidal carbon dioxide, transcutaneous carbon dioxide, esophageal pressure, pH, additional EMG leads, positive airway pressure levels, and leaks. Level I studies are full in-laboratory PSGs that quantify sleep and its stages, and calculate the AHI. All level I studies require a trained technologist to monitor the recording at all times and correct technical problems, address patient issues, and monitor patient behaviors.[2] These studies are therefore called "attended" studies.

Level II, III, and IV studies are completed with portable monitoring devices and are "unattended" by a trained technologist. They may be performed in a sleep laboratory or hospital, but are usually performed at the patient's home (and then sometimes called "out-of-center sleep testing"). Level I and II studies both require recording a minimum of the same 7 channels; hence, the "live monitoring" by a trained technologist is the major difference between a level I and a level II study. Level III studies monitor 4–7 channels and can estimate the AHI or the respiratory disturbance index based on events per hour of recording. Channels do include at least two respiratory channels (measuring airflow and/or respiratory effort), ECG or heart rate, and oxygen saturation (by pulse oximetry). Level IV monitors are also known as "continuous single or dual bioparameter devices" as they may measure as few as 1 or 2 parameters, but no more than 3 parameters. Presently, the American Academy of Sleep Medicine requires that a portable monitor must record airflow, respiratory effort, and blood oxygenation; therefore, it does not recommend the use of level IV devices for the diagnosis of OSA.[2]

Table 15.1 Types of overnight sleep studies

Type of study	Requirements	Required channels	Comments
Level I	• Record a minimum of 7 channels • Attended by a trained technologist • Performed in a laboratory	• EEG • EOG • EMG • Airflow • Respiratory effort • Oxygen saturation • ECG or heart rate	This is a full attended in-laboratory PSG
Level II	• Record a minimum of 7 channels	• EEG • EOG • EMG • Airflow • Respiratory effort • Oxygen saturation • ECG or heart rate	This type of device monitors sleep staging and calculates an AHI
Level III	• Record a minimum of 4 channels	• 2 channels for airflow and/or respiratory movement • 1 ECG/heart rate • 1 oxygen saturation	Most commonly used type of device for out-of-center testing
Level IV	• Record a minimum of 1 channel	• Airflow, and/or • Respiratory effort, and/or • Blood oxygenation	These devices are not recommended for out-of-center testing by the AASM

AASM, American Academy of Sleep Medicine; AHI, apnea/hypopnea index; ECG, electrocardiogram; EEG, electroencephalogram; EMG, electromyogram; EOG, electrooculogram; PSG, polysomnogram.

To understand the differences in information obtained by the various devices, it is best to look at the raw data collected by each of these devices. Figure 15.1 shows the same sleep epochs as they might appear if recorded by level II, III, and IV portable monitors. In Figure 15.1a, the patient's level II study consists of 17 channels and resembles a full level I PSG; however, it was not attended by a technologist so does not meet criteria for a full PSG. Figure 15.1b shows the same two epochs as they might be recorded by a level III monitor. In the level III study, there is no EEG, EOG, and EMG, so sleep cannot be ascertained, and hypopneas cannot be scored using arousal criteria. Therefore, in this case, the level III monitor would have missed both hypopneas that were recorded by the level II device, as the events did not produce a $\geq$ 3% oxygen desaturation, and there would be no EEG to identify arousals. Furthermore,

respiratory effort-related arousals cannot be identified using a level III device. In addition, the AHI in a level III study is calculated by dividing the total number of apneas and hypopneas by the total recording time, instead of the total sleep time as would be standard in type I and II studies. All of these limitations may lead to an underestimation of the AHI by level III monitors. Hence, it is recommended that only patients suspected to have moderate to severe OSA, rather than mild OSA, be tested with portable monitors.

Figure 15.1c and 15.1d reflect what would be recorded from a single parameter level IV study or tri-parameter study, respectively. As is evident from Figure 15.1c, a continuous, single-channel recording cannot diagnose sleep apnea reliably. The 3-channel level IV study in Figure 15.1d may have enough information to allow recognition of OSA, but is subject to the same limitations as the level III study. The Center

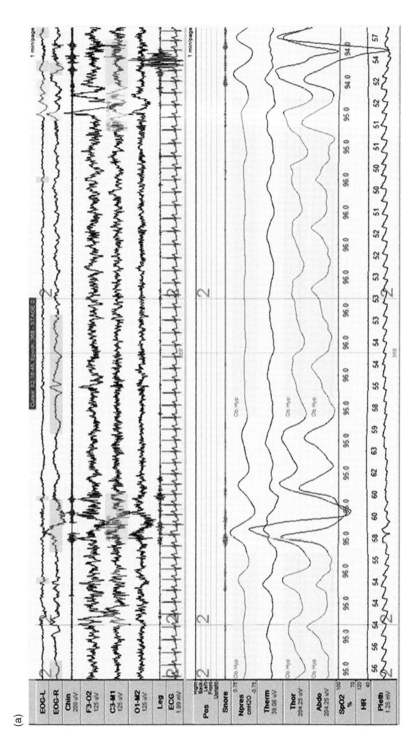

Figure 15.1 (a) Two epochs from the patient's level II sleepy study. (b) The same two epochs from 1 (a) as recorded in a level III study. (c) The same two epochs from (a) as recorded in a level IV study measuring a single parameter. (d) The same two epochs as 1 (a) recorded in a level IV study measuring three parameters.

Abbreviations used in figure: Abdo, abdominal effort; Chin, chin electromyogram; ECG, electrocardiogram; C3-M1, left central –> left mastoid electroencephalogram; F3-O2, left frontal –> right occipital electroencephalogram; HR, heart rate; Npres, nasal pressure (uses pressure as a measure of airflow); O1-M2, left occipital –> right mastoid electroencephalogram; Pleth, inductance plethysmography; Pos, body position; SpO2, oxygen saturation; Therm, naso-oral thermistor (uses temperature as a measure of airflow); Thor, thoracic effort. See plate section for color version.

87

88

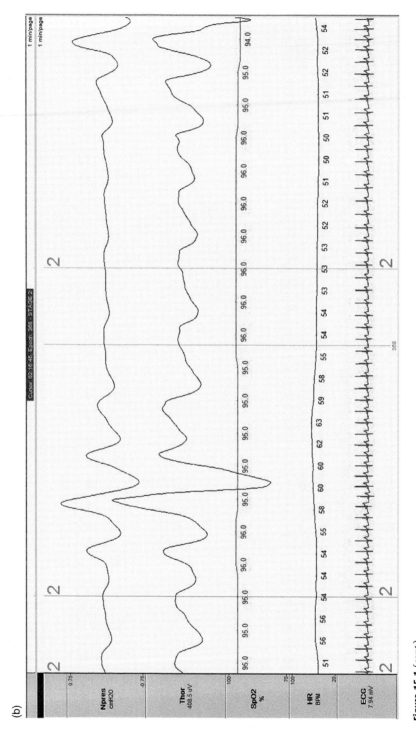

Figure 15.1 (*cont.*)

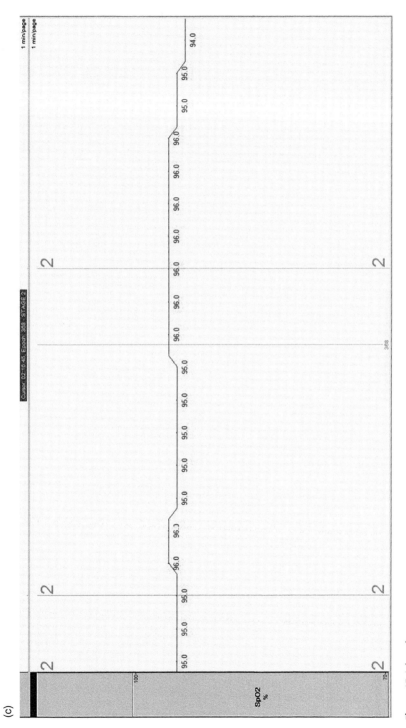

Figure 15.1 (*cont.*)

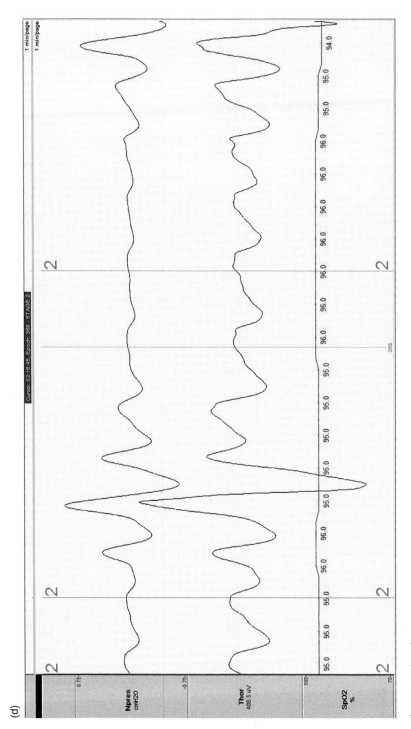

(d)

Figure 15.1 (*cont.*)

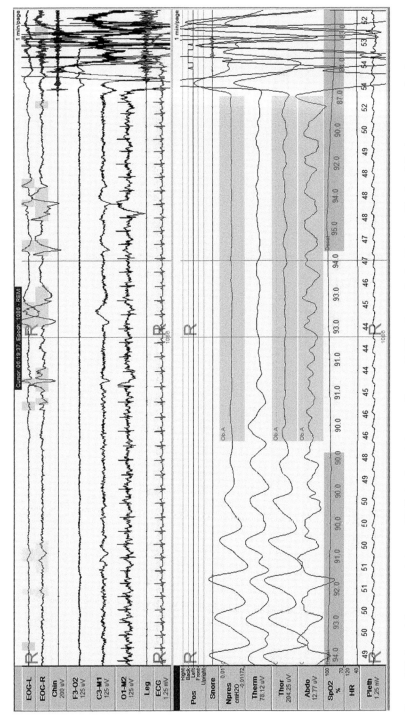

Figure 15.2 Loss of electroencephalogram (EEG) signals and electrocardiogram (ECG) artifact in the O1-M2 channel lead to difficulty in staging the sleep. See Figure 15.1 for abbreviations.

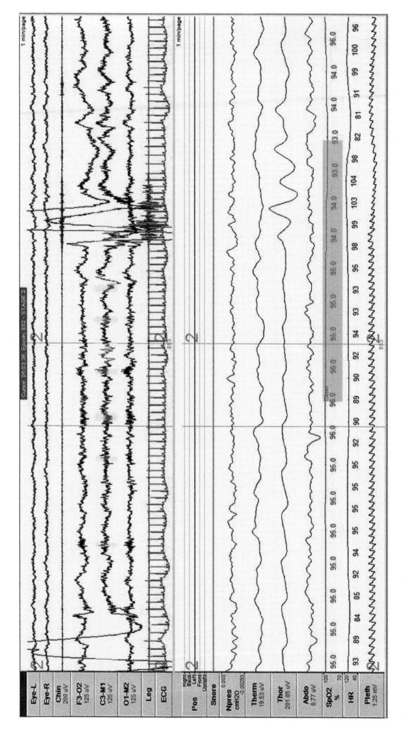

Figure 15.3 Poor signal quality from respiratory channels limits the detection of respiratory events. See Figure 15.1 for abbreviations.

for Medicare and Medicaid Services accepts the diagnosis of OSA by a level IV device only if it records all 3 channels listed in Table 15.1 above.[3]

Lead loss and poor signal quality are additional technical limitations inherent to all sleep studies, but even more so to unattended studies, as corrections cannot occur during the course of the recording. Data loss has been reported to be as high as 18% in level III studies.[4,5] Figures 15.2 and 15.3 demonstrate that poor signal quality and artifacts can affect the interpretation of a study. For example, in Figure 15.3, the heart rate changes (slowing heart rate followed by tachycardia) in conjunction with oxygen desaturation and an arousal suggest the physiologic changes associated with an apnea. However, the respiratory leads (nasal pressure, thermistor, thoracic effort, abdominal effort) cannot be clearly interpreted to clarify the presence or absence of an event.

In detecting an AHI > 5, technically adequate level III portable monitors are often comparable to PSGs. Such **in-laboratory portable monitors** show a sensitivity of 95.3%, specificity of 75%, a positive likelihood ratio (+LR) of 3.8, and a negative likelihood ratio (−LR) of 0.11, while **home-based portable monitors** demonstrate a sensitivity of 96%, a specificity of 64%, a +LR of 2.7, and a −LR of 0.05.[6] As false negative rates for unattended portable monitors can be as high as 17%,[5] if clinical suspicion for sleep apnea is high, and a portable study is negative, the American Academy of Sleep Medicine recommends repeating the procedure with an in-laboratory attended study. Portable monitors should **not** be used as a general screening tool. They should only be used in otherwise relatively healthy patients, without significant medical or sleep comorbidities, who have a high pretest probability of moderate to severe OSA.[2]

REFERENCES

1. Standards of Practice Committee of the American Sleep Disorders Association. Practice parameters for the use of portable recording in the assessment of obstructive sleep apnea. *Sleep* 1994;**17**:372-7.

2. Epstein LJ, Dristo D, Strollo PJ, et al. Adult Obstructive Sleep Apnea Task Force of the American Academy of Sleep Medicine. Clinical guideline for the evaluation, management and long-term care of obstructive sleep apnea in adults. *J Clin Sleep Med* 2009;**5**:263-76.

3. Department of Health and Human Services, Center for Medicare and Medicaid Services. *Decision Memo for Continuous Positive Airway Pressure (CPAP) Therapy for Obstructive Sleep Apnea (OSA)*. CAG#0093R. March 13, 2008.

4. Collop NA, Anderson WM, Boehlecke B, et al. Portable Monitoring Task Force of the American Academy of Sleep Medicine. Clinical guidelines for the use of unattended portable monitors in the diagnosis of obstructive sleep apnea in adult patients. *J Clin Sleep Med* 2007;**3**:737-47.

5. Flemons WW, Littner MR, Rowley JA, et al. Home diagnosis of sleep apnea: a systematic review of the literature. An evidence review cosponsored by the American Academy of Sleep Medicine, the American College of Chest Physicians, and the American Thoracic Society. *Chest* 2003;**124**:1543-79.

6. Tonelli de Oliveira AC, Martinez D, Vasconcelos LF, et al. Diagnosis of obstructive sleep apnea syndrome and its outcomes with home portable monitoring. *Chest* 2009;**135**:330-6.

16

Home cardiopulmonary tests are a useful option, but only under appropriate circumstances

Daniel I. Rifkin

Technological change is like an axe in the hands of a pathological criminal.

Albert Einstein

Despite the availability of limited-channel home cardiopulmonary tests for decades, physicians remain reluctant to use them. Perhaps this is due to the fact that the hundreds of studies on home testing (also known as home sleep tests [HSTs] or "out-of-center" tests [OOCTs]) are performed in homogeneous populations, underpowered with small sample sizes, and essentially lack sufficient rigor in design. Or maybe many studies are funded by those with a vested interest in the outcome of the study, thus creating a real or perceived conflict of interest. Or, those physicians and hospitals performing in-laboratory tests fear a loss of revenue with the utilization of home testing. Despite these concerns, and based on our knowledge to date, limited-channel home cardiopulmonary testing can be an effective alternative to in-laboratory polysomnography in assessment for obstructive sleep apnea (OSA), and can be an important diagnostic tool under appropriate circumstances.

Before ordering a diagnostic test, clinicians should recall the general principle that clinical data obtained by history and examination are often more useful than data obtained from diagnostic tests.[1] To decide whether to order in-laboratory polysomnography or OOCT, the clinician should consider the performance characteristics of the test (likelihood ratio, sensitivity, specificity, and false-positive rate, etc.) to determine whether the outcome of the test is likely to change the pretest probability of disease. Ultimately, diagnostic tests should be selected that affect the clinician's estimate of pretest probability. This is an important concept to remember, as a negative OOCT should truly lead to question either the validity of the test or the clinician's ability to accurately determine the patient's high pretest probability of moderate to severe OSA.

Let us first start with the question: "*What are the different types of OOCT?*"

There are numerous types of OOCTs and they are often classified as follows:[2]

- *Type II* – Comprehensive, unattended, portable polysomnography. Minimum of 7 channels including electroencephalogram (EEG), electrooculogram (EOG), chin electromyogram (EMG), electrocardiogram/heart rate (ECG/HR), airflow, respiratory effort, and oxygen saturation.
- *Type III* – Modified portable sleep apnea testing. Minimum of 4 channels including ECG/HR, oxygen saturation, and at least 2 channels of respiratory movement or respiratory movement and airflow.
- *Type IV* – Continuous single or dual bioparameters, such as airflow and/or oxygen saturation; peripheral arterial tone (PAT) is classified as a type IV monitor.

A more recent classification system proposed by the American Academy of Sleep Medicine, called the SCOPER categorization system (an acronym for **S**leep, **C**ardiovascular, **O**ximetry, **P**osition, **E**ffort, and **R**espiration), allows for a greater description of the

Common Pitfalls in Sleep Medicine, ed. Ronald D. Chervin. Published by Cambridge University Press. © Cambridge University Press 2014.

Table 16.1 Strengths and limitations of home cardiopulmonary testing

Strengths of home cardiopulmonary tests	Limitations of home cardiopulmonary tests
Convenience of home study	Unable to perform split night study in severe apnea
Reduced costs	Unable to correct poor signal
Study in familiar surroundings	Overestimated sleep time
Increased rapid eye movement (REM) sleep	Missed hypopneas and respiratory effort-related arousals (RERAs)
Less patient anxiety	Increased loss of data
Usual body positions	Risk of false negative
Access to care in areas with limited laboratory resources	Different sensors and algorithms to identify respiratory events

measurement of physiologic parameters and how those parameters are being measured.[3]

Whether one decides to use a type III or type IV PAT device or a $S_4C_3O_{1x}P_2E_4R_5$ device, some familiarity with the equipment and the targeted physiologic measures is key to understanding the strengths and limitations of a particular device.

Who should order OOCT?

Patients with a suspected sleep disorder should be evaluated and treated by a provider who is aware of the strengths and limitations of OOCT (Table 16.1). Board certified sleep medicine physicians are often ideal. Sleep-experienced nurse practitioners or physician assistants, usually working on a team led by a sleep medicine physician, can also be knowledgeable about testing options. A growing trend is for primary care providers to recognize, diagnose, and treat OSA. This trend could help to address an important public health challenge, in that the majority of patients with OSA remain undiagnosed, but are most primary care providers ready for this task?

A knowledgeable provider should be able to obtain an adequate history and physical to estimate the pretest probability of OSA, as we know that OOCT is a more appropriate diagnostic tool in patients with a high pretest probability of moderate to severe OSA. But how do we determine if someone has a high pretest probability of moderate to severe OSA? What does that mean exactly? The diagnostic test should be used to increase the pretest probability to a sufficiently high post-test probability to be reasonably certain that

Table 16.2 Common signs and symptoms of obstructive sleep apnea

Common symptoms	Common physical findings
Snoring	Low-lying soft palate
Daytime sleepiness	Class II molar occlusion
Frequent nocturia	Obesity or large neck circumference
Nocturnal diaphoresis	Erythematous post airway
Nocturnal gastroesophageal reflux disease	High narrow hard palate
Excessive drool or dry mouth	Retrognathia
Morning headache	Macroglossia
Decreased libido	Tonsillar enlargement
↓ Concentration or memory	Nasal obstruction

the patient has OSA. The pre- and post-test probability should be sufficiently different to yield a high likelihood ratio.[4] Perhaps an easier way to think about a pretest probability might be as simple as "does the patient have a high likelihood of OSA or not?" And the more symptoms and signs present, the higher the likelihood of OSA (Table 16.2).

Years ago "the obese, middle-aged male, asleep and snoring loudly in the waiting room" was considered the typical patient with a high pretest probability of moderate to severe OSA. However, we now know that a young thin female, with new-onset hypertension, nocturnal reflux, a class II molar occlusion, a shallow anterior-posterior pharyngeal diameter, a markedly erythematous airway, and little or no daytime hypersomnolence or loud snoring, may also have a high pretest probability of OSA. Although both have a high pretest probability for the same condition, will the same OOCT device yield similar results in both patients? How do we know which sensors or "proprietary algorithms" are best suited to uncover the disease? Would in-laboratory polysomnography be a better choice? These are the types of questions, in addition to others, that the clinician must confront to evaluate OSA most effectively.

Case

An 18-year-old woman recently presented to this author's sleep disorders center with a history of attention-deficit/hyperactivity disorder (ADHD) and a chief complaint of difficulty with sleep onset and maintenance, and resultant daytime sleepiness. She tried melatonin and amitriptyline prior to presentation with little or no relief. When asked specifically about her difficulty she stated that she would "doze-off and quickly awaken" repeatedly as she would try to fall asleep. She also reported snoring, nocturnal diaphoresis, holocephalic morning headache, and frequent awakenings with a cough. On examination, she weighed 208 pounds (94 kg), her height was 5 feet, 3 inches (160 cm), and her body mass index was 36.8 kg/m². She had a low-lying soft palate (modified Mallampati Class III) with a Class II molar occlusion. Tonsils were 1+ bilaterally and her tongue was large and scalloped. Where would this adult patient fall in the spectrum of "pretest probability of moderate to severe OSA"? If a "high" pretest probability was chosen and OOCT obtained, then a negative test might result, as occurred in this case (Figure 16.1).

Even though the total recording time might be considered inadequate, notice the periods of decreased flow without associated oxyhemoglobin desaturation or obvious evidence of arousal (Figure 16.2).

Subsequent in-laboratory polysomnography, in contrast, revealed moderate to severe OSA with a respiratory disturbance index of 34 and minimum oxyhemoglobin desaturation of 87% using the current American Academy of Sleep Medicine's manual for the scoring of sleep and associated events.[5]

This example, and perhaps one reason for the discrepancy between the two different tests in the same

patient, speaks to the first major potential pitfall of OOCT: "sleep," per se, is not generally recorded in OOCT unless a type II device is utilized. Certain indirect measures of sleep are instituted at times (actigraphy, PAT, etc.), but OOCT is predominantly a measure of respiratory events that produce a decrease or cessation of airflow lasting at least 10 seconds in duration and associated with a desaturation of oxygen of $\geq 3\%$. So, what happened to the importance of respiratory events associated with arousals of the brain or subcortical arousals (hypopneas and respiratory effort-related arousals)? Even though much of the published literature about OSA focuses on hypoxia as a major risk factor for cardiopulmonary consequences, clinicians must not ignore adverse impact on daytime functioning and alertness in particular as major consequences of OSA. Falling asleep while driving can be just as lethal as myocardial infarction.

How should a clinician interpret the OOCT results?

The absence of any sleep recording is not only a concern because arousals are not identified, as noted above, but also because total sleep time remains unknown. If a patient sleeps for only 1 hour during a total OOCT recording time of 8 hours, the apnea/hypopnea index (AHI; apneas and hypopneas per hour of recording time, since hours of sleep are not known) will be falsely low. For example, if the patient has 30 respiratory events during the 8-hour study, the overall AHI will be 3.8 indicating the absence of OSA based on current guidelines (AHI < 5.0); however, with sleep measured, the AHI becomes 30 apneas or hypopneas per hour of sleep, enough to diagnose **severe** OSA. This pitfall again highlights the importance of recognizing the pretest probability and its relation to the final test result. A negative OOCT should **always** be handled with caution.

Another common concern to consider when interpreting results is that a type IV device that records only one or two biometric parameters cannot often distinguish obstructive from central events, because respiratory effort is not measured.[6] Furthermore, familiarity

Recording

Date:	10/23/2012
Start:	11:28 PM.
End:	1:47 AM.
Duration:	2 h 19 min

Evaluation

Start:	11:38 PM.
End:	1:45 AM.
Duration:	2 h 7 min

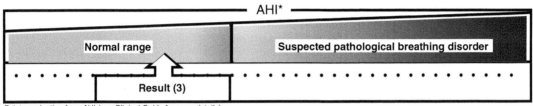

Points evaluation from AHI (see Clinical Guide for more details)

Analysis   (Flow evaluation period: 2 h 7 min / SpO₂ evaluation period: 2 h 9 min)

Indices		Normal	Result	
AHI*:	3	< 5 / h	Average breaths per minute [bpm]:	20.17
RI*:	4	< 5	Breaths:	2555
Apnea index:	0	< 5 / h	Apneas:	0
UAI:	0		Unclassified apneas:	0
OAI:	0		Obstructive apneas:	0
CAI:	0		Central apneas:	0
MAI:	0		Mixed apneas:	0
Hypopnea index:	3	< 5 / h	Hypopneas:	6
% Flow lim. Br. without Sn (FL):	8	< Approx.60	Flow lim. Br. without Sn (FL):	199
% Flow lim. Br. with Sn (FS):	1	< Approx.40	Flow lim. Br. with Sn (FS):	13
			Snoring events:	182
ODI Oxygen Desaturation Index*:	6	< 5 / h	No. of desaturations:	12
Average saturation:	98	94% - 98%	Saturation 90% :	0 min (0%)
Lowest desaturation:	92	-	Saturation 85% :	0 min (0%)
Lowest saturation:	92	90% - 98%	Saturation 80% :	0 min (0%)
Baseline Saturation:	99	%	Saturation 89% :	0 min (0%)
			Saturation 88% :	0 min (0%)
Minimum pulse frequency:	51	50 - 70 bpm		
Maximum pulse frequency:	127	60 - 90 bpm		
Average pulse frequency:	66	bpm		
Proportion of probable CS epochs:	0	0%		

Analysis status: Analyzed automatically

Analysis parameters used (Default)
Apnea [20%; 10ʙ; 80ʙ;1.0ʙ; 20%; 60%; 8%];   Hypopnea [70%; 10ʙ; 100ʙ; 1.0ʙ]; Snoring [6.0%; 0.3ʙ; 3.5ʙ; 0.5ʙ;]; Desaturation [4.0%]; CSR [0.50]

Figure 16.1 In this summary report from a hand-scored type III home study test, the overall respiratory disturbance index does not meet criteria for the presence of obstructive sleep apnea. Abbreviations used in figure: AHI, apnea/hypopnea index; RI, respiratory disturbance index.

with the equipment and the data should be a major emphasis. Learning how to distinguish normative from abnormal data is just as important as recognizing artifact. The interpretation should include mention of technical adequacy as artifact is often recognized in OOCT. For that reason, among others, interpretation should be performed by a board certified or board eligible sleep medicine physician, within a comprehensive sleep medicine

program preferably accredited by the American Academy of Sleep Medicine. At the other end of the spectrum, an OOCT can be ordered on the internet by an individual who may not be a healthcare provider. Clinicians who use OOCT should make sure their patients are studied with approved equipment, not just well-marketed equipment, which is offered and interpreted by ethical and responsible providers.

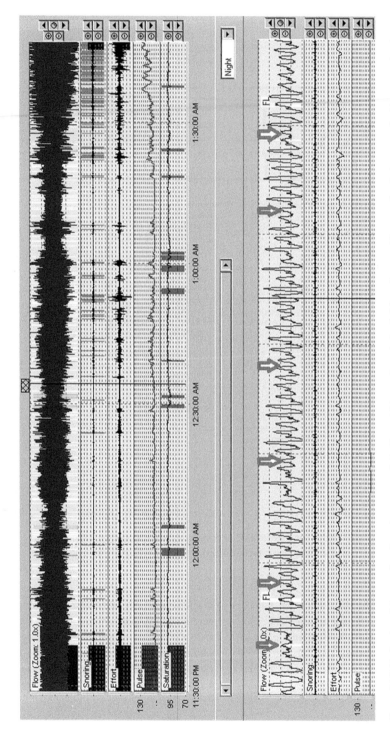

Figure 16.2 Evaluation of the raw data from the same study in Figure 16.1 reveals periods of airflow decrease (downward pointing arrows) without associated oxyhemoglobin desaturation or clear evidence of arousal in the absence of an electroencephalogram (EEG) measurement.

Can we use the positive result of an OOCT to justify auto-PAP in the home instead of a titration study in a sleep laboratory?

Risks arise from incorrect treatment of OSA, from inadequate treatment, or from poor nasal continuous positive airway pressure (CPAP) response. In addition to nasal CPAP, several positive airway pressure (PAP) options are now available for various sleep-related breathing disorders. Such options include, for example, bi-level PAP, bi-level PAP with a back-up respiratory rate, and auto-servoventilation. Automatically adjusting PAP, or auto-PAP, is widely available and is occasionally mandated by certain insurance providers as a first-line home treatment for OSA. In such cases, auto-PAP is used to obviate the need for an expensive in-laboratory CPAP titration study, the more standard approach used to determine an optimal CPAP setting for home use thereafter. Some insurers see auto-PAP as an effective opportunity, for patients initially considered straightforward enough to qualify for a diagnostic OOCT, to completely avoid the high costs of a sleep laboratory. Auto-PAP differs from CPAP in that it uses proprietary algorithms to sense changes in breathing on a continuous, real-time basis. The aim then is to deliver, ideally, only the amount of pressure necessary to keep the airway open at any given moment. Home auto-PAP is not only a treatment but, in an alternative strategy, can also be used as an unattended cardiopulmonary test. Downloaded data from the machine can be used to estimate what fixed CPAP setting should be used at home thereafter. Often, for example, the auto-PAP setting that is chosen for subsequent fixed CPAP use at home is the pressure that appears to have been sufficiently high enough to treat the patient's OSA for 95% of the time during which data were recorded using the auto-PAP machine.

Although some published data exist to support use of these strategies in selected patients, administration of PAP for the first time at home cannot be achieved without potential concern in some cases. For example, many patients judged to have been candidates for home studies because of high pretest probability for moderate or severe apnea do in fact prove to have severe OSA. Such patients, especially if obese, are occasionally at risk for worsened ventilation during the rebound rapid eye movement (REM) sleep, and its attendant atonia, that can occur after chronic REM sleep deprivation in the past. Untreated OSA is often worst in REM sleep and may limit its normal elaboration. Administration of PAP for the first time overcomes the upper airway obstruction and recurrent arousal stimulus that obstructive apneas used to provide. As a result, the drive to breathe may be markedly decreased in certain OSA patients who have experienced years of blunted chemosensitivity to abnormal PaO_2 and $PaCO_2$. With PAP in place, these patients can have significant hypoventilation and oxyhemoglobin desaturation during REM sleep. Prolonged periods of marked hypoxia raise the concern for potential adverse consequences. Figure 16.3 shows, for example, findings from a 61-year-old male patient, without significant comorbidities, who presented to this author's sleep disorders center. This patient's prominent OSA consisted mainly of frank obstructive apneas. A split-night study was performed, in which the second part of the night was used to initiate and titrate CPAP. Upon correction of the obstructive apneas, when the titration reached a pressure of 10 cm of H_2O, the patient started to have REM rebound. His oxygenation plummeted with poor recovery to baseline for an extended period. Frequent premature ventricular contractions were also noted during this time (Figure 16.3). Premature ventricular contractions in themselves are not dangerous, but their elicitation in this patient under hypoxic conditions and knowledge that dangerous arrhythmias including ventricular tachycardia can occur in OSA patients during sleep combine to highlight a potentially consequential "pitfall": risk for adverse impact can arise for certain patients if and when PAP is initiated outside a supervised setting.

Main points

The OOCT and auto-PAP are useful options if used properly in appropriate candidates, and if the

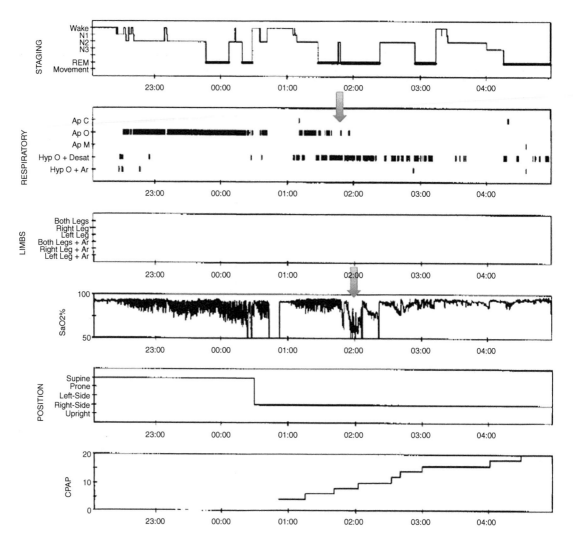

Figure 16.3 A hypnogram of an in-laboratory, attended, split-night polysomnogram with nasal continuous positive airway pressure (CPAP). The downward pointing arrows represent correction of the obstructive apneas with nasal CPAP at 10 cm of water, and a subsequent period of oxyhemoglobin desaturation without recovery to baseline in the setting of persistent obstructive hypopneas.

information generated is interpreted by a clinician with adequate experience in sleep medicine. Cavalier diagnosis and treatment of patients with OSA should be avoided even when the absence of treatment or inadequate treatment can be a major cause of morbidity and mortality.

REFERENCES

1. Sackett DL, Haynes RB, Guyatt GH, Tugwell P. *Clinical Epidemiology: A Basic Science for Clinical Medicine*, Second Edition. Boston, MA: Little, Brown;1991.

2. Ferber R, Millman R, Coppola M, et al. Portable recording in the assessment of obstructive sleep apnea. ASDA standards of practice. *Sleep* 1994;**17**:378–92.

3. Collop NA, Tracy SL, Kapur V, et al. Obstructive sleep apnea devices for out-of-center (OOC) testing: technology evaluation. *J Clin Sleep Med* 2011;**7**:531–48.

4. Jaeschke R, Guyatt G, Sackett DL. Evidence-Based Medicine Working Group. Users' guides to the medical literature. III. How to use an article about a diagnostic test. A. Are the results of the study valid? *JAMA* 1994;**271**:389–91.

5. Berry RB, Brooks R, Gamaldo CE, et al. for the American Academy of Sleep Medicine. *The AASM Manual for the Scoring of Sleep and Associated Events: Rules, Terminology and Technical Specifications*, Online Version 2.0. www.aasmnet.org, Darien, IL: American Academy of Sleep Medicine;2012. (Accessed November 30, 2012)

6. Collop NA, Anderson WM, Boehlecke B, et al. Portable Monitoring Task Force of the American Academy of Sleep Medicine. Clinical guidelines for the use of unattended portable monitors in the diagnosis of obstructive sleep apnea in adult patients. *J Clin Sleep Med* 2007;**3**:737-47.

Positive airway pressure to treat obstructive sleep apnea

Continuous positive airway pressure (CPAP), delivered non-invasively during sleep by a nasal or full face mask, is often a first-line treatment for obstructive sleep apnea and also for central sleep apnea. Equipment used to deliver CPAP has advanced in recent years in many ways. For example, patients who need assistance with ventilation can use bi-level positive airway pressure (PAP) machines that provide a higher pressure on inspiration and a lower but still positive pressure on expiration. Patients who require lower pressure settings for much of the night and higher pressures only at certain times can use automatically titrating PAP. Patients with obstructive sleep apnea who develop PAP-induced central apneas (complex sleep apnea) may benefit from either adaptive servoventilation that seeks to avoid hyperventilation as a trigger for central events, or bi-level PAP with a back-up rate that ensures delivery of the higher inspiratory pressure at fixed intervals, to stimulate a breath if none is initiated by the patient. Other key advances have facilitated objective monitoring by clinicians of

patients' adherence to PAP, and of the effectiveness of the PAP machines. Data can now be collected nightly for many months on machine use, pressures delivered, and machine-estimated control of the sleep apnea. All these advances create opportunity, but they also create more room for pitfalls to avoid in the clinical practice of sleep medicine.

Moreover, technical advances have not obviated the need for clinical strategies to promote adherence, which remains the single largest limiting factor in the effectiveness of PAP therapies. Fortunately, new approaches developed by specialists in behavioral sleep medicine are available to promote adherence to home use of PAP.

The following cases illustrate that a clinician is more likely to provide optimal care for patients with sleep apnea if he or she understands when to use a sleep laboratory, when not to use the laboratory, what can and cannot be achieved by use of specific advances in PAP technologies, and when to request or apply behavioral intervention.

17

Repeated continuous positive airway pressure studies may raise the prescribed pressure above necessary treatment levels

Meredith D. Peters

A 56-year-old single man being treated for obstructive sleep apnea syndrome (OSAS) with bi-level positive airway pressure (Bi-PAP) presents as a new patient to the clinic complaining of new nocturnal awakenings and increasing fatigue despite wearing his Bi-PAP all night, every night. He also has a known history of atrial fibrillation. The patient asks if he needs his Bi-PAP setting "raised again."

The patient was initially diagnosed with obstructive sleep apnea (OSA) 4 years ago by another physician, in the Southwest region of the United States. His presenting symptoms of OSAS had been sleep disruption, frequent nocturia, and excessive daytime somnolence (an Epworth Sleepiness Scale score of 14, on a scale of 0–24). At that time, the patient identified his sleep disruption as "waking every hour, on the hour." He blamed urinary urgency for some of these awakenings, but could not identify a trigger for most. On baseline polysomnography, the patient was found to have severe OSA with a respiratory disturbance index (RDI) of 62 events per hour of sleep associated with oxygen desaturations to a nadir of 72%. The patient's first positive airway pressure titration study was optimal. Bi-PAP at 18/14 cm of water was tested in supine-rapid eye movement (REM) sleep, and the RDI was reduced to 1.8 events per hour. With the initiation of home use of Bi-PAP therapy at 18/14 cm of water, the patient experienced significant improvement in sleep maintenance and daytime somnolence. His nocturia was reduced from three times nightly to once, "if at all."

You review multiple reports from the patient's previous sleep clinic. Following his initial diagnosis and continuous positive airway pressure (CPAP)/Bi-PAP titration, the patient underwent a repeat Bi-PAP titration yearly for the next 2 years. His Bi-PAP setting was increased to 19/15 cm of water and then 20/15 cm of water respectively. He is now treated with Bi-PAP 20/15 cm of water. The patient denies any return of OSAS symptoms or weight change preceding his two repeat Bi-PAP studies. His doctor had advised yearly reevaluation. You observe that each of the patient's retitration studies began with his last prescribed treatment setting. The patient shrugs and tells you that he never felt any further improvement with the increased pressures. Until moving to Michigan earlier this year, the patient had always sustained excellent symptomatic relief with Bi-PAP therapy – the same with all three settings.

Upon questioning, the patient now characterizes his new nocturnal awakenings as four to six brief arousals with a severely dry mouth. "I have jacked up my humidifier to the maximum, and it isn't helping." He did not experience this oral dryness when living in the Southwest. The patient denies awakening with dyspnea, choking, or palpitations. He denies the return of frequent nocturia. He does not feel sleepy in the day and denies dozing off at work or during his evening television programs, like he had prior to starting Bi-PAP therapy. The patient now reports an Epworth Sleepiness Scale score of 7, and scores of 9 or lower are usually considered normal. However, with his sleep being so fragmented, he does endorse some fatigue. You ask about any changes in the patient's chronic medical conditions or medications. He started an over-the-counter oral decongestant "because my nose is stuffed up non-stop since I came to Michigan."

On physical examination, the patient is an obese man in no acute distress. His weight is 222 pounds (101 kg), his height is 5 feet, 6 inches (168 cm), and his body mass index is 34.8 kg/m^2. His neck circumference is 18 inches (46 cm). His head is normocephalic and without retrognathia or midfacial flattening. Nares demonstrate moderate to severe bilateral turbinate hypertrophy with boggy mucosa and clear thick secretions. The nasal septum is straight. Oropharynx demonstrates hypertrophy of the tongue with scalloping. The hard plate appears normal. The soft palate is low lying and elongated with a long, mildly edematous uvula. Tonsils are surgically absent, but there is severe medialization of the posterior pharyngeal tissues. He has a Class I molar occlusion.

Do you order a Bi-PAP retitration for the patient at this time?

In the above case, the patient's initial titration study was characterized as being "optimal." Grading the quality of a positive airway pressure (PAP) titration has been defined by the Positive Airway Pressure Titration Task Force of the American Academy of Sleep Medicine. An abbreviated statement of these grades is as follows: An **optimal** titration reduces RDI < 5 for at least 15-minutes duration and should include supine-REM sleep at the selected pressure. A **good** titration reduces RDI ≤ 10 or by 50% if the baseline RDI < 15 and should include supine-REM. There are also definitions for **adequate** and **unacceptable** titrations.[1]

Clinical guidelines and practice parameters have been published on the initial indications for PAP therapy in treating OSAS, and on the titration of CPAP and Bi-PAP. However, clearly stated standards or protocols for repeating a PAP titration are minimal. Those provided by the Positive Airway Pressure Titration Task Force of the American Academy of Sleep Medicine are as follows:

- A repeat PAP titration should be considered if the initial titration does not achieve a grade of optimal or good (Standard).[1]
- Repeating a polysomnogram after weight loss of 10% or greater is routinely indicated to determine further necessity for PAP therapy or to assess for changes in pressure requirements (Standard).[2]
- A repeat PAP titration may be considered if the patient experiences recurrence of OSAS symptoms or if a patient experiences persistent adherence difficulties.[3]

There is no evidence to support the performance of serial PAP retitration studies, such as the above patient had undergone yearly with his previous provider.[3]

After your interview above, you recommend the patient undergo a repeat Bi-PAP titration, believing that the patient has had recurrence of OSAS symptoms. You request that the repeat titration in your sleep laboratory is started at 16/12 cm of water, lower than the patient's initially prescribed pressure setting, as his weight is unchanged and his symptomatic relief had been equal between 18/14 cm of water and 20/15 cm of water until just recently.

The patient brings his own mask to the retitration study. He wears a nasal cone mask without a chin strap. He tells the technician, "I love my mask. I have been wearing the same model since I started Bi-PAP, and it has always worked really well for me." The patient practices good Bi-PAP supplies maintenance, changing the cushion of his nasal mask every 3 months and replacing the frame and headgear every 6 months. He has never tried a chin strap, to reduce any mouth leak, and has never been offered one. During one of his previous retitration studies in the Southwest, the patient does recall a technician trying to change his interface to a full face mask, which he rejected.

For the present retitration, Bi-PAP was started at 16/12 cm of water using the patient's preferred nasal mask without a chin strap. The setting was increased to Bi-PAP 20/14 cm of water for "persistent hypopneas." At Bi-PAP 20/14 cm of water, the polysomnogram appeared as shown in Figure 17.1.

The technician enters the room and assesses the leak to be a mouth leak (also known as oral venting) and not a mask leak. The technician offers to place a

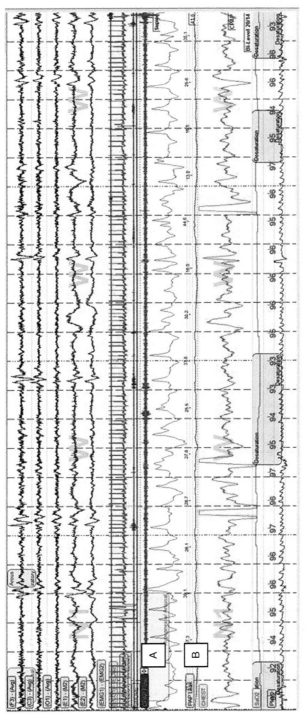

Figure 17.1 Polysomnogram slide of bi-level, positive airway pressure (Bi-PAP) 20/14 cm of water using nasal mask without chin strap. You note that the continuous positive airway pressure (CPAP) flow signal (see **A**) is poor. The waveform above is quite irregular, and the scored hypopnea demonstrates a sine wave of varying amplitude and shape. One would typically expect to see a more uniform sine wave with a hypopnea scored secondary to a persistent amplitude reduction followed by arousal or oxygen desaturation. Such an irregular wave form may be seen in the setting of severe leak, which is confirmed by the CPAP leak signal (see **B**).

chin strap on the patient, and the patient agrees. An immediate and dramatic improvement is noted in the CPAP flow signal, which is sustained as the technician lowers the Bi-PAP setting (Figure 17.2).

Ultimately, complete resolution of snoring, obstructive respiratory events, and excessive arousal is observed with Bi-PAP 17/13 cm of water, tested in supine-REM sleep (optimal study). Four weeks after his Bi-PAP is reduced to 17/13 cm of water with the addition of a chin strap, the patient returns to your clinic. He is no longer awakening with a dry mouth, and he is no longer fatigued. The patient "does not mind that chin strap," but he asks if he will need this new strap indefinitely. His nose remains moderately to severely congested day and night.

Did this patient require a Bi-PAP retitration study?

With the exception of repeating a PAP titration for failure to obtain an optimal or good titration initially, the practice parameters for use of CPAP and Bi-PAP in adults with sleep-disordered breathing first state that "close follow-up for PAP usage and problems in patients with OSA by appropriately trained healthcare providers is indicated to establish effective utilization patterns and remediate problems if needed (Standard)."[4]

Clinic (as opposed to sleep laboratory) follow-up of CPAP and Bi-PAP treatment should include the following comprehensive assessment as well as education, especially if there are complaints or concerns for recurrence of OSAS symptoms.

- Is the patient compliant with PAP?
- Is there leak at the mask interface?
- When was the mask cushion, frame, or headgear last replaced?
- Is the patient experiencing nasal or oral dryness?
- Is there evidence of mouth leak while using only a nasal interface?
- Does the patient have signs or symptoms of mask irritation or pain?
- Can the patient fall asleep with PAP on?

- Does the patient wake during the night feeling the pressure is too high?
- When was the PAP unit last assessed for proper calibration and pressure emission?
- Has the patient gained weight or lost weight?
- Has a new medication been added at bedtime which may exacerbate sleep apnea?
- Does the patient regularly use alcohol at bedtime at home?

In the above case, more careful clinical assessment and remediation of interface problems may have prevented the need for a retitration study. First of all, did the patient really have return of his initial OSAS symptoms? He actually did not. His symptoms were the result of new difficulty with nasal congestion and difficulty with his Bi-PAP mask interface, and differed from his initial presenting symptoms of OSAS. Oral venting was indicated by the patient's severely dry mouth while using a mask that did not cover and provide humidified air to his mouth; and, thus, increasing the humidification setting on his Bi-PAP unit would not correct the symptom.

The patient's history of being offered transition to a full face mask in the past during a titration study suggests that he may have had some mouth leak at that time as well, but it may not have been clinically significant (as it did not result in difficulty with tolerance or symptoms). The patient did not have severely dry mouth waking him until he developed obstructive nasal allergies following his move to Michigan. His fatigue may have been secondary to the leak-induced sleep fragmentation; however, the fatigue may also have suggested that the patient's increased mouth leak resulted in loss of pressure support (which was confirmed during the Bi-PAP retitration you performed).

"PAP mask refit or readjustment should be performed whenever any significant unintentional leak is observed (Consensus)."[1] Realizing the need to treat this patient's new nasal allergies and adding a chin strap or full face mask to control for oral leak may have been a more appropriate first step. If interval follow-up after 1 month demonstrated resolution of the patient's symptoms, a repeat titration study would not have been necessary. Later, successful treatment of the patient's nasal obstruction may allow him to try removing the chin

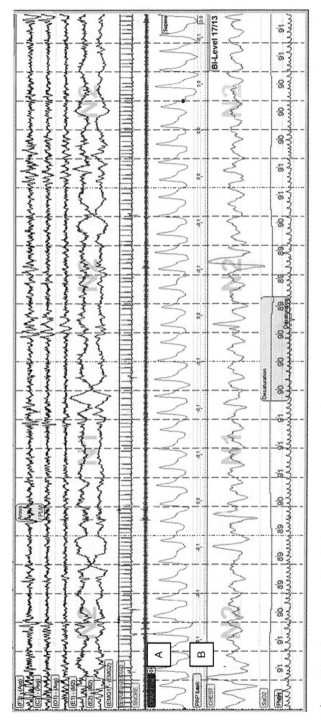

Figure 17.2 Polysomnogram slide of bi-level positive airway pressure (Bi-PAP) 17/13 cm of water using nasal mask with chin strap. Improved uniformity in the continuous positive airway pressure (CPAP) flow waveform (see **A**). Flattening of the CPAP leak signal (see **B**).

strap and return to his original treatment regimen, with which he had remained fully compliant and satisfied.

One last question: why did the patient require higher and higher pressures with his previous yearly titration studies when a lower setting effectively treats his OSA?

During a PAP titration, pressure settings seem almost invariably to increase from the setting at which the study begins. The issue has not been studied adequately, and explanations can only be speculative at this point. The tendency for settings to increase so uniformly during PAP retitrations may arise, for example, secondary to recurrent but physiologic post-arousal hypopneas as the patient transitions to sleep, or from recurrent arousals as the patient attempts to fall asleep in an unfamiliar place. Additionally, the clinical guidelines for titrating CPAP and Bi-PAP provide room for "exploration, increasing the PAP setting up to 5 cm of water above that pressure where control of abnormalities in respiratory parameters is achieved."[1] Though a higher setting may not indicate clear additional benefit, if the same higher setting is the only pressure tested in supine-REM sleep, it may be chosen by the interpreting polysomnographer in order to grade the titration as optimal. Thus, if each retitration were to begin at the patient's currently prescribed PAP setting, it is likely the patient would be prescribed progressively higher CPAP settings. It is also possible, in the above patient's case, that the pressure was increased above his requirements in an attempt to compensate for his oral leak which was not otherwise clinically apparent at that time.

Finally, some studies suggest that in the absence of weight change, a patient's PAP requirement may actually be slightly lower after the first weeks to months of home PAP therapy.[5,6] One reason may be that recurrent irritation of the oropharyngeal mucosa by snoring and apneas causes edema, which subsides once the OSA is treated. When a repeat PAP titration for new or recurrent symptoms is started at a setting lower than the patient's currently utilized setting, the current PAP setting or a lower setting is sometimes found to be effective. This informs the clinician that other potential etiologies for the patient's symptoms should be pursued, and again highlights the importance of a good clinical evaluation.

REFERENCES

1. Kushida CA, Chediak A, Berry RB, et al. Positive Airway Pressure Titration Task Force of the American Academy of Sleep Medicine. Clinical guidelines for the manual titration of positive airway pressure in patients with obstructive sleep apnea. *J Clin Sleep Med* 2008;**4**:157–71.

2. Epstein LJ, Kristo D, Strollo PJ, et al. Clinical guideline for the evaluation, management and long-term care of obstructive sleep apnea in adults. *J Clin Sleep Med* 2009;**5**:263–76.

3. Gay P, Weaver T, Loube D, Iber C. Positive Airway Pressure Task Force, Standards of Practice Committee, American Academy of Sleep Medicine. Evaluation of positive airway pressure treatment for sleep related breathing disorders in adults. *Sleep* 2006;**29**:381–401.

4. Kushida CA, Littner MR, Hirshkowitz M, et al. American Academy of Sleep Medicine. Practice parameters for the use of continuous and bilevel positive airway pressure devices to treat adult patients with sleep-related breathing disorders. *Sleep* 2006;**29**:375–80.

5. Jokic R, Klimaszewski A, Crossley M, Sridhar G, Fitzpatrick MF. Positional treatment vs. continuous positive airway pressure in patients with positional obstructive sleep apnea syndrome. *Chest* 1999;**115**:771–81.

6. Choi S, Mullins R, Crosby JH. Is (re)titration of nasal continous positive airway pressure for obstructive sleep apnoea necessary? *Sleep Med* 2001;**12**:431–5.

18

Patient education and motivational enhancement can make the difference between adherence and non-use of positive airway pressure

Deirdre A. Conroy and Jennifer R. Goldschmied

Research has continuously shown that continuous positive airway pressure (CPAP) is an efficacious treatment for obstructive sleep apnea (OSA).[1-4] Despite its efficacy in research, however, adherence rates from community samples continue to show suboptimal use of CPAP, demonstrating disconnect between its utility and effectiveness. In fact, Kribbs et al.[5] found that less than half of their sample used positive airway pressure (PAP) for 4 or more hours per night, and McArdle et al.[6] found that 25% of patients discontinue treatment within the first year of use. In order for PAP to be useful in eliminating the symptoms and related consequences of OSA, patients must be adherent with the therapy. Adequate PAP-adherence has been defined as at least 4 hours per night on at least 70% of nights.[5,7] However, the choice of this guideline has been driven more by convention than by research per se, and in some respects this has been an arbitrary choice. Despite the efficacy of PAP to control symptoms of OSA, adherence rates in community samples continue to show suboptimal use.

Studies of smoking cessation, weight-loss programs, and other medical intervention have shown that educating patients about the target problem, associated consequences, optimal treatment, and benefits of treatment may increase adherence. Patient education is typically a cost-effective method of increasing patient investment in the intervention as the educational program can generally be administered expediently by the patient care staff. Recently, OSA-specific patient education has been studied to determine its effectiveness at increasing adherence to PAP. Studies have ranged from

patient education to patient-specific models utilizing personalized feedback from full-night polysomnography and PAP-titration studies. Understanding and addressing patient ambivalence regarding therapy initiation has also been explored. These studies suggest that patient education and motivational enhancement can potentially increase PAP adherence.

Case 1

While working on his computer, a 44-year-old man (5 feet, 11 inches [180 cm] tall, weighing 189 pounds [86 kg]) with a history of hypertension and hyperlipidemia suffered a left cerebellar ischemic stroke. At the time of his stroke, he exercised regularly and ate a heart-healthy diet. When asked by his physician, he endorsed snoring, but he was not aware of apneic episodes. He denied depression, anxiety, chest pain, palpitations, or any history of atrial fibrillation.

At the recommendation of his neurologist, a referral for a diagnostic polysomnogram (PSG) was placed. A diagnostic PSG revealed severe sleep apnea characterized by an apnea/hypopnea index (AHI, events per hour of sleep) of 38 and a minimum oxygen saturation of 90%. A CPAP titration study was conducted, to determine an optimal setting for home use, and pressures in the range of 6–10 cm of water were applied. The night was characterized by a long latency to sleep. Stage N1 sleep, the lightest sleep stage, was higher on his diagnostic study (comprising 20% of the night)

Common Pitfalls in Sleep Medicine, ed. Ronald D. Chervin. Published by Cambridge University Press. © Cambridge University Press 2014.

compared to his CPAP titration study (comprising 9% of the night). Oxyhemoglobin saturation was maintained above 90% with CPAP of 10 cm of water. However, the patient encountered difficulty wearing the CPAP device immediately upon receiving it. He was seen in a post-treatment follow-up session with a sleep physician about 2 weeks after his CPAP study, and then was seen by a behavioral sleep medicine specialist approximately 3 weeks after his CPAP study.

When the patient met with the behavioral sleep medicine specialist, the clinician and patient reviewed his sleep study results in detail. They compared his sleep architecture, frequency of apneic events, and SaO_2 saturations with and without the CPAP device. The studies showed that without CPAP his sleep was disrupted and there were frequent fluctuations of his SaO_2 during the night. They discussed the role of sleep apnea as a risk factor for future strokes. The patient was educated about how CPAP would improve his level of oxygen saturation during sleep as well as the quality of his sleep. Next, they discussed adjunctive supplies to increase CPAP comfort, including a CPAP mask liner or a snore pillow, to decrease skin irritation and help him avoid supine sleep.

Finally, the patient's initial reluctance to use the mask was resolved and the clinician introduced the idea of the body's natural response to remove the mask in early CPAP users. The clinician also assessed the patient's motivation and confidence to use CPAP every night. The patient was given a handout about sleep apnea at the conclusion of the session.

When the patient returned to the clinic approximately 6 months after his CPAP study, he reported using CPAP on a nightly basis. A download of his CPAP data card revealed that he was using the device on 98% of nights. The patient expressed a willingness to use CPAP to prevent future strokes.

Discussion

Is patient education sufficient to ensure PAP adherence? Consider individualized motivational enhancement therapy

Patient education is helpful to increase patient adherence to PAP, but additional strategies may also be of benefit. Richards et al.[7] examined the effectiveness of a group intervention utilizing a cognitive behavioral approach to increase adherence to CPAP. This intervention involved two 1-hour sessions over the course of 2 weeks, designed to "correct distorted beliefs and promote a positive outlook to treatment," which was in addition to treatment as usual after the diagnosis of OSA, but before the occurrence of a CPAP-titration study. The sessions included a standardized presentation about OSA and CPAP, a demonstration of relaxation exercises to combat any CPAP-related anxiety, a 15-minute video of CPAP users describing their experiences and benefits from CPAP and the importance of adhering to the treatment despite difficulties, a brochure encompassing more information about CPAP and OSA, and a list of dysfunctional beliefs along with their cognitively restructured counterparts. The results demonstrated that the cognitive behavioral therapy-intervention did decrease attrition, with 8% of the patients randomized to the cognitive behavioral therapy-group refusing CPAP initially, as compared to 30% of the treatment-as-usual group. The authors also found that adherence was increased among those in the cognitive behavioral therapy-group, with 77% using CPAP for at least 4 hours, as compared to 31% of the treatment-as-usual group. The authors highlight the utility of a group intervention and demonstrate that the treatment could be facilitated by an individual without specific psychological training.

Aloia et al.[8] investigated the efficacy of a PAP intervention based on motivational enhancement therapy (MET). The therapy highlights one's readiness to change, perceived importance of change, and confidence in one's ability to change. The ideal time to deliver MET for PAP is shortly after the patient's first PAP study. Ideal candidates for MET are: (i) those who may be struggling with intrinsic motivation and self-efficacy to use the PAP device; and (ii) those who are judged to be good responders to PAP therapy on the titration night. A good responder is someone who showed the following on their PAP titration study: a residual apnea/hypopnea index < 10 events per hour of sleep, resolution of snoring, an arousal index of < 10 per hour of sleep, and a periodic leg movement index of < 15 movements per hour of sleep. The MET may not be indicated in patients with persistent daytime sleepiness or a serious medical condition.[9] The MET does not necessarily need to be delivered by a psychologist or behavioral sleep medicine specialist. Instead, healthcare professionals, such as nurses, physician's assistants, or others who have a background in sleep medicine can be trained sufficiently in a short period of time to use motivational or cognitive strategies to encourage adherence to PAP. For example, MET for PAP therapy has been successfully delivered by nurses with a background in sleep medicine and with specific training for motivational interviewing.

The MET for PAP involves two 45-minute in-person sessions with a trained motivational enhancement therapist, and a 15-minute follow-up phone call designed to enhance "intrinsic motivation" to adhere to PAP use. The sessions involve personalized feedback about the patient's sleep studies and their reactions to having used PAP therapy. The sessions may also provide the opportunity for patients to explore their ambivalence about PAP use. In this study, an education-based intervention was also investigated, which involved the discussion of OSA and PAP for the "typical apnea case." No personalized feedback was given. Results indicated that discontinuation of PAP by the end of the 13-week follow-up period was decreased in the MET for PAP group and the educational group as compared to the treatment-as-usual group. The low adherence rate for the MET for PAP group was 26%; in the educational group this was 30%; whereas in the treatment-as-usual group it was 51%. No differences, however, were found in predicting high adherence rates between the three groups.

In their study, Olsen et al.[1] examined the effects of a motivational interviewing-based intervention that included components of their Health Beliefs Model of PAP adherence. This states that specific health beliefs – including perception of severity, benefits, and risks associated with untreated OSA – affect adherence. This standardized and manualized intervention consists of two 45-minute one-on-one sessions, and one 20-minute booster session prior to PAP titration and initial PAP use, aimed at "addressing the patient's ambivalence and resistance to change." Patients in both groups also completed a standard, 45-minute

education session in the initial phase of the trial. Nurses with background in sleep medicine underwent specific training for motivational interviewing prior to administering the intervention, and had continued supervision throughout the study period.

Results showed that motivational interviewing based intervention increased the rate of initial PAP use over treatment-as-usual at a 3-month follow-up. Subjects who had the motivational interviewing-based intervention showed a 6% rejection rate of PAP, as compared to a 28% rejection rate among those with treatment as usual. The motivational therapy was also shown to increase the number of hours of use at 3 months, compared to treatment as usual. This study suggests that intervening with patients before their initial introduction to PAP may help with future adherence.

Other possible interventions for PAP adherence include exposure therapy for claustrophobic reactions to PAP,[10] and sleep apnea self-management.[11]

Why did the patient return to the sleep disorders center so soon?

The PAP users who are able to use their machine on a daily basis the first 2 weeks after they receive it are more likely to continue to use it after 6 months.[8] Therefore, the first 2 weeks of PAP use may represent a critical time for intervention. When behavioral interventions are initiated after approximately 2 weeks following introduction of PAP, patients may have already developed poor use patterns that are difficult to reverse. Moreover, patients who indicate any ambivalence towards PAP use may especially benefit from early intervention.

Our clinic is busy and we don't have the person-power to provide such individualized feedback. What else could we do to increase PAP adherence in our patients?

Wiese et al.[12] examined the effects of an educational video. The video utilized patient models speaking in lay-language to describe what a diagnosis of OSA means, its causes, potential consequences, and what a treatment that uses PAP may look like on a sample of PAP-naïve OSA patients. The authors found that this educational video, a relatively inexpensive and standardized method that does not require an encounter with healthcare providers, did decrease drop-out rates significantly. Approximately 75% of the patients randomized to the video group remained in treatment at a 1-month follow-up, compared to < 50% of the control group.

Main points

Behavioral intervention aimed at educating or motivating patients to adhere to PAP treatment can decrease the high initial failure rate commonly seen in new PAP users. Each type of intervention has unique elements that contribute to success. Educational videos are low-cost and low-effort to administer, whereas motivational interviewing approaches have shown the greatest efficacy. The timing of behavioral intervention should be considered carefully, because of the sensitive nature of PAP acceptance and tolerance early in treatment.

FURTHER READING

Aloia MS, Arnedt JT, Riggs RL, Hecht J, Borrelli B. Clinical management of poor adherence to PAP: motivational enhancement. *Behav Sleep Med* 2004;**2**:205–22.

REFERENCES

1. Olsen S, Smith SS, Oei TPS, Douglas J. Motivational interviewing (MINT) improves continuous positive airway pressure (PAP) acceptance and adherence: a randomized controlled trial. *J Consult Clin Psychol* 2012;**80**:151–63.

2. Kushida CA, Littner MR, Hirshkowitz M, et al. Practice parameters for the use of continuous and bilevel positive airway pressure devices to treat adult patients with sleep-related breathing disorders. *Sleep* 2006;**29**:375–80.

3. Malhotra A, Ayas NT, Epstein LJ. The art and science of continuous positive airway pressure therapy in obstructive sleep apnea. *Curr Opin Pulm Med* 2000;**6**:490–5.

4. Stepnowsky CJ Jr, Moore PJ. Nasal CPAP treatment for obstructive sleep apnea: developing a new perspective on dosing strategies and compliance. *J Psychosom Res* 2003;**54**:599–605.

5. Kribbs NB, Pack AI, Kline LR, et al. Objective measurement of patterns of nasal CPAP use by patients with obstructive sleep apnea. *Am Rev Respir Dis* 1993;**147**:887–95.

6. McArdle N, Devereux G, Heidarnejad H, et al. Long-term use of CPAP therapy for sleep apnea/hypopnea syndrome. *Am J Respir Crit Care Med* 1999;**159**:1108–14.

7. Richards D, Bartlett DJ, Wong K, Malouff J, Grunstein RR. Increased adherence to PAP with a group cognitive behavioral treatment intervention: a randomized trial. *Sleep* 2007;**30**:635–40.

8. Aloia MS, Smith K, Arnedt JT, et al. Brief behavioral therapies reduce early positive airway pressure discontinuation rates in sleep apnea syndrome: preliminary findings. *Behav Sleep Med* 2007;**5**:89–104.

9. O'Connor CS, Aloia M. Motivational enhancement therapy: motivating adherence to positive airway pressure. In Perlis M, Aloia M, Kuhn B, eds. *Behavioral Treatments for Sleep Disorders*. London, UK: Academic Press;2011.

10. Edinger JD, Radtke RA. Use of in vivo desensitization to treat a patient's claustrophobic response to nasal CPAP. *Sleep* 1993;**16**:678–80.

11. Stepnowsky CJ, Palau JJ, Gifford AL, Ancoli-Israel S. A self-management approach to improving continuous positive airway pressure adherence and outcomes. *Behav Sleep Med* 2007;**5**:131–46.

12. Wiese H, Boethel C, Phillips B, et al. PAP compliance: video education may help! *Sleep Med* 2005;**6**:171–4.

19

A daytime "PAP-Nap" can help new patients adjust to the use of continuous positive airway pressure

Meredith D. Peters and Q. Afifa Shamim-Uzzaman

Introduction

Positive airway pressure (PAP) therapy is the most efficacious treatment for obstructive sleep apnea in a great many patients. However, PAP tolerance and adherence present major hurdles to successful treatment. Although several studies have sought to identify physical and psychosocial predictors for PAP adherence, it is oftentimes difficult to predict which patient will struggle with PAP and which will be successful.

Below, a case is presented in which the patient possesses many characteristics believed to predict good continuous positive airway pressure (CPAP) tolerance and long-term CPAP adherence. The patient has a good understanding of his diagnosis and goals of therapy and is not one whom most treating physicians would have initially considered in need of interventions prior to his CPAP titration study. However, since beginning a trial of CPAP therapy at home, the patient is rapidly failing the compliance requirements set forth by his insurance company. If he does not increase his CPAP usage significantly and within the next month, he risks losing continued coverage for his CPAP equipment.

A daytime abbreviated PAP study, called the PAP-Nap, may improve his tolerance to and success with PAP therapy.

Case

Mr. Green is a well-developed and well-nourished active 62-year-old man with a past medical history of essential hypertension, diagnosed at the age of 45, and new onset paroxysmal atrial fibrillation (PAF). Mr. Green does not have any history of mood disorder and denies any history of claustrophobia. He describes himself as cheerful. He finds his sleep quality is "adequate," and he has been enjoying his retirement with hiking, gardening, and socializing.

In evaluation of his new-onset PAF, work-up for thyroid dysregulation and a treadmill stress test were both negative. A recent 30-day event monitor demonstrated that the majority of Mr. Green's atrial fibrillation episodes begin during the night, specifically during the time Mr. Green has defined as his typical sleep period. The patient's wife accompanied him to a follow-up visit with Cardiology. When the results of the event monitor were being discussed, Mrs. Green reported that her husband has snored very loudly the full 38 years they have been married. Upon further questioning, she has heard both crescendo snoring and pauses in snoring followed by abrupt, loud snorts for many years. Her father had sounded just the same during sleep, and so she had not thought anything of it. The cardiologist ordered a baseline polysomnogram that demonstrated moderate obstructive sleep apnea with an apnea/hypopnea index of 27 events per hour of sleep and oxygen desaturations to a nadir of 78%. Most notably, there was clear evidence that this patient's obstructive sleep apnea may well be triggering his PAF (Figure 19.1).

After his polysomnogram, Mr. Green underwent consultation with a sleep specialist. The majority of

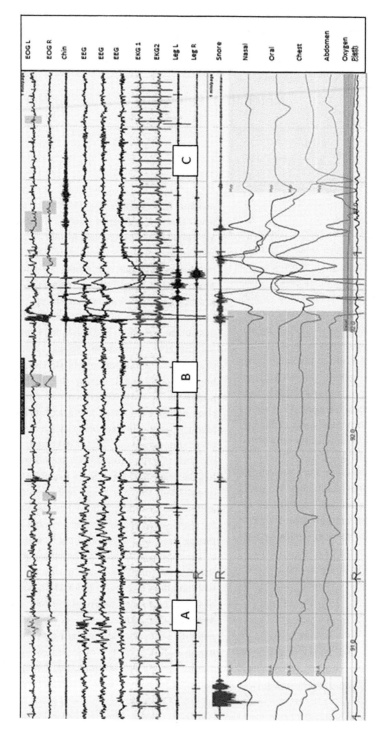

Figure 19.1 This figure highlights the electrocardiogram (ECG) changes observed during an obstructive apnea. Label **A**: Normal sinus rhythm; the rhythm that the patient maintained for the first 2 hours of sleep. Label **B**: Diving reflex is associated with an obstructive apnea and the associated oxygen desaturation. Label **C**: Atrial fibrillation, which began in association with the sympathetic surge that occurred at termination of this obstructive apnea. The patient remained in atrial fibrillation from this time through completion of the polysomnogram. See plate section for color version.

his 45-minute new patient visit was spent counseling the patient on obstructive sleep apnea as well as the treatment options. Continuous positive airway pressure therapy was recommended and discussed in detail. At the end of the visit, Mr. Green expressed motivation to begin CPAP therapy for both symptomatic relief as well as hopeful reduction in the frequency of PAF episodes.

Within 2 weeks, Mr. Green underwent a successful CPAP titration during which he used a full face mask, per his preference, after initially trying on three different masks at the start of the evening. His optimal CPAP setting was 16 cm of water with an expiratory pressure relief of –3. He completed a questionnaire on the morning after his CPAP titration, answering that he felt better upon awakening as compared to a typical morning at home. He maintained sinus rhythm throughout the CPAP study. He reported an initial positive outlook towards therapy.

Due to long wait times at the only sleep medicine clinic in his network, Mr. Green was not able to obtain an appointment for follow-up with his physician until 8 weeks after obtaining his CPAP machine and equipment. Unfortunately, during those 8 weeks, Mr. Green had great difficulty adjusting to CPAP at home.

Complaint after first week: For the first several nights, he was not able to fall asleep with CPAP on due to the excessive pressure sensation. When he called the office, the patient was unable to report on the status of the ramp feature of his machine, designed to start with a low pressure and only gradually raise it to the targeted level. He could not adjust the ramp settings despite verbal instruction.

Intervention: Prescription to durable medical equipment (DME) supplier to assess and re-educate patient on ramp.

Appointment with DME supplier 6 days later: The ramp feature was found to be inactive and was activated to last 45 minutes, according to the therapist working with the patient.

Complaint after second week: Now was able to fall asleep with his CPAP on, but he was waking after 2 hours feeling the pressure was too high. Felt anxious after this awakening, and he would remove the mask to return to sleep, despite the additional use of the ramp.

Intervention: Prescription was sent to temporarily decrease Mr. Green's pressure to 13 cm of water in order to facilitate tolerance.

DME appointment 4 days later: Pressure changed.

Complaint after third week: Now Mr. Green was able to fall asleep and maintain sleep 4.5–5.0 hours per night with CPAP on. However, he woke up each morning though with painful abdominal bloating. The DME supplier had counseled patient towards "tincture of time," but Mr. Green was calling the physician office now because this has not resolved.

Interventions: A wedge pillow was recommended. A prescription was given for mask refit, to replace full face mask with nasal mask and chin strap, as full face masks may be associated with a greater risk for aerophagia.

Durable medical equipment supplier appointment 7 days later: For the preceding 5 nights, Mr. Green had stopped using the CPAP because he was unable to tolerate the aerophagia. One mask was tried during the refit and it was dispensed to the patient. A chin strap was also dispensed.

When Mr. Green was seen in the office after 8 weeks, his first and second 30-day compliance records, downloaded from his CPAP machine data card, were reviewed. During both months, he failed to meet minimum usage requirements required by his insurer. His residual apnea/hypopnea index as estimated by the CPAP unit was 2.9 events per hour over the course of 60 days, suggesting that he may safely remain at CPAP 13 cm of water. Since the last intervention, he had not experienced aerophagia but was having difficulty with mask fit or waking with a severely dry mouth. The simple chin strap he received did not stay in place, and his insurance would not cover a new one for 6 months. Despite Mr. Green's initial motivation and positive outlook, he was becoming progressively pessimistic about his ability to ever tolerate CPAP therapy. In fact, he admitted that he now developed anxiety over the course of the evening in anticipation of putting his CPAP on, which he knows will inevitably lead to discomfort and more interrupted sleep.

The physician expressed her concern with Mr. Green that if he cannot use CPAP for 4 or more hours for over 70% of the remaining 30 nights in his initial 3-month compliance-monitoring period, his insurance would terminate coverage for his CPAP therapy. Because time was limited, the physician recommended a PAP-Nap in order to comprehensively address his physical intolerances and to work on behavioral techniques to address his new anxiety toward therapy. The appointment was urgently scheduled for the next day and would last 3–4 hours.

During the procedure, Mr. Green was able to try on 12 different mask interfaces while lying in bed, as well as 3 different models of chin straps. The respiratory therapist coached him on relaxation techniques and mental imagery to distract from the mask and pressure discomfort. Mr. Green reported sleeping with two "more comfortable" models of nasal masks, along with a more secure chin strap, and leak levels were excellent according to the monitored data. No oral leak was observed, and he denied dry mouth upon awakening. At termination of the study, the patient reported renewed confidence in his ability to tolerate and benefit from therapy. He did not mind paying out of pocket for a new chin strap, given this opportunity to "really try out" the product and to observe his success with it before spending his money. Mr. Green went on to increase his home adherence to CPAP use, above the required threshold, for the remainder of his compliance period.

Discussion

Positive airway pressure non-compliance has been classified into three major categories: (i) psychological factors (especially motivation, claustrophobia, and anxiety); (ii) tolerance problems (such as oronasal dryness, skin breakdown, leak, pressure insensitivity and other side effects of therapy in addition to bed partner intolerance); and (iii) education or follow-up support (or lack thereof) (Table 19.1).[1] Some patients refuse PAP therapy because of its "unattractiveness" in the intimate bedroom environment. Technologic advancements in PAP modalities, mask interfaces, accessories, and pharmaceutic interventions, such as intranasal steroids for nasal congestion or ipratropium bromide for CPAP-induced rhinorrhea, can reduce the side effects of therapy. Behavioral interventions and PAP-Naps can help alleviate psychological factors. As predictors of non-compliance remain elusive, intensive education prior to the start of therapy and close follow-up with early intervention for complications, especially within the first month of therapy initiation, are the keys to success.[2]

A PAP-Nap is an abbreviated cardiorespiratory daytime sleep study to acclimate patients with sleep-disordered breathing to PAP therapy (Table 19.2). Patients prepare for this daytime testing by limiting their sleep the night before and avoiding caffeine and

Table 19.1 Characterizing intolerance and non-adherence to positive airway pressure therapy

Cognitive/behavioral	Tolerance		Psychological
	Equipment	Pressure	
Little understanding of, or belief in the diagnosis (± symptomatic)	Mask leak (sizing, facial structure, wrinkles, beard)	Pressure sensitivity	Motivation
Poor understanding of goals for positive airway pressure therapy	Mask model	Unable to fall asleep due to difficulty breathing with pressure	Claustrophobia
Social obstacles	Headgear	Waking up feeling pressure is too great and removing mask	Anxiety
Excessive confidence in alternative therapies	Mask pain/pressure	Utilizing ramp	Insomnia
	Rash	Aerophagia	
	Nasal/oral dryness		
	Chin strap		
	Tubing		

Table 19.2 The PAP-Nap procedure – abbreviated and amended

1. Introduction of PAP therapy and barrier assessment. This may include:
   - Introduce/review of PAP features patient-adjustable for comfort
     - Ramp
     - Expiratory pressure relief
     - Humidity
   - Comprehensive mask fitting/desensitization
   - Chin strap fitting, if applicable
   - Introduction to CPAP accessories, if applicable
     - Mask liners
     - Padding at the bridge of the nose
     - Differing methods of delivering humidification
   - Pressure desensitization, including a trial of Bi-PAP if the patient has difficulty tolerating CPAP or their previously prescribed CPAP setting
   - Assess and address emotions toward PAP therapy, feelings surrounding PAP use, anxiety
   - Practice mental imagery as a distraction and desensitization technique
2. PAP therapy hook-up with a limited 10-channel montage that monitors physiologic cardiorespiratory parameters, mask leak, and video of the patient and body position
3. PAP therapy testing for 60–120 minutes spent in bed with mask(s) in place and pressure applied. The goal is to help your patient adapt to the PAP therapy sensation via exposure
4. Post-test follow-up. Review

Reproduced with permission from Krakow B, Ulibarri V, Melendrez D, et al.[3]

Bi-PAP, bi-level positive airway pressure; CPAP, continuous positive airway pressure; PAP, positive airway pressure.

naps. However, sleep is not monitored during a PAP-Nap, as this procedure is focused on tolerance and not the efficacy of a PAP setting. Success is measured by the patient's subjective ability to fall asleep while PAP is used, or the patient's ability to tolerate PAP use despite not falling asleep.[3]

PAP-Naps were originally developed for use **prior** to a CPAP titration in patients with psychosocial characteristics that may inhibit them from trying CPAP or predict poor adherence. An article by Krakow et al.[3], who developed the PAP-Nap, demonstrated utilization of these daytime studies to systematically address anxiety or negative preconceptions towards PAP therapy prior to the PAP titration. This tool may also be useful for patients who have previously "failed CPAP," and further research on PAP-Naps is warranted because the serious health consequences of untreated sleep apnea are now widely recognized.

Mr. Green held positive preconceived notions about CPAP therapy, and he lacked concerning psychosocial characteristics. However, after beginning CPAP therapy, Mr. Green experienced common difficulties in tolerance that required hands-on intervention. As may often be the reality, time had quickly passed due to appointment availability at both the DME supplier and physician's office. As the insurance landscape changes dramatically for sleep medicine, DME supplier and physician availability may present a continued challenge. The above case reviews how a PAP-Nap may be useful, in such an environment, to expedite improvement in CPAP tolerance and adherence.

Finally, in patients without complicated comorbidities, some insurance companies across the United States now require the initial use at home of automatically adjusting CPAP (auto-PAP), and its failure, prior to coverage for any sleep laboratory-based, technician-assisted night with CPAP therapy. Such patients do not sleep with CPAP until they are alone, in their home. A study performed through the Veterans Affairs hospital investigated the initiation of auto-PAP outside of the sleep laboratory environment versus traditional in-laboratory titration. Patients who underwent an attended CPAP titration in the laboratory, with the support and education provided by sleep technologists throughout their first night of CPAP, were shown to use CPAP significantly longer and on more nights than those patients whose first exposure to CPAP use was in the home.[4]

When access to an in-laboratory CPAP study is limited in patients without significant comorbidities and without inhibitory psychosocial characteristics, a PAP-Nap may still be useful to promote early adherence to therapy by initial exposure to PAP in a supportive environment prior to overnight home use. Further study will be needed to compare the costs versus gains, both monetary and psychologic, of PAP-Naps in multiple different clinical scenarios.

Main points

Adherence to PAP is critical to successful treatment for obstructive sleep apnea, but establishment of good adherence can be a major challenge, for many reasons that include cognitive preconceptions, maladaptive behavior, difficulty with equipment, and reactions to applied pressure. Particularly in an era when overnight laboratory-based titration studies may not be covered by some medical insurance policies, a daytime PAP-Nap procedure may offer an opportunity, before PAP is used at home, to allay anxiety or proactively reduce chances for subsequent problems. For some patients who have already tried PAP at home, and had difficulties, a PAP-Nap study may offer a cost-effective approach, short of a laboratory-based titration study, to troubleshoot, to

monitor how a patient uses PAP, and to leave a patient more confident that home use can be successful.

REFERENCES

1. Zozulu R, Rosen R. Compliance with continuous positive airway pressure therapy: assessing and improving treatment outcomes. *Curr Opin Pulm Med* 2001;**7**:391–8.
2. Chervin RD, Theut S, Basetti C, Aldrich M. Compliance with nasal CPAP can be improved by simple interventions. *Sleep* 1997;**20**:284–9.
3. Krakow B, Ulibarri V, Melendrez D, et al. A daytime, abbreviated cardio-respiratory sleep study (CPT 95807–52) to acclimate insomnia patients with sleep disordered breathing to positive airway pressure (PAP-Nap). *J Clin Sleep Med* 2008;**4**:212–22.
4. Means MK, Edinger JD, Husain AM. CPAP compliance in sleep apnea patients with and without laboratory CPAP titration. *Sleep Breath* 2004;**8**:7–14.

20

Excessive positive airway pressure can create treatment-emergent central sleep apnea (complex sleep apnea)

Helena M. Schotland

A positive airway pressure (PAP) therapy titration polysomnogram is performed to determine the optimal pressure setting to treat an individual's obstructive sleep apnea (OSA). An optimal PAP setting effectively treats the patient's OSA in all positions and stages of sleep. In most cases, apneas, hypopneas, airflow limitation, and snoring decrease as the PAP pressure is raised. In some patients, higher PAP pressures may actually lead to the development of central apneic events – a condition known alternatively as treatment-emergent sleep apnea or complex sleep apnea. For these select patients, in the words of modernist architect Ludwig Mies van der Rohe, "Less is more." The purpose of this chapter is to review several cases in which excessive PAP may induce central sleep apnea, discuss the proposed mechanisms for this process, and present some strategies for minimizing PAP overtitration.

Case 1

A 44-year-old Caucasian woman with a history of paroxysmal atrial fibrillation and snoring presented to the sleep clinic for evaluation. A baseline polysomnogram revealed severe OSA with an apnea/hypopnea index (AHI, events per hour of sleep) of 32 and an oximetry nadir of 86%. The patient returned to the sleep laboratory for a continuous positive airway pressure (CPAP) titration study. Continuous positive airway pressure was initiated at a pressure setting of 5 cm of water.

Hypopneas and snoring persisted until a CPAP setting of 9 cm was reached. With further increases in CPAP pressure, central apneas emerged and became more prominent as pressures were raised further to a maximum pressure setting of 12 cm of water. The patient was subsequently started on CPAP at 9 cm of water at home and returned to clinic 4 weeks later for follow-up. Download of the patient's CPAP data card revealed an average daily use time of 6 hours and 32 minutes per night, no significant mask leak, and an estimated residual AHI of 0 events per hour.

Discussion

This case demonstrates the development of central apneas as CPAP pressure is raised. In this particular patient, a CPAP pressure of 9 cm of water was effective in treating the patient's sleep apnea. Higher pressure settings did not confer any additional benefit and were, in fact, only problematic. It has been hypothesized that higher CPAP pressure settings may activate pulmonary parenchymal stretch receptors, thus triggering the Hering–Breuer reflex, inhibiting medullary respiratory motor output and causing central apneas.

Case 2

A 62-year-old man presented to clinic with a longstanding history of OSA and CPAP intolerance. The patient was diagnosed with OSA 10 years prior. He

Common Pitfalls in Sleep Medicine, ed. Ronald D. Chervin. Published by Cambridge University Press. © Cambridge University Press 2014.

had had a baseline polysomnogram that revealed an AHI of 22 events per hour of sleep with an oximetry nadir of 88%. A CPAP titration study was performed which demonstrated an optimal pressure setting of 5 cm of water. The patient was unable to tolerate CPAP at that time. He complained that the CPAP machine was noisy and the pressure setting felt "too high." Over the ensuing 10 years, the patient had a 40-pound (18 kg) weight gain and began falling asleep at the wheel of a car while stopped at traffic lights. A repeat baseline polysomnogram now showed an AHI of 46 events per hour of sleep, with an oximetry nadir of 82%. The patient returned to the sleep laboratory for a CPAP titration study. Continuous positive airway pressure was initiated with his prior setting of 5 cm of water and was rapidly titrated upwards to 12 cm of water to eliminate obstructive events, airflow limitation, and snoring. With rapidly increasing CPAP pressures, the patient developed worsening sleep fragmentation and began having central apneic events. A prolonged period of wakefulness occurred in the middle of the study during which the patient felt that the CPAP pressure setting of 12 cm of water was simply "too high" for him and he was not able to fall back to sleep. The CPAP pressure was then reduced to 5 cm for patient comfort, which allowed the patient to fall asleep once more. Once asleep, the CPAP pressure was slowly titrated from 5 cm of water to an optimal setting of 9 cm of water, which was tested in supine rapid eye movement (REM) sleep. On this optimal setting, obstructive apneas and hypopneas were eliminated and no central apneas emerged.

Discussion

In this patient, the rapid titration of CPAP therapy during the initial portion of the polysomnogram led to the development of sleep fragmentation with frequent sleep–wake transitions. Transient central apneas are commonly observed during transitional sleep; this mechanism probably triggered the central apneic events in this patient. A less aggressive CPAP titration during the second half of the study enabled this patient to achieve consolidated sleep with excellent control of his OSA and without the emergence of central events.

Of note, the optimal CPAP setting of 9 cm of water determined during the second half of the study is significantly lower than the pressure setting of 12 cm of water that was used during the first half of the night – an important observation for a patient who has experienced CPAP pressure intolerance.

Case 3

A 39-year-old male truck driver presented to clinic with complaints of loud snoring and witnessed apneas. He denied daytime sleepiness. Physical examination was notable for obesity and markedly enlarged tonsils that significantly occluded the hypopharynx. The patient then underwent a split-night polysomnogram. During the baseline portion of the study, only sleep stages N1 and N2 were observed, with profound sleep fragmentation. There were frank obstructive apneas and hypopneas (AHI of 77 events per hour of sleep) with an oxygen saturation nadir of 70%, consistent with severe OSA. Continuous positive airway pressure was then initiated at a pressure setting of 4 cm of water. With increasing CPAP pressure settings to 12 cm of water, the number of obstructive apneas decreased, but obstructive hypopneas persisted. As the CPAP pressure was raised to 19 cm of water, the number of obstructive hypopneas decreased and central apneas began to emerge. Persistent mask leak was noted on these high CPAP settings. Efforts to reduce the leak included changing the patient to bi-level positive airway pressure (Bi-PAP) with inspiratory PAP of 22–23 cm of water and expiratory PAP pressure settings of 17–18 cm of water. Mask leak decreased significantly. On an optimal Bi-PAP setting of 22/18 cm of water, the patient no longer had obstructive events and his central apneas resolved. Sleep was consolidated on this optimal pressure setting, REM sleep was achieved, and no significant oxygen desaturations were noted.

Discussion

When mask leak occurs with PAP therapy, there is increased washout of carbon dioxide in the proximal anatomic dead space. This decreases the partial pressure of carbon dioxide in the air being inspired by the patient, and can lead to the development of central apneas. This process can also occur in the setting of mouth breathing while a patient is wearing a nasal interface during PAP titration. During this split-night study, the sleep technologist recognized the development of mask leak with increasing pressures and made efforts to reduce the leak, including a change to Bi-PAP therapy. These efforts appeared to eliminate the mask leak with subsequent resolution of the central apneas and effective treatment of the underlying obstructive events.

A change to Bi-PAP, by itself, does not always eliminate or reduce leaks. The transitions from lower to higher pressures with the initiation of each inspiration may at times augment leaks. However, some patients have mouth leak mainly during expiration. In those instances, transition to Bi-PAP settings that permit lower expiratory PAP – lower than the CPAP setting that was problematic – may reduce mouth leaks.

Case 4

A 58-year-old woman presented to the sleep disorders clinic with a 1-year history of snoring and witnessed apneas in the setting of a 30-pound weight gain following a knee injury. Baseline polysomnography revealed severe OSA, with an AHI of 62 events per hour of sleep with an oxygen saturation nadir of 80%. The patient returned to the sleep laboratory for a CPAP titration study that tested pressure settings of 4–16 cm of water. Obstructive events decreased modestly in frequency, but still persisted on higher CPAP settings. Additionally, central apneas that had not been prominent on the baseline polysomnogram emerged at 8 cm of water and increased in frequency as the CPAP was raised further. During the CPAP titration, a total of 240 sleep-disordered breathing events were scored, including 39 obstructive apneas, 61 hypopneas, 8 mixed apneas, and 132 central apneas. Given the large proportion of central apneas – 55% of all events scored – during the CPAP titration study, the patient was asked to return to the sleep laboratory for titration with adaptive servoventilation. Obstructive events as well as central apneas were eliminated on the following adaptive servoventilation settings: maximum pressure 25 cm of water, maximum expiratory PAP 15 cm of water, minimum expiratory PAP 6 cm of water, maximum pressure support 15 cm of water, minimum pressure support 0 cm of water, auto back-up rate, and a rise time of 3 (0.3 seconds). The patient started to use adaptive servoventilation at home and, shortly thereafter, reported complete resolution of her clinical symptoms.

Discussion

This patient had particularly severe OSA, and then treatment-emergent sleep apnea, often referred to as complex sleep apnea, when CPAP was applied. A similar phenomenon can also occur after patients with OSA, particularly when severe, are treated by surgical means. In many patients, during PAP titration studies, use of pressure settings that are higher than necessary will elicit central sleep apnea in a patient who only had OSA at baseline. Use of a lower PAP setting, in such cases, will still offer complete control of the OSA without causing central sleep apnea (as in Case 1, above). However, for some patients, the threshold at which PAP engenders central sleep apnea is lower than the setting needed to resolve OSA. The possibility exists that for some patients continued use of PAP over time, at home, would result in gradual resolution of the central sleep apnea as mechanisms that regulate breathing adapt to the new reality of an unobstructed upper airway each night. However, for other patients the treatment-emergent sleep apnea may not resolve with time. In clinical practice, most sleep specialists seek to treat treatment-emergent sleep apnea, or complex sleep apnea as definitively as possible from the start of home therapy.

Common approaches to treatment of complex sleep apnea include addition of supplemental oxygen to CPAP, adaptive servoventilation, and sometimes Bi-PAP therapy in a spontaneous timed mode. Supplemental oxygen is thought to stabilize the respiratory drive by decreasing the responsiveness of peripheral chemoreceptors. Oxygen supplementation does not treat the underlying tendency for the upper airway to obstruct, and therefore should only be used in conjunction with PAP. In this patient, obstructive apneic events were still seen on higher CPAP pressure settings even after central apneas had emerged; the addition of supplemental oxygen to the CPAP may have ameliorated the central apneas but would not have resolved the remaining OSA. Adaptive servoventilation provides Bi-PAP while analyzing minute ventilation to automatically adjust pressure support throughout the night. This device also has the capability of offering a back-up rate. The algorithm aims to provide more or less ventilatory support (discrepancy between inspiratory and expiratory PAP) when the patient needs it, and overall to avoid the hyperventilation that probably triggers the central sleep apnea when CPAP or regular Bi-PAP is used. In this patient, adaptive servoventilation was first shown to be a highly effective therapy in the sleep laboratory, and the patient then had an excellent clinical response to its use. Bi-PAP ST treats underlying airway obstruction and also provides a back-up respiratory rate for those patients with an impaired respiratory drive. It may be used in patients with complex sleep apnea, though usually after oxygen and ASV have been tried first, as these approaches appear to have more support in published literature on treatment of central sleep apnea.

Main points

Overzealous titration of CPAP, challenges such as mask leaks, and sometimes nothing more than adequate PAP to maintain upper airway patency may result in the development of a form of central sleep apnea called treatment-emergent sleep apnea, or complex sleep apnea, through a number of proposed mechanisms. Strategies to avoid such outcomes include moderation in application of high PAP settings, control of excessive leaks, or use of supplemental oxygen, adaptive servoventilation, or bi-level PAP with a spontaneously triggered back-up rate (spontaneous timed mode). In an era in which costs of assessment and treatment for OSA have increased commensurately with growing realization of the high prevalence of this consequential medical condition, some insurers now limit coverage to automatically adjusting CPAP that is not tested first in a sleep laboratory. The cases in this section illustrate potential pitfalls, with regard to iatrogenic effects of PAP, that could become important for physicians to understand as their patients increasingly use PAP without initial testing under observed conditions in a sleep laboratory.

FURTHER READING

Hoffman M, Schulman DA. The appearance of central sleep apnea after treatment of obstructive sleep apnea. *Chest* 2012;**142**:517–22.

Javaheri S, Smith J, Chung E. The prevalence and natural history of complex sleep apnea. *J Clin Sleep Med* 2009;**5**:205–11.

Malhotra A, Bertisch S, Wellman A. Complex sleep apnea: it isn't really a disease. *J Clin Sleep Med* 2008;**4**:406–8.

21

Appropriate use of automatically adjusting positive airway pressure can enable a patient to use positive airway pressure therapy

Helena M. Schotland

Continuous positive airway pressure (CPAP) therapy for obstructive sleep apnea (OSA) was first described by Colin Sullivan in 1981. This device revolutionized care for patients with this condition, which previously had been treated by weight loss or tracheostomy. Over the years, CPAP has evolved with the development of smaller and quieter machines, the addition of heated humidification, and the development of bi-level therapy, among other advancements. By 1994, a self-setting CPAP machine was being used to deliver variable CPAP pressures to patients with OSA. The development of algorithms analyzing airflow continuously, in real-time, allowed CPAP pressures to be adjusted at home over the course of a night. The use of automatically adjusting positive airway pressure (auto-PAP) therapy has become more popular over the past decade, but not all practitioners of sleep medicine are comfortable with the use of this technology. The purpose of this chapter is to illustrate some of the ways in which auto-PAP can enable a patient to use PAP therapy effectively.

Case 1

A 45-year-old man with a history of hypertension and paroxysmal atrial fibrillation (requiring multiple attempts at cardioversion and catheter ablation) presented with a long history of heroic snoring, witnessed apneas, and daytime fatigue. The patient's Epworth Sleepiness Scale score was evaluated at 15 out of 24

points. A baseline laboratory-based polysomnogram revealed severe OSA, with an apnea/hypopnea index (AHI, events per hour of sleep) of 33 events and an oximetry nadir of 82%. He returned to the sleep laboratory for a CPAP titration study that tested pressures of 4–12 cm of water. On all settings tested, including CPAP at 12 cm of water, the patient had continued hypopneas and airflow limitation. The patient was not interested in returning to the sleep laboratory for a repeat CPAP titration study.

What next?

The patient was started on an auto-titrating CPAP machine with a pressure range of 12–20 cm of water. He returned 4 weeks later, feeling much more refreshed upon awakening. His wife no longer noted snoring or witnessed apneas. A download of the patient's CPAP data card revealed an average daily use time of 7 hours and 30 minutes, an average time with large mask leak per day of only 1 minute, and an estimated residual AHI of 0.2 events per hour.

Take home point: auto-PAP may be an option for patients with an incomplete PAP titration study

During a CPAP titration study, a variety of pressures are tested with the ultimate goal of eliminating sleep-disordered breathing and snoring. An optimal CPAP titration study determines a pressure setting that can

Common Pitfalls in Sleep Medicine, ed. Ronald D. Chervin. Published by Cambridge University Press. © Cambridge University Press 2014.

be used to treat the patient in all positions and stages of sleep, including supine rapid eye movement (REM) sleep, which is often the most vulnerable to obstructive sleep-disordered breathing. However, the best laid plans sometimes go awry and an optimal setting is not able to be determined in the course of a single night. Reasons for difficult or incomplete titration studies include poor sleep efficiency, a delay in or lack of REM sleep periods, and a limited amount of supine sleep, among other variables. A repeat CPAP titration study is sometimes performed, but some patients are unwilling or unable to undergo a repeat CPAP titration study. As in the case report above, auto-PAP can be used effectively for some such patients who have an incomplete CPAP titration, regardless of the reason.

Case 2

A 58-year-old woman with a history of migraine headaches and hypothyroidism presented to the sleep clinic with complaints of excessive daytime sleepiness and witnessed apneas. Her Epworth Sleepiness Scale score was 19 out of a possible 24 points. A baseline polysomnogram revealed severe OSA with an AHI of 50 events per hour of sleep, and an oximetry nadir of 79%. The patient returned to the sleep laboratory for a CPAP titration study, which tested pressure settings of 4–15 cm of water. She did best on a CPAP setting of 15 cm of water, which eliminated all sleep-disordered breathing events (including those in supine-REM sleep). The patient felt more refreshed on the morning after her CPAP titration and she was very excited to start on CPAP therapy. Continuous positive airway pressure at a pressure setting of 15 cm of water was initiated at home.

Two weeks later, the patient called the clinic with complaints that her stomach was painful and bloated every morning after using CPAP. She was "embarrassed by all the belching." The patient usually slept supine and used one pillow for sleep. The patient was advised to sleep in the lateral position with two pillows to see if her aerophagia improved. One week later, the patient called back and stated her aerophagia was no better. She was very disappointed in CPAP and was ready to discontinue therapy.

What next?

The patient was started on an auto-titrating CPAP with a pressure range of 8–15 cm of water. Several weeks later, she returned to the sleep clinic for a routine follow-up visit. The patient felt markedly improved and no longer complained of excessive daytime sleepiness. Her Epworth Sleepiness Scale score was now only 6 out of a possible 24 points (where scores of 9 or less are usually considered normal). She reported that her aerophagia had resolved with the change to the auto-titrating CPAP machine from the fixed pressure CPAP. A download of the patient's CPAP data card revealed an average daily use time of 7 hours per night, no significant mask leak, and an estimated residual AHI of 0.5 events per hour. Her mean CPAP pressure on the data download – the average over time of the pressures that the machine had supplied to her mask – was 11.0 cm of water.

Take home point: auto-PAP can be useful for patients who develop aerophagia on fixed pressure CPAP therapy

Aerophagia is a notoriously troublesome side effect of CPAP therapy resulting in eructation, abdominal pain, bloating, and flatulence. Aerophagia can be so severe and bothersome that some patients are unable to utilize CPAP therapy. A change in sleep position may alleviate symptoms of aerophagia, but is not always effective. As we have discussed above, an optimal CPAP setting is titrated to treat the patient's OSA in the worst possible case scenario. A CPAP setting that is required for a patient in supine REM sleep may be more pressure than what is required in non-supine, non-REM sleep. The higher the CPAP setting, the greater the likelihood of aerophagia. Use of auto-PAP allows the patient to receive, ideally, the lowest possible pressure setting in any given situation, leading to a lower mean CPAP pressure and, in many cases, reduced aerophagia.

Case 3

A 26-year-old morbidly obese male presented to the sleep clinic with the complaint of loud snoring that was disruptive to other members of his household. The patient denied daytime sleepiness. Baseline polysomnography demonstrated severe OSA with an AHI of 65 events per hour and an oximetry nadir of 76%. A CPAP titration study was performed and the patient was titrated to an optimal pressure setting of 19 cm of water. Continuous positive airway pressure therapy was then initiated at home.

Four weeks later, the patient returned for a follow-up visit. He complained that his CPAP machine was waking him up at night. He felt the pressure setting was simply "too high" for him. He was unable to fall back to sleep until he took off his CPAP mask. A download of the data from the patient's CPAP machine revealed an average daily use time of only 55 minutes. His roommates were now asking him to move out since his snoring was as disruptive as ever and the patient was unable to tolerate CPAP therapy.

What next?

The patient was started on an auto-titrating CPAP machine with a pressure range of 10–20 cm of water. He called the sleep clinic 2 weeks later to express his thanks. The patient was now able to sleep through the night using his auto-titrating CPAP machine. He was no longer snoring and his roommates were no longer complaining. Subsequent download of the patient's data card showed an average daily use time of 7 hours and 15 minutes per night, a mean pressure of 14 cm of water, a maximum pressure of 18 cm of water, and a residual estimated AHI of 3 events per hour.

Take home point: auto-PAP may be a helpful option when a patient is intolerant of high fixed CPAP settings

Patients can complain of pressure intolerance when they are started on relatively high CPAP settings. This is seen most commonly in those who are new to CPAP therapy. Use of the ramp feature on the CPAP machine can alleviate this problem for those patients with

sleep-onset insomnia due to CPAP, but does not help patients with sleep maintenance insomnia related to pressure intolerance. The optimal CPAP setting determined during a CPAP titration study treats the patient in the worst possible clinical scenario. However, a sleep apnea patient may not require an elevated pressure setting at all times. Higher CPAP settings may result in sleep fragmentation, nocturnal awakenings, or increased mask or mouth leaks. Auto-PAP algorithms seek to deliver the pressure setting that is required at the time, and not more than is actually needed, which may decrease the number of nocturnal awakenings secondary to pressure intolerance.

If all sleep specialists were convinced that auto-PAP worked perfectly, no need would remain for laboratory-based PAP titration studies or use of fixed PAP settings at home. However, use of a sleep laboratory to assess effectiveness of auto-PAP, when applied for the first time, is often a useful study in place of a standard PAP titration when need for auto-PAP is anticipated. In this author's experience, this night of monitoring on auto-PAP often reveals that auto-PAP does not perform quite as well as fixed pressure determined through a standard titration study. This may be because any auto-PAP algorithm must periodically test lower pressure settings, in order to determine when a decreased pressure may be sufficient. Testing lower settings permits a limited number of hypopneas or episodes of flow limitation to appear. The residual amount of untreated apnea may be small and inconsequential for many patients, or enough to cause concern for some.

Case 4

A 67-year-old woman with a history of diabetes mellitus presented to the sleep clinic with many years of snoring and nocturnal gasping. She also reported daytime sleepiness and had an Epworth Sleepiness Scale score of 14 out of a possible 24 points. A baseline polysomnogram demonstrated moderate OSA with an AHI of 28 events per hour of sleep, and an oximetry nadir of 87%. A subsequent CPAP titration revealed an optimal pressure setting of 10 cm of water, which was tested in supine REM sleep. The patient subsequently started home use of CPAP at 10 cm of water.

The patient returned for her follow-up visit 3 weeks later. She reported that she still had occasional snoring. She felt slightly more refreshed upon awakening, but still required naps every afternoon. Her Epworth Sleepiness Scale score was now 11. A download of the patient's CPAP data card revealed an average daily use time of 8 hours and 10 minutes, with no significant mask leak. The estimated residual AHI was 11 events per hour. The patient did not wish to undergo a repeat CPAP titration study in the sleep laboratory.

What next?

The patient's fixed CPAP was changed to an auto-titrating CPAP machine with pressure settings ranging from 10 to 16 cm of water. She returned to the clinic 4 weeks later and stated she was feeling markedly more refreshed. Her Epworth Sleepiness Scale score was now 6. She no longer needed to nap in the afternoons. A download of the auto-PAP data card revealed an average daily use time of 8 hours and 3 minutes with no significant mask leak. Her estimated residual AHI was now 1.2 events per hour.

Take home point: auto-PAP may be a helpful option when a patient continues to have an increased machine-estimated residual AHI while on fixed-pressure CPAP therapy

A CPAP titration study is conducted over the course of a single night's sleep. In the case of a split night polysomnogram, the titration portion may be conducted over just a few hours. The optimal pressure setting determined is most relevant to the patient's OSA on that particular night. Night-to-night variability of OSA may render a laboratory-determined, optimal CPAP setting suboptimal on another night. An auto-PAP may be especially useful in this setting, particularly when the patient does not accept the more standard approach, which would be to undergo an in-laboratory CPAP retitration study.

Main point

Auto-PAP can play an important role in a variety of scenarios that arise when treating patients with OSA. Auto-PAP has some limitations, but in certain circumstances can provide an alternative to repeat titration studies, or improve CPAP compliance.

FURTHER READING

Berry RB, Parish JM, Hartse KM. The use of auto-titrating continuous positive airway pressure for treatment of adult obstructive sleep apnea. An American Academy of Sleep Medicine review. *Sleep* 2002;**25**:148–73.

Hukins C. Comparative study of autotitrating and fixed-pressure CPAP in the home: a randomized, single-blind crossover trial. *Sleep* 2004;**27**:1512–17.

Ip S, D'Ambrosio C, Patel K, et al. Auto-titrating versus fixed continuous positive airway pressure for the treatment of obstructive sleep apnea: a systematic review with meta-analyses. *Syst Rev* 2012;**1**:20

Krieger J. Therapeutic use of auto-CPAP. *Sleep Med Rev* 1999;**3**:159–74.

Nolan GM, Doherty LS, McNicholas WT. Auto-adjusting versus fixed positive pressure therapy in mild to moderate obstructive sleep apnoea. *Sleep* 2007;**30**:189–94.

Alternatives to positive airway pressure in the treatment of obstructive sleep apnea

Despite all the advances that have been made in positive airway pressure technology and methods to improve adherence, a significant minority of the large numbers of patients with obstructive sleep apnea still do not tolerate use of the machine and mask interface on a nightly basis. Others simply refuse to use it, or to even try it initially. Fortunately, such patients can often be treated through other methods.

As illustrated in this section, some of the most common alternatives to continuous positive airway pressure (CPAP) include surgical procedures and the use of oral appliances during sleep. Surgical interventions such as uvulopalatopharyngoplasty or maxillary and mandibular advancement offer the potential for a "cure" with no remaining need for nightly CPAP. However, these therapeutic options also carry risks without being able to guarantee success in all cases. Oral appliances fabricated by dental sleep medicine specialists are often effective and easier to use than CPAP, but again do not work for every patient.

Other options also exist. Substantial weight loss in a patient who is overweight or obese is difficult to achieve and maintain. Successful weight loss almost always improves obstructive sleep apnea, but less often eliminates the condition completely. For these reasons, weight loss is frequently recommended, but rarely relied upon as the sole approach to treat obstructive sleep apnea. Some medications, such as tricyclic antidepressants and selective serotonin reuptake inhibitors, may increase tone of the genioglossus muscle and show mild tendency to reduce obstructive sleep apnea. Behavioral intervention can include avoidance of supine sleep, which tends to elicit the worst sleep apnea, and avoidance of evening alcohol, which can exacerbate sleep-disordered breathing. In most instances, however, these types of approaches are used in an adjunctive rather than primary manner, except when treatment by CPAP, surgery, or oral appliances are each completely ineffective or unsuitable for a given patient.

The following cases provide examples of primary approaches taken for specific patients when CPAP is not an option to treat obstructive sleep apnea. One recurring theme is that a multidisciplinary strategy is often necessary. Since 1999, the University of Michigan Sleep Disorders Center has maintained a unique Multidisciplinary Alternatives to CPAP Clinic. On a single afternoon visit, patients have extensive evaluations by multiple services, along with any necessary assessment procedures. A conference at the end of the day allows clinicians from each service to combine their findings and opinions, and formulate consensus recommendations for each patient. This program has been highly successful, and although it still may be unique in the United States, it illustrates what can be accomplished in other locations when specialists with complementary knowledge and understanding of sleep and the upper airway combine their skills to address the needs of some of the most challenging sleep apnea patients.

22

Some patients with sleep apnea who are intolerant to continuous positive airway pressure can be treated most effectively with a mandibular advancement device

Emerson Robinson

Introduction

The author practices, in part, as a member of a Multi-disciplinary Alternatives to CPAP Clinic at a major university hospital. This clinic can refer patients who are unable to tolerate continuous positive airway pressure (CPAP) therapy to the School of Dentistry for treatment with an oral appliance. Before patients are referred, they go through extensive evaluations by a team of clinicians composed of a neurologist, otolaryngologist, oral-maxillofacial surgeon, and a dentist who specializes in dental sleep medicine.

After all the patients are seen in the Alternatives Clinic on a given day, this group of clinicians meet to determine how to advise the patients with regard to treatment options. The young man described below was reluctant to continue using CPAP because he was claustrophobic and had problems associated with wearing different masks. He was referred by the Alternatives to CPAP team to the School of Dentistry for treatment of his OSA with oral appliance therapy.

Case history/diagnosis

This patient, a 27-year-old man, presented to the Multidisciplinary Alternatives to CPAP Clinic seeking an alternative to his use of CPAP. The patient had a several-year history of significant snoring, excessive daytime sleepiness, as well as witnessed apneic episodes. He most often woke up not feeling refreshed.

When he used CPAP, he stated that it felt like it was not doing any good. Upon awakening in the morning he still felt tired and unrefreshed. The patient wore a bite splint for bruxism. His prior medical history was significant for anxiety, depression, asthma, and hay fever.

He presented at 5 feet, 7 inches (170 cm) tall, weighing 152 pounds (69 kg) with a calculated body mass index of 24 kg/m^2, and a neck circumference of 15 inches (38 cm). He presented with an intact dentition and a Class I molar occlusion bilaterally. He had an inter-incisal distance of 46 mm, an overbite of 2 mm, and an overjet of 2 mm. The hard palate was narrow and mildly elevated. He had no complaints regarding teeth, muscles, or joints. He showed a maximum protrusive range of 12 mm.

An intranasal exam showed that his nasal passages were patent except for a deviated nasal septum to the right. The tonsils had not been surgically removed and were a plus-1 in size. The soft palate and uvula were not elongated. The patient had a Friedman Class I airway. Flexible fiber optic laryngoscopy showed mild baseline narrowing at the level of the palate with quiet expiration and moderate (< 75%) closure with forced inspiration. At the retrolingual level, there was moderate baseline narrowing and severe (> 75%) reduction in the area with forced inspiration.

Cephalometric radiography showed a Sella Nasion Subspinale (SNA) of 84 degrees and a Sella Nasion Supramentale (SNB) of 77 degrees, advancing to 80 degrees with protrusion. The posterior airway space was 2 mm (normal is 11 mm) and this increased

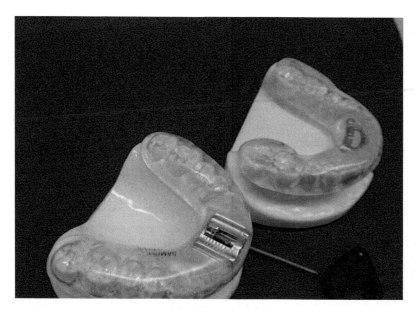

Figure 22.1 Thornton Adjustable Positioner appliance.

to 4 mm with mandibular protrusion. The palatal length was 36 mm (normal is 35 mm) and the hyoid-to-mandibular plane distance was 26 mm (normal is 15 mm) with a decrease to 21 mm on mandibular protrusion.

A diagnostic nocturnal polysomnogram was performed in a sleep laboratory. It showed obstructive sleep apnea (OSA) with a respiratory disturbance index of 27 apneic events per hour of sleep and a minimum oxygen desaturation to 81%. The baseline polysomnogram was interpreted as showing OSA, predominantly in the form of hypopneas and worse in the supine position.

A CPAP titration study was performed in the sleep laboratory. This study showed that the OSA was well treated at 8 cm of water. The patient had now been using the CPAP machine regularly but did miss a few days intermittently. Although he noted significant improvement in his daytime sleepiness while using CPAP, he indicated that he felt claustrophobic with the mask on his face. He tried both a standard nasal mask interface and nasal pillows, but neither was helpful in preventing his feeling of claustrophobia at night.

In the Alternatives to CPAP conference following an afternoon of evaluations by the different specialists, a

consensus emerged that a reasonable alternative approach in treating this patient's OSA would be a mandibular advancement device. He was therefore referred to the School of Dentistry.

Selecting appropriate patients for oral appliance therapy is important for a good outcome. First and foremost, the patient must have a sufficient number of teeth (eight in each arch) to retain the appliance during usage. He or she must have teeth that are not compromised by periodontal disease, and must not have limited mandibular range of motion.

Treatment

After evaluation for oral appliance therapy, a custom-made Thornton Adjustable Positioner (TAP) was fabricated and placed in the patient's mouth. The TAP is an anterior mandibular positioner (Figure 22.1). The specific appliance was the TAP 3 TL, an intraoral appliance worn during sleep to manage the patient's snoring and OSA. This appliance can be an effective alternative to surgery or the use of CPAP while sleeping. This appliance keeps the airway open by holding the mandible

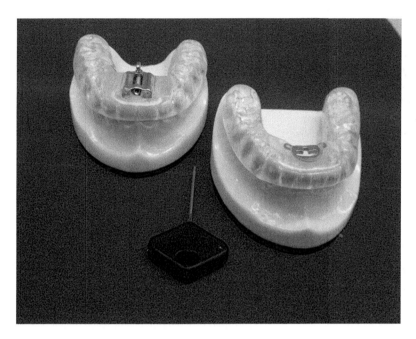

Figure 22.2 Thornton Adjustable Positioner appliance.

comfortably in a forward position, pulling the tongue anteriorly, and minimizing or eliminating snoring and obstructive apneas. The patient continues to breathe naturally and easily through the nose or mouth.

The TAP 3 TL device consists of an upper tray that fits over the upper teeth and a lower tray that fits over the lower teeth (Figure 22.2). A hook mechanism attached to the upper tray fits into a socket attached to the lower tray, which advances the lower jaw forward to prevent the soft tissue of the throat from collapsing and obstructing the airway. An adjustment key for the appliance permits the patient to modify the protrusion of the lower jaw to achieve the most effective and comfortable position. The hook moves forward and back by using the adjustment key to dial the adjustment screw clockwise or counter clockwise. Each 180-degree turn is a 0.25 mm adjustment. The maximum advancement of the hook mechanism is 8 mm.

The hook mechanism is controlled with the adjustment key by turning it counter clockwise (towards the left ear) to advance (protrude) the mandible until the

patient begins to feel discomfort in the temporomandibular joint or in the facial muscles (**maximum mechanical protrusion** or MMP). The hook is dialed back until the patient's teeth are end-to-end. This is the starting position. The patient then advances the appliance forward by two 180-degree turns, which equal 0.5 mm, every 2 days. This is continued until the snoring has stopped.

The patient described above could be passively advanced to 8 mm. The appliance was then adjusted gradually to maximize subjective therapeutic effect. **Maximum therapeutic protrusion** with the appliance in place is defined as the point when a patient stops snoring and subjective symptoms are resolved.

Self-titration was performed by the patient with incremental advancements of a half-turn (equaling 0.25 mm) every 2 days, without discomfort. At a follow-up appointment 4 weeks after he received the appliance, he reported that he had responded quickly to the oral appliance therapy. His significant other reported that he had stopped snoring and had no observed pauses in his breathing. He was aware that he was at last getting a full night's sleep. He had no difficulty getting used to the oral appliance. He did experience some temperomandibular joint discomfort at 20 half-turns (5 mm protrusion). However, he retruded his mandible back to 4 mm protrusion by adjusting the appliance back from 20 half-turns to 16 half-turns. This resolved the discomfort.

The patient was referred back to his sleep physician for retesting. He had a diagnostic polysomnogram performed with the oral appliance in place. This repeat polysomnogram showed resolution of his OSA, with an apnea/hypopnea index of 1.1 events per hour of sleep, and a minimum oxygen saturation of 91%. His sleep physician reminded him of the necessity for follow-up evaluations at 6 months, 1 year, and then at additional time points as recommended by the dentist treating him for his sleep apnea.

The patient was seen at 6 months, and again at 1 year. He indicated that he was starting to make sounds when he was sleeping – as told by his significant other. He had advanced the appliance as far as possible (8 mm). To move it further, the patient was shown how he could advance his mandible so that the upper mechanism (hook) engaged behind the lower plate to gain additional protrusion.

This procedure resolved his problem, and the patient has done very well since this time. The patient has continued to follow-up with his therapy for the last 6 years with annual reevaluations. He continues to be adequately treated with the TAP appliance, though he had advanced his device to 9 mm protrusion. During this time, his occlusion has remained stable. He has had no pain or dysfunction of his stomatognathic system.

Discussion

Oral appliance therapy for the treatment of OSA is becoming more than an occasional alternative to positive airway pressure (PAP) treatment.[1] Oral appliance therapy has been shown to be an effective treatment for mild or moderate OSA, and in some cases for severe OSA. In many cases oral appliance therapy is a first-line alternative to CPAP. The American Academy of Sleep Medicine's "Practice parameters for the treatment of snoring and OSA with oral appliances: an update for 2005," recommendation 3.3.3, states that, "Oral appliances [OAs] are indicated for use in patients with mild to moderate OSA who prefer OAs to CPAP, or who do not respond to CPAP, and are not appropriate candidates for CPAP."[2]

The author's position is that all patients should try CPAP initially, as it is the gold standard for OSA treatment and it has proven successful in maintaining a patent upper airway. Success with CPAP, when used, is a good indication that oral appliance therapy should also work by similarly opening the airway. A temporary trial of CPAP may assist, in this manner, in identification of candidates for the use of oral appliances.

The type and number (50–75) of oral appliances is extensive and still growing. Currently, there are two major groups – the mandibular advancement device (MAD) and the tongue-retaining device (TRD). The TRD is used very seldom, mainly when dental reasons preclude use of a MAD. The TRD has a bulb that uses a vacuum to hold the tongue forward. The MAD is the most common type of oral appliance used today. These devices can be fixed (protrusive distance cannot be changed) or the variable (protrusion can be increased or decreased). Each of the two types of oral appliances has a primary effect on either the tongue or the tongue and mandible together. The TRD has a direct effect on tongue posture.

In some cases oral appliance therapy may not be successful in controlling OSA. A primary adjunct to increase the success of oral appliance therapy may be uvulopalatopharyngoplasty surgery. With surgical excision of the uvula, posterior soft palate, tonsils, and redundant lateral pharyngeal tissue, significant obstructions are removed. This improves opening of the upper airway with the oral appliance in place.

Numerous studies[3] have been carried out validating the effectiveness of MADs. Ferguson et al.[4] conducted an evidence-based review of the literature on use of oral appliances in the treatment of OSA from 1995 to 2006. Some 87 articles were suitable for inclusion in their evidence-based review, which substantiated the efficacy in the treatment of OSA with oral appliances. Oral appliances are effective to varying degrees and appear to work as a result of an increase in airway space that is achieved by advancing the mandible. In contrast to CPAP adherence that can be monitored electronically, long-term compliance data for oral appliances are limited at present, and mostly based on patient report.

Most dentists who practice dental sleep medicine are not affiliated with a clinic such as the Multidisciplinary Alternatives to CPAP Clinic described above. Furthermore, some sleep physicians still do not include in their practice use of oral appliance therapy as an alternative for the treatment of sleep apnea patients. Consequently, the need still exists for the development of symbiotic relationships between sleep physicians and dentists who practice dental sleep medicine. By working together, they are often better able to address the needs of OSA patients who are intolerant to CPAP.

In most cases, successful treatment of a chronic disease such as OSA requires a patient to continue treatment indefinitely. Since sleep apnea can often progress over time, it is important that patients also return to their treating sleep physicians for regular follow-up. If they do not do so, there is a high likelihood that they will not be adequately treated in the long term.[5]

The case above is an example of a patient who had moderate OSA, bordering on being severe, but he was intolerant of CPAP. The eventual success with an oral appliance can be attributed to a specific management algorithm. The first step is to obtain a diagnosis from a sleep physician. The choice of an appliance for any patient should be based on independent peer-reviewed literature, preferably comparing the specific oral appliance to the gold standard CPAP. Almost all oral appliances are different, based on the mechanism for protrusion, amount of protrusion, patient adjustability to the appliance, retention, ease of fit, and skill level of the dental practitioner.

With the described approach taken by the Multidisciplinary Alternatives to CPAP Clinic, the team was able to determine an effective treatment option that allowed for adequate resolution of the patient's OSA. Collaboration between members of the multidisciplinary team was key to the successful treatment of this patient.

REFERENCES

1. Aarab G, Lobbezo F, Hamburger HL, Naije M. Oral appliance therapy versus nasal continuous positive airway pressure in obstructive sleep apnea: a randomized placebo-controlled trial. *Respiration* 2011;**81**:411–19.
2. Kushida CA, Morgenthaler TI, Littner MR, et al. Practice parameters for the treatment of snoring and obstructive sleep apnea with oral appliances: an update for 2005. *Sleep* 2006;**29**:240–3.
3. de Almeida FR, Lowe AA, Tsuiki S, et al. Long-term compliance and side effects of oral appliances used for the treatment of snoring and obstructive sleep apnea syndrome. *J Clin Sleep Med* 2005;**1**:143–52.
4. Ferguson KA, Cartwright R, Rogers R, Schmidt-Nowara W. Oral appliances for snoring and obstructive sleep apnea: a review. *Sleep* 2006;**29**:244–59.
5. Thornton WK. In IT for the long run. *Sleep Rev* 2012;**13**:24–7.

23

Inadequate preoperative assessment risks ineffective surgical treatment of obstructive sleep apnea

Jeffrey J. Stanley

Case

A 56-year-old woman was referred to the Multidisciplinary Alternatives to CPAP Clinic at the University of Michigan Hospital for assessment and treatment of obstructive sleep apnea (OSA). In this clinic, patients with sleep-disordered breathing who are unable to tolerate continuous positive airway pressure (CPAP) therapy are seen by physicians from Sleep Medicine, Otolaryngology, Dentistry, and Oral and Maxillofacial Surgery. Evaluation includes a complete review of outside polysomnogram results and physicians' notes. All patients undergo a thorough head and neck physical examination including flexible pharyngoscopy as well as cephalometric analysis via cone beam computed tomography (CT).

The patient had experienced a 10-year history of heroic snoring, excessive daytime sleepiness and witnessed apneic episodes. She also had a long-standing history of depression and was being treated for hypertension, diabetes, asthma, and gastroesophageal reflux. Current medications included atenolol, furosemide, verapamil, metformin, albuterol and omeprazole.

Polysomnography performed 8 years earlier documented the presence of OSA. The overall apnea/hypopnea index (AHI, events per hour of sleep) at that time was 26 with an oxygen saturation nadir of 79%. The patient slept in the supine position throughout the study. No additional details regarding variation in severity with sleep stage, rapid eye movement (REM)

versus non-rapid eye movement (NREM) sleep, were available. The patient underwent uvulopalatopharyngoplasty (UPPP) with tonsillectomy (Figure 23.1[1]) 2 years following the initial OSA diagnosis, but reported minimal improvement in her daytime symptoms. She discontinued driving a year later due to concerns regarding drowsiness.

Repeat diagnostic polysomnography performed 1 year prior to her current evaluation revealed persistent OSA with an AHI of 23 events per hour of sleep (NREM AHI of 11 and REM AHI of 75) with an oxygen saturation nadir of 81%. Again, the patient slept in the supine position throughout the study. The patient's Epworth Sleepiness Scale score at that time was 15 (normal < 10). No significant weight change since the initial polysomnogram was reported.

A subsequent CPAP titration study showed resolution of respiratory events at a positive airway pressure of 9 cm of water, used with a feature ("C-Flex" set at 3) that lowers the pressure transiently at the very onset of expiration, to make positive airway pressure (PAP) more tolerable. However, she was still unable to tolerate CPAP at home because of ongoing severe claustrophobia. Despite attempts at desensitization, the patient remained CPAP intolerant. In summation, she reported the intermittent use of CPAP for a total of 4 months during the past 8 years since her initial diagnosis of OSA.

On physical examination, the patient was 5 feet, 3 inches (160 cm) tall and weighed 242 pounds (110 kg) with a body mass index (BMI) of 42 kg/m^2.

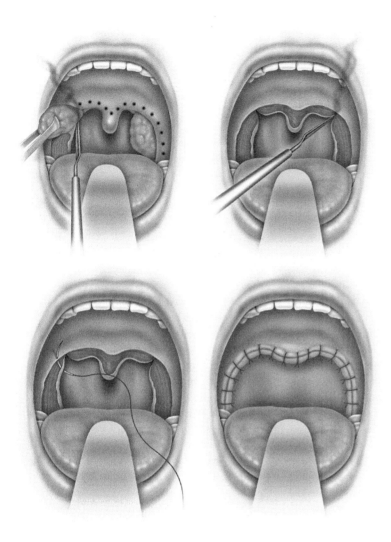

Figure 23.1 Uvulopalatopharyngoplasty with tonsillectomy. Reproduced from Katsantonis GP,[1] with permission of Elsevier.

Her neck circumference was 15 inches (38 cm) and her blood pressure was 132/72 mmHg. Her cranial nerves were intact and there was no sinus or temporomandibular joint tenderness. Intranasal exam revealed a rightward deviated nasal septum and significant inferior turbinate hypertrophy bilaterally with associated nasal airway obstruction. The tongue was hypertrophied with prominent scalloping along the lateral borders. She had a Friedman tongue position III. The palatine tonsils had been surgically removed. The soft palate was well healed with evidence of previous UPPP. There was no evidence of posterior pharyngeal narrowing or nasopharyngeal stenosis. There was no significant redundant posterior pharyngeal tissue.

The maxilla was edentulous and the patient had limited mandibular dentition.

Flexible fiberoptic pharyngoscopy (with Müller's maneuver) showed minimal ($<$ 25%) baseline narrowing at the level of the palate at quiet expiration, and minimal further closure with forced inspiration. At the retrolingual level, there was moderate (50%) baseline narrowing and severe ($>$ 75%) reduction in cross-sectional area with forced inspiration.

Computed tomography imaging documented a cranial base angle (Ba-S-N) of 136 degrees with a Sella Nasion Subspinale (SNA) of 81 degrees (normal 82) and a Sella Nasion Supramentale (SNB) of 80 degrees (normal 80). The posterior airway space was 3 mm (normal 11 mm), palatal length (PNS-P) was 18 mm (normal 35 mm), and the hyoid mandibular plane (H-MP) distance was 20 mm (normal 15 mm). The minimal airway volume was determined to be 23 mm^3 with the site of maximal obstruction identified at the level of the tongue base.

The patient was determined not to be a candidate for use of a mandibular advancement device due to lack of dentition. The patient deferred further consideration of maxillomandibular advancement due to concerns regarding a potentially significant change in her facial profile.

Following a thorough discussion regarding the risks, benefits, and alternatives, a decision was made to proceed with mandibulotomy with genioglossus muscle advancement, hyoid suspension, nasal septoplasty, and cauterization of the inferior turbinates bilaterally. This was accomplished uneventfully and she was discharged on postoperative day 1. Her clinic evaluations 2 and 6 weeks later revealed normal healing. Repeat diagnostic polysomnography was performed 4 months later. Despite an initial weight loss of 10 pounds (5 kg), there was no interval change in her BMI at that time. This polysomnogram revealed an AHI of 8 events per hour of sleep (vs. 23 preoperatively); an NREM AHI of 4 (vs. 11 preoperatively) and an REM AHI of 25 (vs. 75 preoperatively) with an oxygen saturation nadir of 86% (vs. 81% preoperatively). The patient slept in the supine position throughout the study. The proportion of REM sleep (20% postoperatively) was similar to that observed during her preoperative polysomnogram

(19%). The patient's Epworth Sleepiness Scale score following surgery was 8 (vs. 15 preoperatively) and the patient reported a marked improvement in her daytime sleepiness.

Discussion

Inadequate preoperative assessment increases the risk of ineffective surgical treatment of OSA. It is important to recognize that OSA frequently results from obstruction at multiple anatomic sites including the nose, oropharynx and hypopharynx. Fujita characterized the different levels of anatomic obstruction in patients with OSA nearly 3 decades ago.[2] Fujita class I, II, and III were used to describe patients with obstruction at the oropharynx only, oropharynx and hypopharynx, and hypopharynx only, respectively. Greater than 50% of patients had multilevel obstruction and such was suspected to be the cause of UPPP failure. Subsequent case series[3] and a recent meta-analysis of nearly 2000 patients[4] confirmed that the majority of patients undergoing surgical treatment of OSA have multilevel obstruction. During the preoperative assessment of patients with OSA, sites of obstruction are typically determined by a combination of physical examination, the Müller's maneuver and cephalometry.

The Friedman tongue position (FTP) is a valuable grading system used to identify potential sites of obstruction (Figure 23.2[5]).[6] The FTP describes the position of the tongue, in a relaxed position within the mouth, relative to the tonsils and tonsillar pillars and also the uvula, soft palate, and hard palate. The FTP provides an indirect assessment of hypopharyngeal obstruction and has been correlated with the posterior airway space as measured objectively by cephalometry. Friedman tongue position I allows for visualization of the tonsils, tonsillar pillars, and the entire uvula. Friedman tongue position IIa allows for visualization of the uvula but not the tonsils and tonsillar pillars. Friedman tongue position IIb allows for visualization of the base of the uvula and most of the soft palate, but not the tonsils, tonsillar pillars, and tip of the uvula. Friedman tongue position III allows for visualization of a portion of the soft palate, but not the

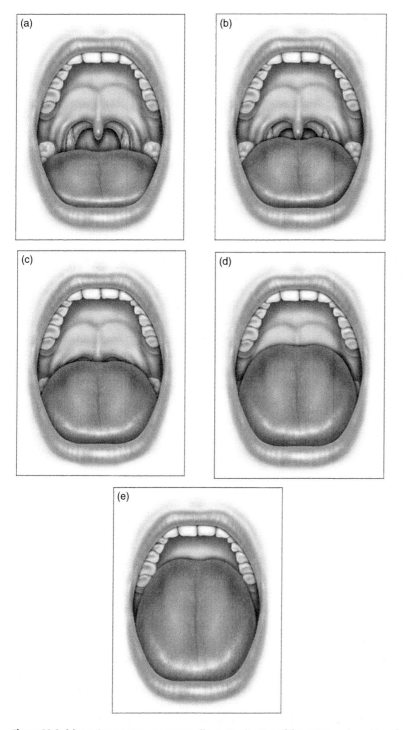

Figure 23.2 (a) Friedman tongue position I allows visualization of the entire uvula and tonsils/pillars. (b) Friedman tongue position IIa allows visualization of most of the uvula, but the tonsils/pillars are absent. (c) Friedman tongue position IIb allows visualization of the entire soft plate to the base of the uvula. (d) In Friedman tongue position III some of the soft palate is visualized but the distal structures are absent. (e) Friedman tongue position IV allows visualization of the hard palate only. Reproduced from Friedman M,[5] with permission of Elsevier.

distal soft palate, uvula, tonsils, or tonsillar pillars. Friedman tongue position IV allows for visualization of the hard palate only. A higher FTP score predicts a lower likelihood of improvement following UPPP only. The FTP grade combined with tonsil size and BMI is the basis of the Friedman staging system, which has been shown to be highly predictive of surgical outcomes following UPPP.[7]

The Müller's maneuver is commonly used in the preoperative assessment of patients with OSA. This maneuver utilizes flexible fiberoptic endoscopy to evaluate the upper airway during forced inspiration against a closed airway. It allows for an individual estimate of airway collapsibility at both the oropharynx and hypopharynx. Because this is a subjective assessment and relies on patient effort with regards to forceful inspiration, this test is rarely used in isolation.

Cephalometric analysis is also frequently used in the preoperative evaluation of patients with OSA. The SNA and SNB measurements can help detect maxillary or mandibular deficiencies. In addition, a posterior airway space (PAS) < 8 mm has been shown to correlate with failure of isolated palatal surgery. An increase in the mandibular H-MP length is also predictive of a hypopharyngeal site of collapse.

More recently, sleep endoscopy has been employed to determine sites of obstruction in patients with OSA. This technique combines fiberoptic pharyngoscopy with drug-induced unconsciousness (e.g. with propofol) to assess the retropalatal and hypopharyngeal areas that collapse. This approach has the distinct advantage over conscious endoscopy (Müller's maneuver) in that it allows for evaluation of upper airway collapsibility in the setting of decreased muscle tone, a critical component of OSA.

Historically, surgical treatment of OSA has focused on single-site oropharyngeal procedures. Uvulopalatopharyngoplasty with or without tonsillectomy has been the mainstay of therapy following its introduction in the early 1980s. This surgical technique was designed to specifically address the retropalatal area of collapse observed in OSA. The overall success rate of UPPP, arbitrarily defined as a reduction in AHI of at least 50%, and a final overall AHI < 20 among unselected patients with OSA is approximately 40%.[7]

Although usually not curative, this procedure was previously thought more likely to be effective in the treatment of patients with mild to moderate disease. Increasing evidence now suggests that the severity of disease is not as predictive of surgical success as is proper identification and treatment of all anatomic sites of obstruction.[8,9] Modifications of the UPPP technique, including the uvulopalatal flap, Z-palatopharyngoplasty, and expansion sphincter pharyngoplasty have led to improved success rates for isolated palatal procedures and a reduction in postoperative complications, but still fail to address the problem of hypopharyngeal obstruction.

Limited improvement following oropharyngeal surgery alone, coupled with the identification of additional anatomic sites of obstruction, prompted the development and implementation of multiple procedures to address nasal and hypopharyngeal sites of obstruction. Improved surgical outcomes with multilevel procedures have been well documented.[3,4,10] The importance of nasal obstruction in patients with OSA has received considerable attention. Nasal obstruction has a direct effect on the critical closing pressure (Pcrit) of the oropharynx and hypopharynx (collapsible segments). Increasing nasal resistance leads to an increase in the Pcrit of the downstream segments and worsens obstruction.[11] Common causes of nasal obstruction include nasoseptal deviation, turbinate hypertrophy, and nasal polyposis. Although nasal surgery alone is rarely curative, it is frequently performed in conjunction with other procedures of the oropharynx and hypopharynx to maximize surgical improvement. Isolated nasal surgery has also been performed to improve CPAP compliance by reducing CPAP pressure requirements and improving tolerance of nasal pillow/nasal mask use.[12]

In the past two decades, there has been an increasing emphasis on multilevel surgery in the treatment of OSA, with a particular focus on hypopharyngeal procedures. In one of the largest case series of patients undergoing surgery for OSA, directed by site of obstruction, Riley et al.[3] reported an overall success rate of 61%. Success rates were higher for those with mild and moderate disease, 78% and 71%, respectively. A recent meta-analysis of 1978 patients who underwent multisite surgery reported an overall success rate of 66%.[4] Those benefiting from surgery exhibited significant improvements in both AHI and oxygen saturation levels. These and other studies suggest that surgical treatment based on adequate preoperative assessment of potential sites of obstruction yield better outcomes than isolated oropharyngeal procedures, such as UPPP.

Despite this knowledge, surgical practice patterns in the United States have been slow to change. Data from the 2006 Nationwide Inpatient Sample, State Ambulatory Surgery Database, and State Inpatient Database revealed that of the > 35 000 outpatient and inpatient operations performed for the treatment of OSA that year, 75% were isolated palatal procedures. In total, 93% included oropharyngeal procedures and only 19% included hypopharyngeal procedures.

It is clear that fewer hypopharyngeal operations are performed than would be expected based upon the known prevalence of multilevel obstruction in patients with OSA. A thorough preoperative assessment is critical to identify all potential sites of obstruction in order to maximize the improvement that can be achieved with sleep surgery. Inadequate preoperative assessment risks suboptimal surgical treatment of OSA.

REFERENCES

1. Katsantonis GP. Uvulopalatopharyngoplasty. In Friedman M (ed.) *Sleep Apnea and Snoring: Surgical and Non-Surgical Therapy*. Philadelphia, PA: Saunders Elsevier;2009, pp. 178, 181.
2. Fujita S. UPPP for sleep apnea and snoring. *Ear Nose Throat J* 1984;**63**:227–35.
3. Riley RW, Powell NB, Guilleminault C. Obstructive sleep apnea syndrome: a review of 306 consecutively treated surgical patients. *Otolaryngol Head Neck Surg* 1993;**108**:117–25.
4. Lin HC, Friedman M, Chang HW, Gurpinar B. The efficacy of multilevel surgery of the upper airway in adults with obstructive sleep apnea/hypopnea syndrome. *Laryngoscope* 2008;**18**:902–8.
5. Friedman, M. Friedman tongue position and the staging of obstructive sleep apnea/hypopnea syndrome. In Friedman M, ed. *Sleep Apnea and Snoring: Surgical and Non-Surgical Therapy*. Philadelphia, PA: Saunders Elsevier;2009, p. 106.
6. Friedman M, Ibrahim H, Bass L. Clinical staging for sleep-disordered breathing. *Otolaryngol Head Neck Surg* 2002;**127**:13–27.
7. Sher AE, Schechtman KB, Piccirillo JF. The efficacy of surgical modifications of the upper airway in adults with obstructive sleep apnea syndrome. *Sleep* 1996 **19**:156–77.
8. Senior BA, Rosenthal L, Lumley A, et al. Efficacy of uvulopalatopharyngoplasty in unselected patients with mild obstructive sleep apnea. *Otolaryngol Head Neck Surg* 2000;**123**:179–82.
9. Friedman M, Vidyasagar R, Bliznikas D, Joseph N. Does severity of obstructive sleep apnea/hypopnea syndrome predict uvulopalatopharyngoplasty outcome? *Laryngoscope* 2005;**115**:2109–13.
10. Friedman M, Ibrahim H, Lee G, et al. Combined uvulopalatopharyngoplasty and radiofrequency tongue base reduction for treatment of obstructive sleep apnea/hypopnea syndrome. *Otolaryngol Head Neck Surg* 2003;**129**:611–21.
11. Cole P, Haight JS. Mechanisms of nasal obstruction in sleep. *Laryngoscope* 1984;**94**:1557–79.
12. Friedman M, Tanyeri H, Lim JW, et al. Effect of improved nasal breathing on obstructive sleep apnea. *Otolaryngol Head Neck Surg* 2000;**122**:71–4.

24

Genioglossus advancement and hyoid suspension carries risks and may not obviate the need for subsequent use of continuous positive airway pressure

Sharon Aronovich and Joseph I. Helman

Case

A 49-year-old man presented to the Multidisciplinary Alternatives to CPAP Clinic at the University of Michigan Medical Center with the objective to further investigate surgical options for the management of his obstructive sleep apnea (OSA).

Past medical history was consistent with seasonal allergies, hyperlipidemia, and hypertension. He was treated with diphenhydramine, simvastatin, and beta-blockers.

His evaluation by a sleep medicine physician noted that the patient reported significant daytime sleepiness and previous intolerance to continuous positive airway pressure (CPAP) due to claustrophobia. His body mass index (BMI) was 32 kg/m^2, his apnea/hypopnea index (AHI, events per hour of sleep) was 35, and his minimum oxygen saturation (Min.% SpO$_2$) was 85%. He had cephalometric X-rays performed, in addition to pharyngoscopy, and was also seen on the same day by a prosthedontist, an oral and maxillofacial surgeon, and an otolaryngologist, each with experience and particular interest in devices or surgical approaches to control OSA. A conference at the end of the afternoon included input from all specialists, review of the results of the X-rays and pharyngoscopy, and a joint decision about potential options for the patient.

Subsequent discussion with the patient of surgical options included (i) maxillomandibular advancement (also called MMA or bimaxillary advancement), or (ii) multilevel airway surgery that could include uvulopalatopharyngoplasty (UPPP), tonsillectomy, and genial advancement and hyoid suspension (GAHS). The patient elected to undergo UPPP, tonsillectomy, and GAHS.

The procedure was performed without any complications. Immediate postoperative complications included difficulty swallowing and paresthesia of the mental branch of the left inferior alveolar nerve. Although the paresthesia soon improved, the changes in swallowing did not.

Three months after the procedure, the patient perceived a "snap" in the region of the anterior neck. Further radiographic investigation demonstrated a fracture of the paramedial aspect of the hyoid bone, which did not require additional treatment.

Postoperative polysomnography was performed 1 year after surgery. His BMI was 31.4 kg/m^2, his AHI was 55 events per hour of sleep (up from 35 previously), and his minimum oxygen saturation (Min.% SpO$_2$) was 82%. The patient was referred for further surgery, namely MMA.

Discussion

Most studies recognize that adult patients with OSA have multilevel obstruction that may involve the nasal passages, nasopharynx, oropharynx, and hypopharynx. When CPAP therapy is not tolerated, or simply refused outright, surgical treatments may be offered based on a thorough assessment of the patient's airway and

Common Pitfalls in Sleep Medicine, ed. Ronald D. Chervin. Published by Cambridge University Press. © Cambridge University Press 2014.

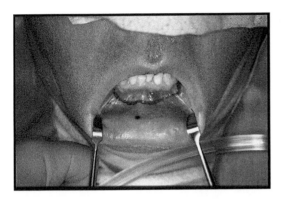

Figure 24.1 At the start of a genioglossus and hyoid suspension (GAHS), an incision is planned in the labial mucosa about a centimeter labial to the attached gingiva.

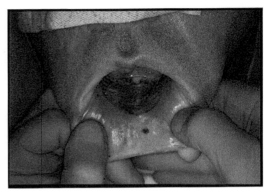

Figure 24.2 The incision is then performed through mucosa, submucosa, mentalis muscle, and periostium, while leaving a cuff of muscle attached to the occlusal aspect of the mucosa in order to facilitate closure of the soft tissues.

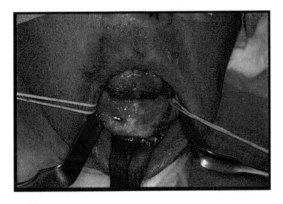

Figure 24.3 The periostium is elevated from the bone and the chin is completely exposed. Both mental nerves are identified and protected. In the picture a vessel loop has been passed around the mental nerves (clearly obvious on the patient's left side).

disease severity as determined by objective assessments, such as the clinical exam, radiography, and polysomnography, and subjective assessments such as the Epworth Sleepiness Scale (see Chapter 23). When a suitable surgical candidate is identified, surgical options must be presented with their respective cure rates, expected postsurgical course, and risks of temporary or permanent complications. Several surgical procedures have been advocated for the treatment of OSA. One of them is GAHS. This procedure is also referred to as inferior sagittal mandibular osteotomy and also genioglossal advancement with myotomy and suspension.

The goal of GAHS is to increase the patency of the retroglossal and hypopharyngeal airway. Genioglossus advancement (GAA) is typically performed transorally. An incision is planned in the labial mucosa about a centimeter labial to the attached gingiva (Figure 24.1). The incision is carried through mucosa, submucosa, mentalis muscle, and periosteum. An adequate cuff of mentalis muscle must remain attached to proximal mucoperiosteum to facilitate soft tissue closure (Figure 24.2). A subperiosteal dissection is performed exposing the anterior aspect of the mandible and bilateral mental nerves (Figure 24.3). The osteotomy is designed to include the genial tubercles with its genioglossus attachments and carried out with a reciprocating or sagittal saw (Figure 24.4). Several anatomical studies have identified landmarks for complete inclusion of the genioglossus muscle bundles.[1-3] Once the osteotomy is completed, the segment of bone is mobilized anteriorly with its lingual muscle attachments (Figure 24.5). The buccal cortex and medullary bone is removed, allowing advancement of the lingual cortex to the level of the adjacent facial cortex for fixation with a titanium plate and screws (Figure 24.6). To expose the hyoid bone, a 3 cm horizontal incision is

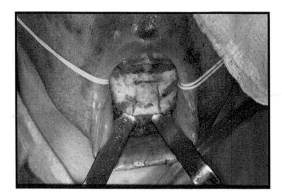

Figure 24.4 The outline of the osteotomy is performed. In this case the shape has been a quadrangular design which includes both genial tubercles on the lingual aspect of the osteotomy.

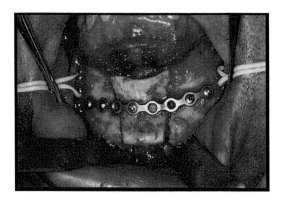

Figure 24.6 In this specific design of the osteotomy, the buccal and medular bone are removed and the lingual cortical bone is plated in continuity with the labial cortical bone, generating an average of about 13 mm advancement of the genial tubercles. Some other authors advocated a rectangular or a cylindrical design of the osteotomy with the same objective of advancing the genial tubercles.

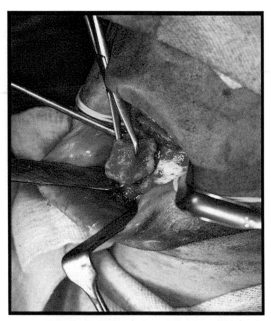

Figure 24.5 The osteotomy is finalized with a reciprocating saw and the segment of bone is mobilized. The segment of bone contains the genial tubercles in the lingual aspect of the mandible.

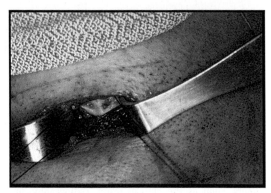

Figure 24.7 The anterior aspect of the hyoid bone is dissected and a myotomy is performed by dividing the stylohyoid ligament which allows for a larger advancement of the hyoid.

placed in a neck crease. After dissection to reach the hyoid, a myotomy of the stylohyoid ligament is performed to allow anterior and superior repositioning (Figure 24.7). The hyoid bone may be suspended to the chin using sutures with or without a strip of fascia from the lateral thigh (Figure 24.8). Alternatively, the hyoid may be suspended inferiorly to the thyroid cartilage.

Beyond an accurate diagnosis of the sites of obstruction, there are several things to consider when interpreting the literature. Success has been typically defined as a respiratory disturbance index (RDI) < 20

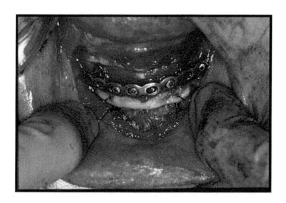

Figure 24.8 With either sutures or fascial strips the hyoid is suspended to either the chin or the thyroid cartilage in a subplastysma layer.

apneic events per hour of sleep, and a decrease in RDI (or AHI) by at least 50%. Follow-up polysomnography is typically obtained at 6-12 months postoperatively without further long-term data, and multiple variations of these procedures may limit direct comparisons. We present results of cases done at our institution and review the literature on these procedures with respect to variables measured, details of the procedure, effectiveness in treating OSA, and complications.

Twenty-two consecutive patients with OSA underwent GAHS and UPPP at the authors' institution. Significant changes were noted in comparisons of preoperative and postoperative polysomnography results and cephalogram measurements. The RDI decreased from 46 ± 29 to 22 ± 18. Lowest oxygen saturation (LSAT) increased from 83 ± 6% to 88 ± 6%. Posterior airway space increased from 1.9 ± 1.2 mm to 4.0 ± 1.7 mm. Hyoid to mandibular plane distance decreased from 25.9 mm to 16.6 mm consistent with anterior and superior suspension. While the results of GAHS and UPPP showed marked improvements, only 26% of patients had a postoperative RDI that did not warrant further therapy with CPAP.

Hendler et al.[4] retrospectively evaluated the results of surgical treatment in 40 patients. In their protocol, 33 patients with an RDI of 9-130 (mean 60) underwent UPPP and mortised GGA. Their modified genioplasty technique included a broad muscular pedicle consisting of geniolossus, geniohyoid, mylohyoid, and digastric muscle attachments with a 10 mm advancement. Patients had a mean age of 47 years (28 males, 5 females) and mean BMI of 32.6 kg/m². At 6 months follow-up, 29 of 33 patients showed improvement with an overall mean RDI of 29 (50% decrease in RDI). Fourteen patients with baseline RDI < 50 had 71% success while 19 patients with RDI > 50 had 32% success. Overall, patients with an RDI between 21 and 40 had an 86% success. Normal or mildly elevated BMI (< 30 kg/m²) was associated with increased success.

Yin et al.[5] treated 18 patients with GAHS for severe OSA (AHI > 40). The GGA was performed as described by Dattilo[6] and the hyoid bone was suspended anteriorly and superiorly after division of the infrahyoid muscles. The mean age was 44 years and mean preoperative AHI was 64 ± 16 with an LSAT of 72%. At 6 months post surgery, the mean AHI was 21 ± 20 with an LSAT of 81%. The success rate was 67% at the 6 months follow-up. Preoperative factors that distinguished responders and non-responders were younger age (39 vs. 53 years), fewer oxygen desaturations below 90% (19 vs. 38), a larger posterior airway space (8.3 vs. 6.8 mm), and lower BMI (27.6 vs. 30.7 kg/m²).[5]

Neruntarat[7] treated 31 patients with GAHS and UPPP under local anesthesia at Vajira Hospital in Thailand. Genioglossus advancement was performed with a rectangular osteotomy of the anterior mandible and rotation of the lingual cortex over the adjacent frontal surface of the mandible. The hyoid bone was released from the stylohyoid ligaments, advanced anteriorly and inferiorly, and secured over the thyroid cartilage with four permanent sutures. Patients had a mean age of 46.2 years, 90% were male, and their BMI ranged from 27.4 to 30.2 kg/m². Preoperative RDI and LSAT were 48% and 82% respectively. Postoperative measurements obtained at a mean of 8.3 (6-10) months demonstrated significant improvements with RDI and LSAT to 15% and 89% respectively. There were also statistically significant improvements in percentage REM sleep, sleep efficiency, Epworth Sleepiness Scale score (from 14.9 to 8.2), and snoring scale (from 8.1 to 3.4). The overall success rate was 70%.

Miller et al.[8] retrospectively analyzed 24 cases treated with GGA and UPPP. Twenty-one were male, with a mean age of 43 years, and a mean BMI of 30.5 kg/m^2. Follow-up polysomnograms were obtained at 3–6 months postoperatively. The GGA was performed using the circular trephine system of 12 or 14 mm diameter. Thirteen patients in this group had hyoid suspension but details of this procedure were not provided. Significant improvements were detected on follow-up RDI (from 53 to 16), AHI (from 20 to 6), LSAT (from 80% to 88%) and posterior airway space (from 7.9 to 12.6). The overall success rate was 67%. The success rate was 88% in patients with a preoperative RDI < 40, and 56% for those with RDI > 40. Success rate was not influenced by hyoid suspension. In a similar study looking at 26 patients with severe OSA, Yi et al.[9] showed a reduction in AHI from 66 to 30 with an overall success rate of 46% at 6 months. Despite a small sample size, they were able to show that Friedman stage III is correlated with significantly worst outcomes. Surprisingly, there was no change in the posterior airway space after surgery.[9]

Altman et al.[10] investigated the effect of UPPP with GAHS (hyoid to thyroid) on swallowing function in OSA patients. Fifteen patients without a history of preoperative swallowing issues filled out a swallowing questionnaire and underwent a modified barium swallow 6–26 months after surgery. The modified barium swallow was used to assess velopharyngeal function, tongue base movement, laryngeal elevation, epiglottic movement, and laryngoesophageal opening. Of note, objective findings did not correlate with subjective symptoms. Five out of nine patients with abnormal objective findings on modified barium swallow reported normal swallowing. The findings included premature spillage over tongue base, nasopharygeal reflux, pooling in vallecula, aspiration, incomplete epiglottic inversion, and bolus partition. On the other hand, of the six patients with normal findings on modified barium swallow, five noted subjective changes in their swallowing. The latter group complained of food going down the wrong tube, food getting stuck in the throat, difficulty with swallowing, and nasopharyngeal reflux symptoms.

In a prospective study, Stuck et al.[11] used magnetic resonance imaging (MRI) to examine the effect of hyoid suspension on the upper airway in 15 patients. The hyoid was released and suspended inferiorly to the thyroid cartilage as described by Riley et al.[12] The mean age was 47.3 years and the mean BMI was 27.5 kg/m^2. Fourteen patients completed the study with postoperative MRI and polysomnogram at 8.7 (6–14) weeks. Mean RDI changed from 35 ± 19 to 27 ± 26. Six patients had no significant change in RDI while one patient deteriorated. Although mild improvements in daytime sleepiness were observed, there were no significant changes in upper airway measurements on MRI or lateral cephalogram.[11]

A study by Baisch et al.[13] examined 83 patients undergoing multilevel soft tissue surgery with or without hyoid suspension. While a change was noted in the mean AHI (from 36 to 19), there was no significant benefit in AHI reduction for the group that had additional hyoid suspension. In another study evaluating the outcomes of hyoid suspension, Bowden et al.[14] demonstrated poor outcomes with the technique described by Riley et al.[15] Patients had a mean BMI of 34.1 kg/m^2 and a mean AHI of 37. There were no significant changes noted in the LSAT or the Epworth Sleepiness Scale score. Only 5 out of 29 (17%) met success criteria. Overall, there was no change in AHI with 10–30% worsening in the mild OSA group. Complications included transient dysphagia lasting 3–4 days and postoperative neck hematoma.[14]

In 1997, Riley et al.[16] looked at the intraoperative risks and postoperative complications of 182 patients undergoing various upper airway operations including UPPP and maxillofacial procedures. A total of 210 procedures were performed. Thirty-nine patients (18.6%) had difficult intubations with two episodes of transient airway obstruction after extubation. Rare postoperative complications included bleeding, infection, seroma, arrhythmia, angina, and loss of skeletal fixation. Most patients required active management of perioperative hypertension. Recently, Pang et al.[17] carried out a similar retrospective review of 487 cases involving multilevel soft tissue operations including tongue base radio-frequency and hyoid suspension. There was an overall complication rate of 7.1%. Six patients with severe OSA required treatment for oxygen desaturations within the first 3 hours after surgery, 15 patients had perioperative hypertension, and another 15 had late hemorrhage. Nine patients had tongue edema and one patient had to be re-intubated. Negative pressure pulmonary edema was also a rare complication. These studies highlight the importance of optimizing the patient's comorbidities preoperatively and underscore the need for vigilant postoperative management in a monitored unit.

In a literature review on hypopharyngeal surgery, Kezirian and Goldberg[18] found that most existing studies are case series or retrospective reviews (level 4 evidence). While there is evidence of improved outcomes with surgery, careful patient selection can significantly affect the success of treatment. The authors correctly state that multicenter randomized controlled trials are needed to compare surgical treatments and identify prognostic factors.[18]

Several complications have been reported after multilevel airway surgery including GAHS. This includes infection, mandibular fractures (10%), floor of mouth hematoma, wound dehiscence, exposed hardware requiring removal, dysphagia, hypertrophic scarring requiring scar revision, drooling, transient paresthesia or hypoesthesia in the mental nerve distribution, persistent paresthesia of the mandibular incisor teeth, and occasional cases of dysesthesia involving the mental nerve region. Pain after surgery was rated as mild to moderate (visual analog scale [VAS] of 4–7; mean 5.2) being worst on day 3 and resolved by day 7.

Vilaseca et al.[19] published dismal outcomes after UPPP and GAHS with a preoperative AHI of 60 and a postsurgical AHI of 45. Bowden et al.[20] reported their results after performing GAHS in 29 patients. The preoperative AHI was 37 and the postoperative AHI was 38.

Main points

In short, although some early reports on GAHS, particularly in combination with UPPP, suggested that for appropriate candidates good results could be achieved, a broader consideration of accumulated literature at this point, in combination with the authors' own experience, suggest that the success rate of GAHS

is not high and that significant morbidity is associated with the procedure. Although OSAS often improves, the outcome that is often most important to the patient – not having to use CPAP anymore – is not likely to be achieved. Risks may not justify the gain for many patients, and the case presented above serves as one example of why a critical reassessment of this technique should be considered, in the opinion of the present authors, before further implementation of GAHS.

REFERENCES

1. Silverstein K, Costello BJ, Giannakpoulos H, et al. Genioglossus muscle attachments: an anatomic analysis and the implications for genioglossus advancement. *Oral Surg Oral Med Oral Pathol Oral Radiol Endod* 2000;**90**:686–8.

2. Yin SK, Yi HL, Lu WY, et al. Anatomical and spiral computed tomographic study of the genial tubercles for genioglossus advancement. *Otolaryngol Head Neck Surg* 2007;**136**:632–7.

3. Li KK, Riley RW, Powell NB, et al. Obstructive sleep apnea surgery: genioglossus advancement revisited. *J Oral Maxillofac Surg* 2001;**59**:1181–4.

4. Hendler BH, Costello BJ, Silverstein K, et al. A protocol for uvulopalatopharyngoplasty, mortised genioplasty, and maxillomandibular advancement in patients with obstructive sleep apnea: an analysis of 40 cases. *J Oral Maxillofac Surg* 2001;**59**:892–7.

5. Yin SK, Yi HL, Lu WY, et al. Genioglossus advancement and hyoid suspension plus uvulopalatopharyngoplasty for severe OSAHS. *Otolaryngol Head Neck Surg* 2007;**136**: 626–31.

6. Dattilo DJ. The mandibular trapezoid osteotomy for the treatment of obstructive sleep apnea: report of a case. *J Oral Maxillofac Surg* 1998;**56**:1442–6.

7. Neruntarat C. Genioglossus advancement and hyoid myotomy under local anesthesia. *Otolaryngol Head Neck Surg* 2003;**129**:85–91.

8. Miller FR, Watson D, Boseley M, et al. The role of the genial bone advancement trephine system in conjunction with uvulopalatopharyngoplasty in the multilevel management of obstructive sleep apnea. *Otolaryngol Head Neck Surg* 2004;**130**:73–9.

9. Yi HL, Sun XQ, Chen B, et al. Z-palatopharyngoplasty plus genioglossus advancement and hyoid suspension for obstructive apnea hypopnea syndrome. *Otolaryngol Head Neck Surg* 2011;**144**:469–73.

10. Altman JS, Halpert RD, Mickelson SA, et al. Effect of uvulopalatopharyngoplasty and genial and hyoid advancement on swallowing in patients with obstructive sleep apnea syndrome. *Otolaryngol Head Neck Surg* 1999;**120**:454-7.

11. Stuck BA, Neff W, Hormann K, et al. Anatomic changes after hyoid suspension for obstructive sleep apnea: an MRI study. *Otolaryngol Head Neck Surg* 2005;**133**:397-402.

12. Riley RW, Powell NB, Guilleminault C. Obstructive sleep apnea and the hyoid: a revised procedure. *Otolaryngol Head Neck Surg* 1994;**111**:717-21.

13. Baisch A, Maurer JT, Hörmann K. The effect of hyoid suspension in a multilevel surgery concept for obstructive sleep apnea. *Otolaryngol Head Neck Surg* 2006;**134**:856-61.

14. Bowden MT, Kezirian EJ, Utley D, et al. Outcomes of hyoid suspension for the treatment of obstructive sleep apnea. *Arch Otolaryngol Head Neck Surg* 2005;**131**:440-5.

15. Riley RW, Powell NB, Guilleminault C. Obstructive sleep apnea and the hyoid: a revised surgical procedure. *Otolaryngol Head Neck Surg* 1994;**111**:717-21.

16. Riley RW, Powell NB, Guilleminault C, et al. Obstructive sleep apnea surgery: risk management and complications. *Otolaryngol Head Neck Surg* 1997;**117**:648-52.

17. Pang KP, Siow JK, Tseng PT. Safety of multilevel surgery in obstructive sleep apnea. *Arch Otolaryngol Head Neck Surg* 2012;**138**:353-7.

18. Kezirian EJ, Goldberg AN. Hypopharyngeal surgery in obstructive sleep apnea. *Arch Otolaryngol Head Neck Surg* 2006;**132**:206-13.

19. Vilaseca I, Morello A, Monserrat JM, Santamaria J, Iranzo A. Usefulness of uvulopalatopharyngoplasty with genioglossus and hyoid advancement in the treatment of obstructive sleep apnea. *Arch Otolaryngol Head Neck Surg* 2002;**128**:435-40.

20. Bowden MT, Kezirian EJ, Utley D, Goode RL. Outcomes of hyoid suspension for the treatment of obstructive sleep apnea. *Arch Otolaryngol Head Neck Surg* 2005;**131**:440-5.

25

Maxillary and mandibular advancement offers an effective surgical approach to severe obstructive sleep apnea, but is not appropriate for all potential candidates

Sharon Aronovich and Joseph I. Helman

Case

A 32-year-old man presented to the Alternatives to CPAP Clinic at the University of Michigan searching for a permanent solution to his obstructive sleep apnea (OSA). He was diagnosed a year earlier mainly as a result of his loud snoring, which disturbed his bed partner. The patient's apnea/hypopnea index (AHI, events per hour of sleep) was 20 and his minimum oxygen saturation was 88%. He was initially treated with continuous positive airway pressure (CPAP) at a setting of 10 cm of water, which afforded complete resolution of his symptoms. However, as a result of pressure intolerance and aerophagia, he decided to seek a surgical solution.

> *Medical history*: mild hypertension; mild OSA; body mass index (BMI), 26 kg/m^2.

> *Examination findings*: Mallampati Class III with a long soft palate and long uvula.

One year after his initial exam, the patient underwent an uvulopalatopharyngoplasty (UPPP), tonsillectomy, septoplasty, and bilateral turbinate reductions. Transient postoperative complications included pain and difficulties swallowing. A postoperative polysomnogram, performed 6 months after the UPPP, showed an AHI of 40 and oxygen desaturation to 85%. At this stage the patient decided to try again CPAP with nasal pillows, but again experienced aerophagia and could not demonstrate good adherence to the therapy.

Two years after his UPPP, a maxillomandibular advancement (also called MMA or bimaxillary advancement) consisting of a Le Fort I maxillary osteotomy and a bilateral mandibular sagittal split osteotomy was performed, with an overall advancement of 11 mm of both jaws. His postoperative airway was maintained by keeping the patient intubated overnight in the Intensive Care Unit. Extubation was performed on postoperation day 1. The patient was discharged from his hospitalization 3 days after the operation. Postoperative complications were significant for pain, swelling, and infection in the site of the left mandibular osteotomy as well as decreased sensation on both sides of the lower lip. Maxillomandibular wiring was maintained for 8 weeks, in addition to internal rigid fixation to maximize the stability of the occlusion. Six months after the MMA, a postoperative polysomnogram was performed. This study demonstrated an AHI of 6 and a minimum oxygen saturation of 90%. The return of sensation was reported by the patient to be 80% of normal.

Discussion

Untreated OSA has been associated with cardiovascular disease and has a deleterious effect on quality of life.[1,2] Weight-loss strategies (e.g. lifestyle and dietary alterations), commonly recommended for the treatment of OSA, are rarely sustained and relapse often occurs. Also, a significant proportion of patients with severe OSA are unable to tolerate nasal CPAP. Although nasal surgery such as septoplasty and

Common Pitfalls in Sleep Medicine, ed. Ronald D. Chervin. Published by Cambridge University Press. © Cambridge University Press 2014.

(a)   (b)

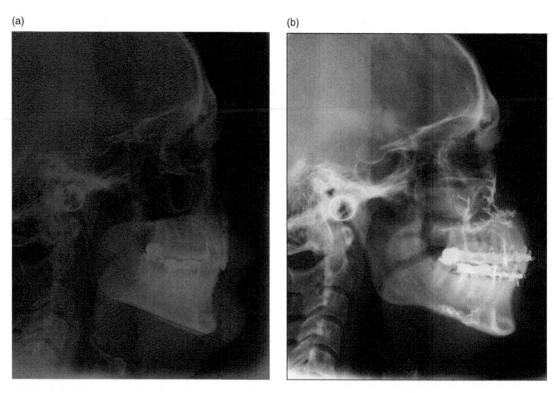

Figure 25.1 (a) Preoperative cephalometric X-ray. (b) Postoperative cephalometric X-ray. Note the increase in posterior airway space after maxillomandibular advancement.

turbinectomy may improve compliance to CPAP in select cases, patients frequently seek other surgical options designed to enlarge the upper airway.

Commonly sought surgical options such as UPPP and genioglossus advancement with hyoid suspension have a high failure rate for obese adult patients with severe sleep apnea (AHI > 30). Patients treated by these procedures frequently remain dependent on positive airway pressure therapy after surgery while being subjected to possible surgical complications such as velopharyngeal insufficiency, paresthesia of the mental nerve distribution, mandible fracture, and dysphagia.[3] Another surgical option is tracheostomy. While highly effective in curing OSA, tracheostomy has significant morbidity and low acceptance rate as a permanent solution.[4,5] Similarly, although bariatric surgery has been shown to improve objective

measures of OSA in some studies,[6-8] it also carries significant morbidity. For instance, after gastric bypass surgery, OSA patients may have a significant risk of airway complications secondary to anesthesia, opioid use, and unchanged airway dimension postoperatively. In addition, use of CPAP may disrupt the gastrojejunal anastomosis.[9] For those reasons, some patients must undergo upper airway surgery prior to bariatric intervention. Currently, MMA surgery is recognized as one of the most efficacious treatment options in the management of severe multilevel OSA (Figure 25.1).

Review of the literature on MMA suggests a reduction in AHI by 84-95%, and a success rate of 93-98%.[10-13] In a study of 15 patients, Lye et al.[14] found a success rate of 87% by polysomnography and 93% based on objective success criteria (AHI decrease by 50%

and < 20) and quality of life assessment using the Functional Outcomes of Sleep Questionnaire (FOSQ > 18). Two patients in their sample, while significantly improved from baseline, continued to have hypopneas and central apneas postoperatively. Goodday and Bourque[15] assessed subjective outcomes of 116 patients via questionnaires administered before and after surgery. Based on preoperative Epworth Sleepiness Scale (ESS) scores, 33 (28%) of the patients were not sleepy (ESS < 10), 37 (32%) were sleepy (ESS 10–16), and 46 (40%) were very sleepy (ESS > 16). Postoperatively, 104 (90%) of the patients were not sleepy, with 11 (9%) patients in the sleepy category, and one being very sleepy (< 1%). They found an 83% reduction in snoring and 94% reduction in witnessed apneas. It is interesting to note that while 96% of patients using CPAP before surgery no longer required CPAP, 89% felt the surgery was worthwhile and 95% would recommend it to other patients with OSA. Despite the high patient satisfaction, a few patients are expected to remain unsatisfied.

Maxillomandibular advancement, or telegnathic surgery, is a form of major reconstructive facial surgery that should only be offered to patients who are medically and psychologically stable. It is comprised of a Le Fort 1 maxillary osteotomy to mobilize and advance the maxilla, and a bilateral sagittal split osteotomy for advancement of the distal or tooth-bearing portion of the mandible. The bones are repositioned anteriorly and carry with them all associated muscles and soft tissue attachments including the parapharyngeal tissues, tongue, and suprahyoid musculature. In addition, this procedure carries the advantage of familiarity to the oral and maxillofacial surgeon who performs orthognathic surgery. Several differences must be noted, however. Orthognathic surgery is usually performed in conjunction with orthodontics to correct a significant malocclusion or abnormal bite for a predominantly adolescent population. In contrast, telegnathic surgery patients are typically adults with comparatively normal occlusion that must be maintained postoperatively. In addition, while the surgery is considered low-risk with a 1-night hospitalization for the former group, the latter group may have higher risks of complications, requirements for a higher level of postoperative monitoring, a more difficult recovery, and a 2–5-day hospitalization.

A retrospective review of 76 patients (BMI 31 ± 7 kg/m², age 45 ± 10 years) by Boyd[16] found a 5% rate of blood transfusion, a hospitalization of 2.6 ± 1.7 days, 8% wound infections treated with local measures and antibiotics, and no deaths of cardiac events perioperatively. Objective measures of OSA were significantly reduced (AHI 54 ± 27 to 13 ± 12 and minimum oxygen saturation 78–84%) consistent with other studies reviewed. In the authors' experience, the need for perioperative blood transfusion is very low.

Several transient early postoperative issues may be quite bothersome to patients in the immediate postoperative period. Moderate to severe facial edema with or without bruising is visible immediately after surgery and may be alleviated with perioperative intravenous corticosteroid administration. There is a 75% reduction in overall edema at 2 weeks postoperatively. Low-grade epistaxis and nasal congestion are common to all patients, with some experiencing subjective dyspnea. These symptoms are typically alleviated with vasoconstrictor nasal sprays such as oxymetzoline, saline sprays, and most reliably, time. Postoperative nausea and vomiting is common, with one study finding a 75% incidence on day 1, and 43% of patients experiencing such symptoms beyond the first 24 hours after surgery.[17] Blood swallowed during orthognathic surgery is recognized as a potent irritant leading to nausea and vomiting. Use of intraoperative throat pack and gastric evacuation with an oro-gastric tube may prevent postoperative nausea and vomiting in some cases.

The postoperative course typically includes 2–8 weeks of maxillomandibular fixation (MMF, or also known as teeth wired together) to help reduce the chances of a fibrous union. The duration is variable according to surgeon experience. Maxillomandibular fixation may not be well tolerated by some patients. William and Cawood[18] found a significant increase in upper airway resistance in a group of healthy volunteers undergoing pulmonary function testing with and without MMF. Their forced expiratory volume in 1 second (FEV_1) decreased by 23% and their peak expiratory flow (PEF) decreased to 52% of baseline.

This may be troublesome in the setting of postsurgical facial edema, if symptoms of nausea and vomiting arise, and in patients with baseline chronic obstructive pulmonary disease.

Maxillomandibular fixation also limits temperomandibular joint (TMJ) movement and synovial fluid dynamics needed for normal joint homeostasis, delays rehabilitation to normal mouth opening, and limits oral hygiene. Consequentially, accumulation of thick bacterial biofilm predisposes patients to gingival and periodontal inflammation, caries, and fetor oris. Lastly, MMF has a transient negative impact on patient's quality of life.[19] Dietary modifications include a liquid or blendarized diet that is gradually advanced to soft diet over several weeks. In addition, patients must refrain from strenuous physical activity, and may be unable to return to work while an immature bony callous is forming.

Significant complications of telegnathic surgery include wound infection, bleeding including epistaxis, unfavorable osteotomy (bad split), malocclusion, neurosensory deficits, infected hardware requiring removal, non-union of bony segments, TMJ disorders, unfavorable facial appearance, and need for additional surgery. Waite et al.[20] reported a 44% incidence of minor malocclusion that required occlusal equilibration. Patients may occasionally require orthodontic treatment for larger postoperative occlusal discrepancies. While this may seem like a minor issue, orthodontics treatment with full fixed appliances may be cost prohibitive and lengthy (months to years).

A common late complication of MMA is neurosensory deficit in the trigeminal distribution. Hypoesthesia or paresthesia of the infraorbital nerve region is typically a temporary deficit that arises secondary to retraction of this nerve. However, a higher rate of permanent neurosensory deficits has been observed in the inferior alveolar nerve (IAN) distribution after sagittal split osteotomy (SSO) of the mandible. This leads to drooling in the first few weeks. Walter and Gregg[21] found an 84% incidence of neuropathy in patients undergoing SSO, while Riley et al.[10] documented 12.5% of cases with permanent IAN anesthesia. Bruckmoser et al.[22] found subjectively abnormal sensation in 25% at 6 months and 23% at 12 months after SSO. Overall, studies of postoperative IAN deficit

generally suggest a frequency of 5–40%, and the risk increases with patient age. This finding is related to a progressive decrease in marrow space within the mandible and reduced capacity for nerve regeneration with increasing age. In the authors' opinion, most patients who experience permanent hypoesthesia or areas of anesthesia do not find these to be significantly noticeable or bothersome at 6–12 months postoperatively. Dysesthesia however is poorly tolerated.

Changes in facial appearance may represent a substantial concern in patients undergoing MMA. Specifically, patients may develop excessive protrusion of the lower face with undesirable over-rotation of the nasal tip. Li et al.[23] evaluated subjective perception of facial appearance (visual analog scale [VAS] score 0–10) in 44 patients via questionnaires 6–12 months after surgery. Twenty-four (55%) of the patients reported favorable changes in their facial appearance and 14 were neutral. However 4 (40%) of 10 patients with preoperative skeletal protrusion based on cephalometric norms felt they were less attractive after surgery. This information can be used to warn patients that they are at risk for unfavorable facial changes.

Large gaps between proximal and distal bone segments of the repositioned maxilla and mandible may put patients at risk of developing non-union or a fibrous union. Gregoire[24] retrospectively reviewed 145 cases (from 1994 to 2006) with a mean maxillary and mandibular advancement of 8.7 mm and 9.5 mm, respectively. Four (3%) developed non-union of the maxilla and one (0.7%) developed non-union of the mandible. These were successfully treated with autologous bone grafting. The author[24] concluded that routine bone grafting during MMA is not warranted. Risk factors for non-union include age, the amount of advancement and gap size, rigidity of fixation applied, bone quality and quantity, postoperative infection, postoperative radiation, patient compliance with dietary restrictions, and duration of postoperative MMF.

Main points

Patients who have moderate to severe OSA and do not tolerate CPAP may be candidates for MMA. The efficacy of MMA is supported by numerous retrospective and cohort studies that demonstrate significant improvement in objective and subjective parameters. Given the extensive nature of this treatment, treating providers must carefully weigh the risk-to-benefit ratio to ensure proper patient selection. Patients must be well informed of the expected postoperative course, and significant complications that may arise. When unrealistic expectations are combined with any postoperative complications, patient dissatisfaction is guaranteed.

Although the patient described in this chapter had a typical positive outcome from MMA, our experience has shown a lower success rate with morbidly obese patients who have an AHI above 70. In this specific population, the cure rate for OSA by MMA has been about 60%. On the other hand, our patients with a BMI below 32 and an AHI below 70 have had a cure rate of 92% after MMA.

Presently we recommend a larger advancement in the subgroup of patients who are morbidly obese and have very severe OSA. The advancement is performed through bimaxillary distraction osteogenesis of 25 mm over a period of a month. After the initial distraction, the MMF by wiring the upper and lower dental arches together continues for an additional period of 3 months. The cure rate has been close to 100%, but the emotional and physical toll of such a long treatment is significant and requires considerable professional attention as well as a very motivated patient who clearly understands the length of treatment and the potential complications of the procedure.

REFERENCES

1. Parish JM, Somers VK. Obstructive sleep apnea and cardiovascular disease. *Mayo Clin Proc* 2004;**79**:1036–46.
2. Lye KW, Waite PD, Meara D, et al. Quality of life evaluation of maxillomandibular advancement surgery for treatment of obstructive sleep apnea. *J Oral Maxillofac Surg* 2008;**66**:968–72.
3. Boyd SB, Walters AS, Song Y, et al. Comparative effectiveness of maxillomandibular advancement and uvulopalatopharyngoplasty for the treatment of moderate to severe obstructive sleep apea. *J Oral Maxillofac Surg* 2013;**71**:743–51.
4. Conway WA, Victor LD, Magilligan DJ, et al. Adverse effects of tracheostomy for sleep apnea. *JAMA* 1981;**246**:347–50.
5. Thatcher GW, Maisel RH. The long-term evaluation of tracheostomy in the management of severe obstructive sleep apnea. *Laryngoscope* 2003;**113**:201–4.
6. Rasheid S, Banasiak M, Gallagher SF, et al. Gastric bypass is an effective treatment for obstructive sleep apnea in patients with clinically significant obesity. *Obes Surg* 2003;**13**:58–61.
7. Kalra M, Inge T, Garcia V, et al. Obstructive sleep apnea in extremely overweight adolescents undergoing bariatric surgery. *Obes Res* 2005;**13**:1175–9.
8. Sarkhosh K, Switzer NJ, El-Hadi M, et al. The impact of bariatric surgery on obstructive sleep apnea: a systematic review. *Obes Surg* 2013;**23**:414–23.
9. Deutzer J. Potential complications of obstructive sleep apnea in patients undergoing gastric bypass surgery. *Crit Care Nurs Q* 2005;**28**:293–9.
10. Riley RW, Powell NB, Guilleminault C. Obstructive sleep apnea syndrome: a review of 306 consecutively treated surgical patients. *Otolaryngol Head Neck Surg* 1993;**108**:117–27.
11. Dattilo DJ, Drooger SA. Outcome assessment of patients undergoing maxillofacial procedures for the treatment of sleep apnea: comparison of subjective and objective results. *J Oral Maxillofac Surg* 2004;**62**:164–8.
12. Hochban W, Conradt R, Bradenburg U, et al. Surgical maxillofacial treatment of obstructive sleep apnea. *Plast Reconstr Surg* 1997;**99**:619–26.
13. Prinsell JR. Primary and secondary telegnathic maxillomandibular advancement, with or without adjunctive procedures, for obstructive sleep apnea in adults: A literature review and treatment recommendations. *J Oral Maxillofac Surg* 2012;**70**:1659–77.
14. Lye KW, Waite PD, Meara D, et al. Quality of life evaluation of maxillomandibular advancement surgery for treatment of obstructive sleep apnea. *J Oral Maxillofac Surg* 2008;**66**:968–72.
15. Goodday R, Bourque S. Subjective outcomes of maxillomandibular advancement surgery for treatment of obstructive sleep apnea syndrome. *J Oral Maxillofac Surg* 2012;**70**:417–20.
16. Boyd S. Adverse outcomes after maxillomandibular advancement for treatment of obstructive sleep apnea. *J Oral Maxillofac Surg* 2011;**69**(Suppl.):e25–6.
17. Arbon J, Turvey, Blakey G III, et al. Evaluation of postoperative and post-discharge nausea and vomiting in orthognathic surgery patients. *J Oral Maxillofac Surg* 2011;**69**(Suppl.):e25–6.

18. William JG, Cawood JI. Effect of intermaxillary fixation on pulmonary function. *Int J Oral Maxillofac Surg* 1990;**19**:76–8.

19. Bertolini F, Russo V, Sansebastiano G. Pre- and postsurgical psycho-emotional aspects of the orthognathic surgery patient. *Int J Adult Orthodon Orthognath Surg* 2000;**15**:16–23.

20. Waite PD, Wooten V, Lachner J, et al. Maxillomandibular advancement surgery in 23 patients with obstructive sleep apnea syndrome. *J Oral Maxillofac Surg* 1989;**47**:1256–61.

21. Walter JM Jr., Gregg JM. Analysis of postsurgical neurologic alteration in the trigeminal nerve. *J Oral Surg* 1979;**37**:410–14.

22. Bruckmoser E, Bulla M, Alacamlioglu Y, et al. Factors influencing neurosensory disturbance after bilateral sagittal split osteotomy: retrospective analysis after 6 and 12 months. *Oral Surg Oral Med Oral Pathol Oral Radiol* 2013;**115**:473–82.

23. Li KK, Riley R, Powell NB, et al. Patient's perception of the facial appearance after maxillomandibular advancement for obstructive sleep apnea syndrome. *J Oral Maxillofacial Surg* 2001;**59**:377–80.

24. Gregoire CE. The need for concomitant bone grafting during maxillomandibular advancement for the treatment of obstructive sleep apnea syndrome. *J Oral Maxillofac Surg* 2007;**42**:e1–2.

Diagnosis and treatment of chronic insomnia

Occasional insomnia is part of the human experience, but chronic insomnia is unfortunately also a common, costly, and often suboptimally addressed morbidity. About one-third of individuals experience prolonged periods of insomnia at some point in their lifetimes, and the cross-sectional prevalence is estimated at about 10%. Many patients do not realize that they can bring complaints of insomnia to clinicians. Those who do so often receive assistance, but rarely the same type of assistance that they would receive if they saw a sleep specialist. Some non-sleep specialists assume that a sleep laboratory study should be informative for a patient with chronic insomnia. The most commonly offered solution to insomnia, in primary care, is prescription hypnotics. Although chronic use of a hypnotic may not be the initial intention, a good number of insomnia patients end up using pharmacologic means to control their insomnia for months or years on end.

Sleep specialists, in contrast, infrequently request sleep studies for patients with chronic insomnia, unless sleep apnea is suspected as the underlying cause, or initial strategies to control insomnia have been unsuccessful and the cause of the insomnia remains unclear. Furthermore, sleep specialists in comparison to other clinicians are often less likely to prescribe hypnotics. When sleep specialists do prescribe hypnotics, the plan almost always envisions

a limited time course, for example during adjustment-related insomnia that occurs after the death of a family member, or particular stress at work. Longer-term approaches to insomnia instead involve diagnosis and treatment of any underlying medical contributions; diagnosis and understanding of psychological contributors to the chronic insomnia; and cognitive behavioral therapy for insomnia (CBT-I) delivered over several sessions. Abundant literature, including randomized controlled trials, now supports the efficacy of CBT-I. Short-term outcomes are as good as those achieved by hypnotics, and longer-term outcomes may be better.

Nonetheless, pitfalls exist even for clinicians who see many patients with sleep complaints and take advantage of CBT-I. Some clinicians may assume that insomnia arising in the context of other medical or psychiatric morbidity must be treated by addressing that morbidity first. Although this approach is sometimes advisable, effective and timely treatment of insomnia can be particularly important for some patients with past or present alcohol dependence, depression, or certain medical complaints. The following chapters highlight cases of patients for whom missed opportunities to recognize and treat their insomnia could have led to years of unnecessary suffering from distinct – yet to a surprising extent, related – medical and psychiatric issues.

26

A sleep study is often unnecessary in a patient with chronic insomnia

Scott M. Pickett and J. Todd Arnedt

Insomnia is among the most frequent complaints in primary care, where patients with sleep problems usually first present for assistance.[1] Primary care physicians must make decisions about insomnia treatment, often while also dealing with other health concerns, during a brief office visit. Many physicians opt to obtain more diagnostic information about insomnia complaints by ordering an overnight polysomnogram (PSG). This chapter focuses on situations when such a diagnostic study may not be of value, and offers alternative suggestions for obtaining key information about an insomnia complaint that can help to guide treatment planning.

The following example illustrates a case where PSG was used following primary complaints of difficulties maintaining sleep at a primary care visit.

Case: use of PSG to confirm insomnia diagnosis

Diane was a 40-year-old woman who presented to her primary care doctor complaining of difficulties staying asleep at night. She estimated that she woke up several times each night and had trouble returning to sleep once awake. Occasionally, she also had difficulty falling asleep. Diane reported experiencing these symptoms for about the last 3 years, attributing their onset to starting a new stressful job. As a perceived result of her nighttime sleep problems, she complained of significant fatigue and lack of energy during the daytime, which in turn interfered with her work performance.

On physical exam, Diane was 5 feet, 4 inches (163 cm) tall and weighed 160 pounds (73 kg). Her blood pressure was 140/90 mmHg and her pulse rate was 72 beats per minute. She was in no acute distress and the remainder of the physical exam was unremarkable. Medical history was significant for hypertension and depression, currently managed with lisinopril and citalopram, respectively.

On the basis of Diane's report, the physician ordered an overnight sleep study, which is summarized in Table 26.1.

The sleep study was consistent with a diagnosis of insomnia, but was negative for a sleep-related breathing disorder or periodic limb movements during sleep. Diane's subjective complaints were largely confirmed, with an increased amount of stage N1 sleep (20%), elevated wake time after sleep onset (middle of the night insomnia) of 150 minutes, and reduced sleep efficiency (total sleep time/time in bed*100) of 64%. The patient's sleep latency (22 minutes), stage N3 percentage (12%), and REM percentage (18%) all were within normal limits for her age. On the basis of the sleep study results, the physician initiated a trial of controlled-release zolpidem 12.5 mg nightly to address the sleep maintenance difficulties. Diane returned to the clinic after 6 weeks, and reported substantial improvements in her difficulties with sleep maintenance and daytime fatigue.

Common Pitfalls in Sleep Medicine, ed. Ronald D. Chervin. Published by Cambridge University Press. © Cambridge University Press 2014.

Table 26.1 Summary statistics from diagnostic polysomnogram for patient

Sleep analysis			
Lights out	22:40	Wake after sleep onset (min./%TST)	150/49.5
Lights on	06:15	Stage N1 sleep (min./%TST)	60.6/20
Total recording time (TRT, mins)	475.0	Stage N2 sleep (min./%TST)	151.5/50
Total sleep time (TST, mins)	303.0	Stage N3 sleep (min./%TST)	36.4/12
Latency to sleep (mins)	22.0	Stage REM sleep (min./%TST)	54.5/18
REM latency (mins)	82.5	Sleep efficiency (TST/TRT*100)	63.8

Respiratory analysis			
Apnea/hyponea index (AHI)	1.3	Mean sleep%SpO$_2$	93
NREM AHI	1.1	Min.%SpO$_2$	91
REM AHI	2.0		
Respiratory disturbance index (RDI)	1.6		

Leg movement analysis			
Periodic leg movements (PLMs) during sleep (no.)	12	PLM index	0.3
Periodic limb movements during sleep with arousals (no.)	2	PLM arousal index	0.1

NREM, non-rapid eye movement sleep; REM, rapid eye movement sleep.

Discussion

The case above is a good example depicting the unnecessary use of a PSG for a patient complaining of insomnia. Although the patient's self-report of insomnia was objectively verified on PSG, there are several important considerations when deciding on the utility of a diagnostic sleep study for patients complaining of insomnia.

Insomnia is a *subjective* complaint and PSG is not routinely indicated unless suspicion for an organic sleep disorder is high

A key diagnostic requirement for insomnia is a *subjective* complaint of sleep disturbance.[2] Specifically, a patient must self-report difficulties initiating or maintaining sleep, or describe a pattern of sleep that is non-restorative. Additionally, perceived distress regarding the sleep disturbance or impairment in daytime activities due to the consequences of the sleep disturbance must be reported.[2] No objective verification is necessary for the diagnosis. Thus, the determination of an insomnia diagnosis should be based initially on the patient's experience, with consideration given to the need for PSG only under certain circumstances. The necessary information can typically be gathered from a patient during a short interview focused on current complaints and the history of those complaints. In addition, a few brief questions can be used to determine whether another sleep disorder may be present that might warrant overnight PSG. A series of questions aimed at an appropriate diagnosis and need for diagnostic PSG are presented in Table 26.2.

In the case example above, the primary care physician may have decided to order a sleep study to rule out an organic cause for insomnia, such as sleep apnea, because the patient reported multiple nighttime

Table 26.2 Sample assessment questions for confirmation of insomnia diagnosis

Diagnostic criteria	Initial diagnostic question	Possible follow-up questions
Problematic sleep pattern	Describe your sleep pattern over a typical week	What does a bad night of sleep look like? A good night of sleep? How many bad nights do you have in a typical week?
		How long does it typically take you to fall asleep?
		How many times do you wake up in the night? How much time do you spend awake during the night?
		How many hours of sleep do you obtain on a typical night?
		When did your sleep problem begin? Was there any specific trigger to your sleep problem?
Poor quality of sleep	How would you describe the quality of your sleep?	Is your sleep refreshing?
		Is the quality of your sleep adequate?
		Do you feel rested when you wake up?
		Restless?
Distress about sleep pattern	How do you feel about your sleep pattern?	Do you feel dissatisfied? Nervous/worried? Frustrated/angry?
		How concerned are you about your sleep problem?
Impaired daytime functioning	What daytime impact do you notice due to your sleep pattern?	As a result of your sleep pattern:
		Do you feel irritable?
		How is your mood?
		Do you feel tired? Sleepy?
		How is your concentration? Memory?
		How is your work/school performance?
Sleep-related breathing disorders	Do you or has anyone else noticed pauses in your breathing during sleep?	Do you snore loudly?
		Do you wake up gasping or choking?
Restless legs syndrome or periodic limb movements during sleep	Do you feel the overwhelming urge to move your legs that are accompanied by strange sensations, like creepy crawly feelings? Do you have leg twitches during sleep?	Do you have difficulty keeping your legs still?
		What time of day are the strange leg sensations most common?
		Are your legs relieved with movement?
		Are your leg sensations worse when you are at rest?
		Are you a restless sleeper at night?
Parasomnias	Do you have strange or disruptive behaviors during sleep?	What do you do?
		What time of night do these typically occur?
Narcolepsy	Do you fall asleep when you do not want to or without warning?	When does this happen?
		Do you notice transient weakness when you experience an intense emotion, like when you laugh, get angry, or you are startled/surprised?
		Do you ever see or hear things that aren't there when you are falling asleep?

awakenings, daytime fatigue, and a history of hypertension. However, there were several missed opportunities to ask follow-up questions that could have clarified the necessity for a PSG. For example, the patient indicated that she woke "several times each night and had trouble returning to sleep once awake" and that "occasionally, she also had difficulty falling asleep." Follow-up questions regarding the frequency and duration of the sleep disturbances could have provided the necessary information for treatment choice (e.g. the need for a longer acting sleep medication to help with sleep maintenance problems) and the responses would have been more consistent with a diagnosis of insomnia than sleep apnea. Specifically, sleep maintenance complaints in patients with sleep apnea typically include multiple, *brief* awakenings during the night, not the more extended awakenings reported in the case example. Moreover, sleep apnea patients rarely present with sleep initiation complaints, yet Diane reported that she occasionally had trouble falling asleep. Diane was also able to identify a specific trigger to her insomnia complaints, which is more consistent with a diagnosis of insomnia than sleep apnea. In Diane's case, additional symptoms suggestive of a sleep-related breathing disorder – such as loud snoring, witnessed apneas, or self-reported nocturnal gasping or choking – would be necessary to warrant overnight PSG.

A PSG may also be appropriate in instances where a patient has failed to respond to first-line insomnia treatments. In these situations, PSG is used to determine whether an occult underlying sleep disorder, for which there was low suspicion at baseline, may in fact underlie the insomnia complaints. Recent research evidence suggests that sleep-related breathing disorders can often cause insomnia symptoms, even among individuals who deny cardinal symptoms of sleep-disordered breathing on initial presentation.[3]

Polysomnogram findings can confound the insomnia diagnosis

If a PSG is ordered in the absence of symptoms suggestive of an organic sleep disorder, PSG results are likely to mirror subjective complaints, although how closely the subjective estimates and objectively derived sleep parameters correspond varies considerably among insomnia patients. In the case example, Diane's PSG revealed sleep maintenance difficulties consistent with her self-report, with a total wake after sleep onset of 150 minutes. Sleep onset fell within normal limits, but difficulty with sleep onset had been reported as occasional. Indeed, PSG research findings in people with insomnia indicate that, compared to good sleepers, they have greater difficulties with sleep continuity, such as increased sleep onset latency and time awake after sleep onset, in addition to decreased sleep efficiency and total sleep time (see, for example, Morin and Espie[4]). Further, the PSG patterns of individuals with insomnia are indicative of heightened electroencephalogram (EEG) arousal around sleep onset and during sleep, resulting in lighter, non-restorative sleep.[5]

In certain instances, the PSG may confound the insomnia diagnosis. For example, some research suggests that PSG assessments may misrepresent the experience of a patient with insomnia, because some patients may show little evidence of objective sleep abnormalities on PSG. This may occur because insomnia patients sometimes paradoxically sleep better in a novel environment, such as a sleep laboratory (the so-called reverse first night effect); the pattern of sleep disturbance is variable among insomnia sufferers, so isolated nights can be of good quality; or PSG does not adequately capture the EEG hyperarousal characteristic of many patients with insomnia. Further, patients with insomnia may appear to have better objective sleep patterns than healthy sleepers given that there is such variability in PSG data, resulting in significant overlap of the PSG distributions of good and poor sleepers.[4] If a patient's subjective complaints of sleep disturbance are dismissed in favor of reliance on PSG findings, a patient may be misrepresented as "healthy" and not receive an appropriate diagnosis or treatment.

Evidence-based assessment tools other than PSG exist to characterize subjective insomnia complaints more fully

In addition to PSG frequently being unnecessary in the diagnosis of insomnia, the sleep laboratory test is an inefficient and costly method for gathering sleep

SLEEP DIARY

Session: __/__/__ @____am/pm
(mm/dd/yy)

Fatigue	0	25	50	75	100
Rating Scale	extremely fatigued	moderately fatigued	mildly fatigued	somewhat energetic	very energetic

COMPLETE AT NIGHT in reference to today   **COMPLETE IN MORNING** in reference to previous night

Day and Date	Fatigue rating	Naps (Start and end times)	Sleep meds or alcohol (Name & dose)	Time you went to bed and turned out the lights	How long it took you to fall asleep for the first time	Number of times you woke up after falling asleep	How long you were awake during the night	Time you woke up this morning for the last time	Time you got up for good	Total sleep time	Quality rating: 1=very poor 2=poor 3=fair 4=good 5=excellent	Restfulness rating: 1=not at all 2=slightly 3=somewhat 4=rested 5=well rested
TU 8-9	50	none	R(15)10³⁰ R(15)2³⁰	10³⁰	30 min	2	1 hr	5³⁰	6³⁰	5½	2	2
Wed 8.9	50	none	R(15)10⁵⁰ R(15)11³⁰	10³⁰	1½ hr	2	2 hrs	6⁰⁰	6³⁰	4	2	2
TH 8.10	25	none	R(15)10⁵⁵ R(15)12²⁵	10³⁰	2 hr	1	15 min	7³⁰	7³⁰	6½	3	2
FR 8.11	40	1ᵖᵐ- 1³⁰ᵖᵐ	R(15)10⁵⁵ R(15)½12	10⁴⁵	1 hr	1	1 hr	8⁰⁰	8¹³	7¼	3	2
SAT 8-12	70	none	R(15)10⁴⁰ R(15)11⁴⁵	10⁴³	2½	2	1 hr	7⁰⁰	7⁰⁰	5¾	2	2
SUN 8.13	50	none	R(30)10⁴⁵	11¹⁵	15 min	3	2 hr	7³⁰	7⁴⁰	5-6	2	3
MON 8.14	70	none	R(30)10:15	10¹⁵	15 min	1	1 hr	7⁰⁰	7⁰⁰	7½	3	3

Figure 26.1 Sample 1-week sleep–wake diary for a patient with insomnia and taking medication (mirtazapine 15 mg twice per night).

information in insomnia patients. Given the night-to-night variability in insomnia symptoms, assessment over multiple nights is preferred, to generate stable and representative sleep information. Such assessment is typically accomplished with daily sleep–wake diaries. These are simple, self-report measures that provide night-to-night information on sleep pattern, quality, and relevant daytime behavior. An example of a sleep diary completed by an insomnia patient is shown in Figure 26.1. Recently, consensus was reached by an expert panel of insomnia researchers about the specific information that should be included in a sleep–wake diary.[6]

The primary advantage of sleep–wake diaries over PSG is that they provide prospective, subjective assessments of sleep patterns over multiple nights, in the home environment. Patients typically maintain a diary daily for at least 2 consecutive weeks, during a time when they expect to be engaged in their normal daily activities. During the initial assessment period, patients are discouraged from adjusting any of their habits, but instead are asked to maintain their nightly routines. The sleep–wake diary can be especially helpful for characterizing the nature, frequency, and severity of sleep problems at baseline and then can be used as a tool to monitor progress during treatment. Sleep information is typically summarized with averages over an assessment period for the following sleep parameters: bedtime, rise time, sleep onset latency, frequency of nighttime awakenings, wake after sleep onset, total sleep time, sleep efficiency, and sleep quality. Sleep–wake diary assessments provide integral information to inform both medication and non-medication insomnia treatments.

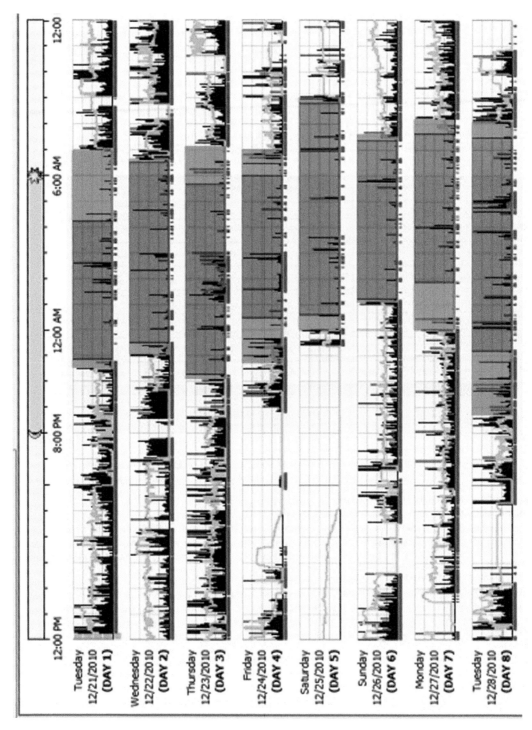

Figure 26.2 Sample 8 days of actigraphy from a patient with insomnia. Twenty-four hour activity data are presented from 12:00 PM on one day to 12:00 PM the following day. Black vertical bars represented activity and the yellow line represents light levels. Cyan shaded areas represent time in bed according to sleep diary information; blue shaded areas indicate estimated sleep periods according to the actigraphy analysis software. Note the variability in the bedtimes and rise times (particularly the early bedtime on the last day) and the significant wakefulness each day during the attempted sleep period. See plate section for color version.

Validated global self-report scales also exist to evaluate insomnia complaints. The best known and most widely used of these scales is the Insomnia Severity Index,[7] a seven-item questionnaire that assesses the nature, severity, and impact of sleep problems. This scale has been used in several randomized controlled treatment trials of insomnia and, recently, definitions of insomnia treatment response and remission have been developed,[8] providing another gauge of treatment progress and facilitating clinical decisions about the need for ongoing treatment.

Aside from PSG, another alternative objective measure of sleep and wake is actigraphy. Actigraphs are small watch-like devices that are worn on the nondominant wrist. Actigraphs provide continuous information on activity levels over several days to weeks. Validated software algorithms evaluate the activity and provide estimates of sleep and wake activity during the assessment period. Sleep episodes can be reliably identified when actigraphy information is considered along with other measures of sleep and wake, such as a concurrent sleep–wake diary. An example of actigraphy results for an insomnia patient is shown in Figure 26.2.

Compared to PSG, actigraphy is a low-cost alternative that can provide objective information over several days to weeks. It is important to note, however, that actigraphy yields only an indirect measure of sleep. The actigraphy scoring software also has difficulty differentiating sleep from quiet wakefulness, so the correspondence of actigraphy with PSG-measured sleep is higher for good sleepers than for sleep-disordered populations. Nevertheless, current practice guidelines indicate that actigraphy can be useful in the assessment of insomnia, particularly when a circadian rhythm sleep disorder is suspected to be causally related to the insomnia complaints, and in evaluation of treatment response after insomnia interventions.[9]

Main points

- Subjective complaints of sleep disturbance and related impairments are key to an insomnia diagnosis.

- The use of PSG may confound an insomnia diagnosis by misrepresenting a patient's experience.
- Differential diagnosis assessment questions can help to determine whether the use of PSG is necessary.
- The most common reason to obtain a PSG, for a patient with insomnia, is to evaluate the possibility as suggested by relevant symptoms that obstructive sleep apnea could contribute to the sleep disturbance.
- Several validated measures of insomnia are available to corroborate clinical interview findings.
- Given the variability of insomnia symptoms on a night-to-night basis, the use of a sleep diary and actigraphy may be helpful to assess a patient's experience across time (e.g. a 2-week period).

REFERENCES

1. Simon GE, Von Korff M. Prevalence, burden, and treatment of insomnia in primary care. *Am J Psychiatry* 1997; **154**:1417–23.
2. American Academy of Sleep Medicine. *International Classification of Sleep Disorders. Diagnostic and Coding Manual*, Second Edition. Westchester, IL: American Academy of Sleep Medicine;2005.
3. Krakow B, Romero, E, Ulibarri VA, Kikta S. Prospective assessment of nocturnal awakenings in a case series of treatment-seeking chronic insomnia patients: a pilot study of subjective and objective causes. *Sleep* 2012;**35**:1685–92.
4. Morin CM, Espie CA. *Insomnia: A Clinical Guide to Assessment and Treatment*. New York, NY: Kluwer Academic/Plenum Publishers;2003.
5. Perlis ML, Merica H, Smith MT, Giles DE. Beta EEG activity and insomnia. *Sleep Med Rev* 2001;**5**:1–12.
6. Carney CE, Buysse DJ, Ancoli-Israel S, et al. The consensus sleep diary: standardizing prospective sleep self-monitoring. *Sleep* 2012;**35**:287–302.
7. Morin CM. *Insomnia: Psychological Assessment and Management*. New York, NY: The Guilford Press;1993.
8. Morin CM, Belleville G, Bélanger L, Ivers H. The insomnia severity index: psychometric indicators to detect insomnia cases and evaluate treatment response. *Sleep* 2011;**34**:601–8.
9. Morgenthaler T, Alessi C, Friedman L, et al. Practice parameters for the use of actigraphy in the assessment of sleep and sleep disorders: an update for 2007. *Sleep* 2007;**30**:519–29.

27

Chronic use of hypnotics is unnecessary and can be counterproductive

Leslie M. Swanson and Todd Favorite

Case

A 59-year-old married Caucasian female presented with a 17-year history of difficulty falling asleep and frequent nighttime awakenings. Her medical history was significant for diabetes, obesity, and obstructive sleep apnea. She reported good adherence to continuous positive airway pressure (CPAP). The patient's insomnia treatment history included use for 6 years of an over-the-counter sleep aid, which the patient discontinued in favor of zolpidem (Ambien) 5 mg as recommended by her primary care physician. During 1 year of nightly use, the zolpidem 5 mg became less effective and she required a larger dose to fall asleep. Her physician increased the dose to 10 mg and referred her to behavioral sleep medicine for a trial of cognitive behavioral therapy for insomnia (CBT-I) because of concern that she had developed tolerance to zolpidem.

During her intake evaluation for CBT-I, the patient stated "I can't fall asleep without medication." When she used zolpidem, her self-reported sleep onset latency was around 60 minutes; without it, her sleep onset latency was at least 120 minutes, and often longer. Exploration of the patient's thoughts about sleep revealed a firmly entrenched belief that she would not be able to sleep without a hypnotic medication.

During the first treatment session, the patient was instructed to follow stimulus control rules (e.g. to leave the bed in favor of engaging in quiet, relaxing activities in another room if she was unable to sleep), and to reduce the frequency of her zolpidem use to every other night.

She was prescribed a 6-hour time-in-bed schedule (sleep restriction). Her habitual bedtime was delayed by 2 hours to achieve the restricted time-in-bed schedule.

When the patient returned for her next session 2 weeks later, her sleep diaries showed poor adherence to the prescribed sleep schedule, and continued nightly use of zolpidem. When queried about her difficulties with adhering to the prescribed interventions, it became apparent that her preoccupation with her need for sleep medication was a major barrier. For example, she stated, "I can't go to bed that late because I take my Ambien much earlier and it puts me to sleep. I don't want to take Ambien later in the evening because I might be groggy in the morning." The patient remained resistant to numerous efforts to increase her adherence, including psychoeducation and motivational enhancement techniques. The patient expressed doubt about the effectiveness of CBT-I, stating "I know Ambien will put me to sleep even if I wake up during the night. I don't know if your strategy will help me to fall asleep and it sounds more difficult than just taking medication."

After four subsequent sessions of treatment focused on helping the patient to engage in treatment, she was still unable to adhere to sleep restriction and stimulus control. Although she made a few improvements in her sleep hygiene, such as reducing her caffeine intake and limiting her food intake during the night, she remained resistant to other changes in her sleep environment and continued to use zolpidem nightly. Treatment was terminated with little improvement in the patient's insomnia, and minimal change in the

Common Pitfalls in Sleep Medicine, ed. Ronald D. Chervin. Published by Cambridge University Press. © Cambridge University Press 2014.

patient's sense of self-efficacy regarding her ability to improve her sleep without medication.

Discussion

What are the risks and benefits of pharmacologic treatment for insomnia?

Pharmacotherapies are commonly used to treat insomnia. Frequently used over-the-counter agents include antihistamines, melatonin, and herbal supplements such as valerian. Limited data exist to support the effectiveness of over-the-counter medications for chronic insomnia. Prescribed hypnotic medications include benzodiazepines, benzodiazepine receptor agonists, sedating antidepressants, sedating antipsychotics, and anticonvulsants. Of the pharmacotherapies for insomnia, benzodiazepines and benzodiazepine receptor agonists have the most research to support their efficacy.[1] However, the majority of these studies are conducted over short periods, and scant data have been generated to support long-term (i.e. longer than 6 months) efficacy and safety. Thus, guidelines for management of chronic insomnia state that hypnotic medications are indicated for short-term use only.[2]

The major benefit of hypnotics is immediate symptom relief produced with very little effort on behalf of the patient. Hypnotics may be most useful when prescribed for short periods in patients with acute insomnia (i.e. symptoms have been present for < 4 weeks), particularly when the insomnia is associated with a specific, transient stressor. When initiated before insomnia becomes chronic, hypnotic medications theoretically prevent factors that perpetuate insomnia from taking hold. Patients with insomnia often engage in behaviors to manage their sleep loss, such as spending a long amount of time in bed in the hope that they will make up for lost sleep, napping, "sleeping in" on the weekends, and excessive caffeine or alcohol use. In many cases, these behaviors actually perpetuate the insomnia by weakening sleep drive, dysregulating circadian rhythms, and increasing hyperarousal.[3,4] For example, patients who spend long amounts of time in bed while they are awake may develop conditioned arousal to the bedroom, such that the bed and

bedroom environment become a stimulus for wakefulness, and not sleep. Thus, short-term prescription of a hypnotic early in the course of insomnia, before the perpetuating behaviors begin, may prevent the development of these behaviors and stop the insomnia from progressing to a chronic disorder.

As in the case described above, most patients who present for insomnia treatment have developed a chronic condition. The persistent nature of insomnia, coupled with the tendency for patients to relapse when they discontinue a hypnotic, leads to long-term hypnotic use for many patients who initiate a medication for sleep. Risks of chronic hypnotic use include side effects (e.g. daytime sedation, anterograde amnesia, increased risk for falls, and complex sleep-related behaviors), tolerance, dependence, and abuse or misuse. This case illustrates a common clinical trajectory, whereby a patient begins an over-the-counter medication for sleep, switches to a prescribed hypnotic after consulting a physician for treatment, develops tolerance over time, and must use an increasingly higher dose to treat the symptoms. Eventually, tolerance can develop even to the maximum safe dosage, and patients may be left with suboptimal options of either a new medication that may again lead to tolerance, or discontinuation of the drug, often accompanied by a relapse to insomnia.

In patients who have developed chronic insomnia, with symptoms that have persisted for a month or longer, long-term hypnotic use may lead to the development of hypnotic-dependent insomnia.[5] A chain of events leading to hypnotic-dependent insomnia can be triggered by withdrawal symptoms that occur upon discontinuation of the medication. Rebound insomnia, which may represent physiologic withdrawal, is often a consequence of abrupt discontinuation of hypnotics that have been used for a long period.[6] Rebound insomnia may manifest as recrudescence or a transient exacerbation of the original condition. Some cases result in insomnia symptoms that are far worse than what the patient had experienced prior to using the medication. The return of insomnia symptoms after discontinuation of the hypnotic often increases anxiety for the patient. The heightened anxiety may in turn maintain insomnia symptoms even after the physiologic withdrawal effects have dissipated. Feeling anxious and unable to sleep, the patient resumes the hypnotic, or requests a different medication for sleep. Use of the medication immediately alleviates the insomnia and sleep-related anxiety. This process powerfully reinforces medication use. The reinforcement increases the likelihood that the patient will continue regular use of the hypnotic. It also further strengthens the patient's belief that sleep will not occur without medication, and a psychological dependence on the drug may develop.

As abrupt discontinuation of a hypnotic is associated with withdrawal symptoms, a supervised gradual taper of medication dose and frequency is recommended in patients who are using a hypnotic regularly.[5] This can be achieved by reducing the dose by small increments over several days, and/or lengthening intervals between medication administration to every other or every third night. Although the process may take several weeks or longer, it is generally more tolerable for patients than abrupt discontinuation.

What non-pharmacologic treatment options should be considered for chronic insomnia?

When considering interventions for chronic insomnia, established guidelines state that behavioral interventions should be first-line treatments; further, even patients who are prescribed a short-term hypnotic should be referred for behavioral interventions when possible.[2] Behavioral interventions for insomnia are often implemented within the multicomponent therapy of CBT-I.[7] Cognitive behavioral therapy typically includes several behavioral strategies such as sleep restriction, stimulus control, and relaxation training, and may also include cognitive components such as identification and restructuring of maladaptive beliefs about sleep. The treatment directly targets the factors that perpetuate insomnia. Sessions are typically 30–60 minutes long. The course of treatment is relatively brief, lasting between four and eight sessions, with most patients completing treatment in six sessions.

The efficacy of CBT for primary insomnia and comorbid insomnia has been well-established through numerous studies.[8] Comparisons between CBT and hypnotics generally show that the treatments are equally effective in the short term. However, CBT is superior to medications in the long term, as patients who have completed CBT often maintain insomnia remission for years after treatment has been completed, whereas many patients who use medications relapse upon discontinuation.

Unlike a medication, CBT-I requires significant effort on behalf of the patient, and treatment gains will be minimal if the patient does not adhere to the program. Some of the elements of CBT-I that are critical to success (e.g. sleep restriction, stimulus control) can be challenging to implement and have transient side effects, such as increased daytime sleepiness, that are difficult for some patients to tolerate. Thus, the patient's motivation is important. As illustrated by the case above, chronic use of hypnotics may

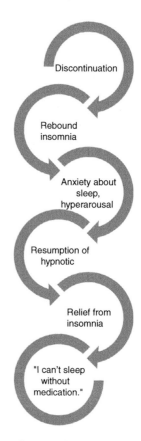

Figure 27.1 Development of hypnotic dependence.

compromise patients' ability to adopt the more challenging aspects of treatment, and may render patients
less willing to endure the uncomfortable, though transient, side effects.

Nevertheless, CBT can provide an effective treatment option for patients who attempt to discontinue
a medication for sleep.[9] Higher rates of successful
hypnotic discontinuation are observed when CBT is
added to a systematic hypnotic taper program relative
to taper alone. Furthermore, using CBT during a hypnotic taper is associated with improved subjective
sleep relative to taper alone. Some patients who are
using hypnotics while receiving CBT spontaneously
reduce their hypnotic usage on their own. However,
combining CBT with a structured, supervised hypnotic
taper program is associated with the best outcomes
with respect to long-term remission of insomnia.

Main points

Pharmacotherapies are commonly used to treat
chronic insomnia. However, they are not curative and
long-term use is associated with risk for tolerance and
dependence. Hypnotic-dependent insomnia can
emerge from chronic hypnotic use (Figure 27.1). Non-
pharmacologic treatment options should often be considered as first-line interventions for chronic insomnia.

REFERENCES

1. Krystal AD. A compendium of placebo-controlled trials of
   the risks/benefits of pharmacological treatments for
   insomnia: the empirical basis for US clinical practice. *Sleep
   Med Rev* 2009;**13**:265–74.
2. NIH State-of-the-Science Conference Statement on manifestations and management of chronic insomnia in adults.
   NIH Consensus State Sci Statements 2005;**22**:1–30.
3. Morin CM. *Insomnia: psychological assessment and management.* New York, NY: Guilford;1993.
4. Jefferson C, Drake C, Scofield H, et al. Sleep hygiene practices in a population-based sample of insomniacs. *Sleep*
   2005;**28**:611–15.
5. Bélanger L. Management of hypnotic discontinuation in
   chronic insomnia. *Sleep Med Clin* 2009;**4**:583–92.
6. Licata SC, Rowlett JK. Abuse and dependence liability of
   benzodiazepine-type drugs: $GABA_A$ receptor modulation
   and beyond. *Pharmacol Biochem Behav* 2008;**90**:74–89.
7. Spielman AJ, Caruso LS, Glovinsky PB. A behavioral perspective on insomnia treatment. *Psychiatric Clin North Am*
   1987;**10**:541–53.
8. Mitchell M, Gehrman P, Perlis M, Umscheid C.
   Comparative effectiveness of cognitive behavioral therapy
   for insomnia: a systematic review. *BMC Fam Pract*
   2012;**13**:40.
9. Morin CM. Randomized clinical trial of supervised tapering
   and cognitive behavior therapy to facilitate benzodiazepine
   discontinuation in older adults with chronic insomnia. *Am
   J Psychiatry* 2004;**161**:332–42.

28

Overlooking insomnia in a depressed patient can interfere with effective treatment for the mood disorder

Edward D. Huntley and J. Todd Arnedt

Approximately half of all Americans will fulfill diagnostic criteria for a mental disorder at some point in their life. The lifetime prevalence estimate for depression is 16.2%.[1] Individuals who experience depression and insomnia generally fare worse than do people with depression only, and patients commonly continue to report insomnia even after successful treatment of their depression.[2] Therefore, insomnia is a significant risk factor for new onset,[3] relapse, and recurrence of depression.[4] The following case examples highlight common clinical scenarios in which depression treatment was optimized by appropriately considering insomnia in patients presenting with comorbid depression and insomnia.

Case 1: treatment of insomnia can effectively reduce depression symptoms

A 30-year-old Caucasian female presented with a 7-month history of depression with features of anxiety and insomnia. The patient was referred to the Behavioral Sleep Medicine clinic after she discontinued cognitive behavioral therapy (CBT) for depression due to minimal symptom relief. She attributed the onset of her current depressive episode to moving cross-country to begin a new job, which she found stressful, and she reported few new social supports since moving. She also reported difficulty coping with stressors related to the new job because of difficulty concentrating, low motivation, and excessive fatigue. She attributed these symptoms primarily to her difficulty sleeping through the night. She was generally healthy but in the past 7 months reportedly gained 20 pounds (9 kg) after she stopped exercising due to fatigue and anhedonia. She reported excessive guilt associated with her current job performance, and her weight gain contributed to a negative appraisal of her body image.

Despite the patient's prominent sleep disturbance complaints, no assessment of these complaints had been undertaken at her initial psychiatric consultation. On evaluation at the Behavioral Sleep Medicine clinic, the patient described nightly poor sleep quality with difficulties maintaining sleep. She reported an average of nearly 3 awakenings per night with a mean wake after sleep onset time of over 90 minutes (Table 28.1). Although she denied current difficulty initiating sleep or early morning awakenings, she indicated that she fell asleep on her couch nearly every night while watching television because she would feel "more awake" and unable to relax in her own bedroom. When awake during the night, she reported remaining in bed, clock-watching, and feeling physically restless and bored, ruminating about being awake and how she would feel the next day. On nights after a poor night of sleep, she would typically attempt to initiate sleep earlier than her habitual bedtime. On the weekends, she would "sleep in" late into the morning in an effort to "catch up" on lost sleep.

The patient dated the onset of her insomnia difficulties to her early childhood, stating, "I've always been a

Common Pitfalls in Sleep Medicine, ed. Ronald D. Chervin. Published by Cambridge University Press. © Cambridge University Press 2014.

Table 28.1 Summary sleep diary data and self-reported symptom inventories

	Week of intervention							
	Baseline	1	2	3	4	5	6	4-week follow-up
SOL (min)*	28.6 (13.8)	21.4 (7.8)	14.3 (5.3)	12.1 (8.9)	7.1 (6.5)	5.7 (4.6)	6.4 (2.4)	9.4 (3.8)
FNA*	2.7 (1.4)	2.5 (1.3)	2.0 (0.8)	1.4 (0.9)	0.7 (0.8)	0.7 (0.8)	1.5 (1.2)	0.4 (0.9)
WASO (min)*	91.4 (70.5)	61.4 (18.7)	39.6 (49.3)	25.7 (17.9)	13.6 (9.8)	5.0 (5.8)	8.6 (6.3)	3.0 (6.7)
TIB (hours)*	8.4 (2.2)	7.4 (1.1)	6.7 (0.7)	6.7 (1.2)	7.1 (1.5)	7.4 (0.9)	7.1 (0.9)	7.8 (1.3)
TST (hours)*	6.4 (1.9)	6.0 (1.2)	5.8 (0.9)	6.1 (1.0)	6.8 (1.6)	7.2 (0.9)	6.8 (0.9)	7.6 (1.3)
SE%*	76.3 (12.5)	80.8 (5.8)	86.9 (10.5)	90.9 (4.4)	94.7 (3.5)	97.6 (1.4)	96.5 (1.5)	97.3 (2.1)
ISI	25		16		9		4	4
PHQ-9	19		11		5		4	2
GAD	12		9		7		4	3

Note: * indicates mean (standard deviation). SOL indicates sleep onset latency. FNA indicates frequency of night awakenings. WASO indicates wake after sleep onset time. TIB indicates time in bed. TST indicates total sleep time. SE indicates sleep efficiency. ISI indicates insomnia severity index (scale range: 0–28; scores $\geq$ 11 fall in the clinical range). PHQ-9 indicates Patient Health Questionnaire 9-item scale (scale range: 0–27; scores $\geq$ 5 fall in the clinical range). GAD-7 indicates Generalized Anxiety Disorder 7-item scale (scale range: 0–21; scores $\geq$ 5 fall in the clinical range).

bad sleeper." These sleep problems reportedly resolved by her early twenties after she completed graduate school and started her career. She experienced a recurrence of her insomnia symptoms shortly after starting her new job, and her symptoms continued to increase in severity as she struggled with the daytime impairments caused by her insomnia. She began to experience symptoms of depression a month after her difficulty sleeping had reappeared.

Aside from insomnia, the patient denied symptoms of other sleep disorders such as obstructive sleep apnea, restless legs syndrome, and circadian rhythm sleep disorders. Her medical history was unremarkable and her psychiatric history, other than the depression diagnosis, was negative.

The initial diagnostic consideration was psychophysiologic insomnia, as suggested for example by the sleep-focused ruminations and an apparent association between bedroom stimuli and arousal. In addition, her poor sleep hygiene practices, including excessive time in bed and an inconsistent sleep schedule, likely contributed to the maintenance of her insomnia complaints. Given her history of insomnia in childhood, a diagnosis of idiopathic insomnia was also considered. A 6-week course of cognitive behavioral therapy for insomnia (CBT-I) was initiated, with

sleep restriction and stimulus control therapy, supplemented by sleep hygiene psychoeducation. Cognitive therapy addressed her tendency to ruminate. The patient had a favorable response after 6 weeks of treatment and maintained this initial treatment response at 1-month follow-up (Table 28.1).

Discussion

Poor sleep is reported in up to 90% of people diagnosed with depression.[5] Therefore depression and insomnia occurring together is a common presentation for psychiatric referrals. However, it is a common mistake for clinicians assessing depression to assume that a complaint of insomnia would be subsumed by a diagnosis of depression rather than representing a primary comorbid diagnosis. This may have been the assumption that the initial clinician made, which may explain why the patient's insomnia was not an initial focus of treatment. A simple timeline (Figure 28.1a) can be utilized during the initial evaluation to chart the onset and intensity of depression and insomnia symptoms. The timeline can provide a sense of how independent the two problems are, or how they covary over time. For example, this patient's insomnia symptoms had an earlier onset and greater severity relative

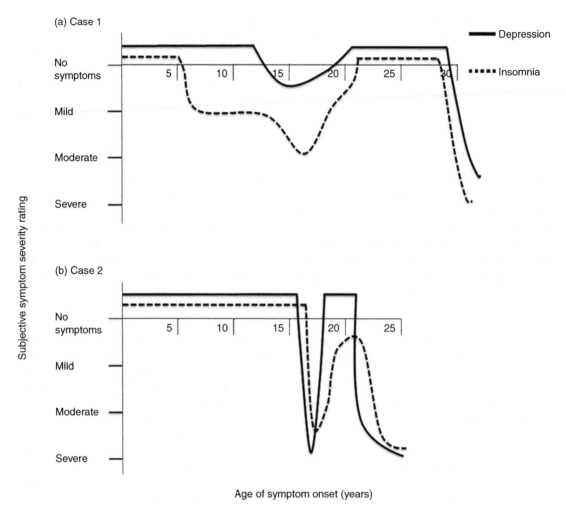

Figure 28.1 Timeline of depression and insomnia symptom onset and self-reported symptom severity for (a) Case 1 and (b) Case 2.

to her depression symptoms, making her insomnia a salient target for intervention. In addition, the patient's former course of insomnia was overlooked as a predisposing factor that increased vulnerability to the development of depression. This case example highlights that an accurate assessment of the trajectory of psychiatric symptoms is critical to the diagnosis and subsequent treatment planning. In addition, sleep problems first presenting in adolescence may persist into adulthood; therefore this case highlights that a complete history of a patient's sleep difficulties and

associated daytime impairments is warranted when insomnia symptoms are present.

Determining the sequencing of interventions when co-occurring diagnoses such as depression and insomnia are present is an important step in treatment planning. This patient's initial entry into therapy was focused on her depression rather than sleep. Yet she remained fatigued and she attributed this symptom to her low motivation and subsequent ambivalence about therapy. As the patient's insomnia and frequent night wakings predated her depression symptoms, interventions to target her sleep would have been an alternative starting point for therapy. Given that the patient had discontinued a previous course of therapy, it was critical to engage her actively in identification of treatment goals and to assess her motivation to address her depression and sleep concerns. The patient indicated that her sleep and fatigue were most salient to her. These were the symptoms she wanted to address initially. However, if the patient's history of insomnia symptoms had revealed that they coincided with the onset of depression symptoms and remitted once depression improved, a reasonable approach would have been to target the depression symptoms initially or the depression and sleep disturbances concurrently.

The failure of this client's initial course of therapy also highlights the importance of ongoing assessment throughout the course of therapy. Had the initial clinician included symptom inventories relevant to the client's presenting concerns, her ongoing sleep concerns and daytime functioning might have been identified and incorporated into the treatment plan. Therefore, it is highly recommended that clinicians treating co-occurring depression and insomnia utilize daily sleep dairies to monitor subjective sleep estimates as well as evidence-based self-reported symptom inventories such as the Patient Health Questionnaire (PHQ-9), Generalized Anxiety Disorder 7-item scale (GAD-7), and insomnia severity index (ISI). In the present case, as seen in Table 28.1, the client had a positive response to behavioral interventions, with significant reductions in mood symptoms achieved by focusing on insomnia. Cognitive behavioral therapy for insomnia has demonstrated efficacy for reducing depression[6] and for improving both insomnia and depression in patients with comorbid insomnia and mild to moderate depression.[7] The patient's sleep diaries did indicate significant variability in her sleep efficiency and wake after sleep onset (WASO) over the initial course of treatment. After review of the client's GAD-7 score, which indicated a moderate level of worry (total scores < 5 fall within normal limits), cognitive interventions were initiated to reduce cognitive arousal after nighttime awakenings. Thus, ongoing assessment permits evaluation of treatment gains and, at the same time,

can provide critical indications to change the course of treatment. If a response to insomnia interventions is evident without a corresponding mood response, for example, further assessment of mood may be indicated and the course of clinical intervention should be reevaluated.

Case 2: augmenting antidepressant treatment with CBT-I improves outcomes in patients with comorbid depression and insomnia

A 22-year-old, African-American female nursing student presented to the Behavioral Sleep Medicine Clinic with chief complaints of difficulties both initiating and maintaining sleep. She dated the onset of her insomnia to her first episode of depression during her junior year of high school. During that episode, she described difficulties both initiating and maintaining sleep, which continued periodically despite subsequent resolution of her depression symptoms. During the last 6 months, she reported a recurrence of depression symptoms, triggered by the death of a close relative. Her insomnia symptoms also returned and both the depression and insomnia had become progressively worse. In the fall, she stopped attending nursing school to focus on recovery. Since that time, sleep initiation and maintenance difficulties continued to worsen, and she now reported obtaining only about 2–3 hours of sleep each night. She endorsed depression rumination when unable to sleep, with some sleep-specific concerns. The patient reported that she was very inactive during the day, spending most of the time in her room in bed. She described low energy and a lack of desire to interact with her friends and family. She denied caffeine, alcohol, smoking, exercising, or current substance use. Apart from depression and insomnia, the patient reported no other chronic medical conditions.

The patient initiated depression treatment with a community psychiatrist and therapist a month prior to presenting to the Behavioral Sleep Medicine Clinic. She was started on bupropion 100 mg daily, trazodone 25 mg nightly, and alprazolam 0.25 mg as needed.

A referral to the Behavioral Sleep Medicine clinic was initiated for further evaluation and consideration of cognitive-behavioral treatment for insomnia.

On evaluation, the patient described current difficulties both initiating and maintaining sleep. She denied early morning awakenings. Primary daytime symptoms attributed to the sleep complaints included extreme fatigue and low energy, and worsening depression symptoms after particularly bad nights of sleep. She denied symptoms suggestive of other sleep disorders. Physical exam was within normal limits. She described her mood as "depressed" and noted no response to either the mood or sleep medications.

The initial diagnostic consideration was insomnia due to a mental disorder. The initial treatment recommendations included increasing trazodone from 25 mg to 50 mg with reassessment of treatment response after a month. Cognitive behavioral therapy for insomnia was recommended once depression symptoms were more improved. The patient was encouraged to focus diligently on better mood management.

The patient returned after a month and reported significant improvement in both her insomnia and depression symptoms. She had increased her daytime activity and was more engaged with friends and family. She was participating actively in her depression treatment. At this point, in collaboration with the psychiatrist, the patient was slowly weaned from trazodone 50 mg and a trial of CBT-I was initiated. She completed a 6-week course of CBT-I with good treatment response.

Discussion

As seen in Figure 28.1b, this patient's depression and insomnia co-varied closely over time, which illustrates the importance of a complete history of insomnia. For this patient, depression symptoms were more severe and warranted greater attention as the initial target of treatment. In addition, the use of an antidepressant medication with hypnotic effects (trazodone) improved the patient's sleep quality until her depression symptoms improved, at which point initiating CBT-I was feasible. Cognitive behavioral therapy for insomnia has been utilized to augment antidepressants, contributing to higher rates of remission of depression and insomnia relative to antidepressant therapy alone.[8] In many cases, CBT-I is contraindicated in patients with co-occurring insomnia and depression when depression symptoms are unstable or severe. In the example above, the patient presented with significant vegetative symptoms that would likely limit her level of engagement in therapy and her ability to adhere to interventions like sleep restriction and stimulus control therapy, which require a high level of motivation and organization to initiate and utilize consistently. Therefore, in presentations where depression symptoms are unstable or motivation is perceived to be low, it is often best to sequence interventions with an initial focus on stabilizing depression symptoms before addressing symptoms of insomnia. If focus on insomnia is desired, hypnotic medication when safe may be preferable to CBT-I given concerns about adherence with cognitive and behavioral sleep recommendations. In addition, it is worth noting that some aspects of CBT-I, most notably those strategies likely to induce sleep deprivation, can exacerbate symptoms of depression in certain patients.

Main points

- A thorough history of sleep problems is critical in comorbid depression and insomnia to set appropriate treatment goals and sequence clinical interventions.
- For some patients, treating insomnia alone can lead to clinically significant reductions in depression symptoms.
- For other patients, depression treatment should be prioritized when symptoms are severe or unstable, even in the presence of clinically significant insomnia symptoms.
- Cognitive behavioral therapy for insomnia can be used to augment antidepressant therapy concurrently or after depression-focused treatment, and in comparison to depression treatment alone, may produce higher rates of remission of depression and insomnia.

REFERENCES

1. Kessler RC, Berglund P, Demler O, et al. The epidemiology of major depressive disorder: results from the National Comorbidity Survey Replication (NCS-R). *JAMA* 2003;**289**:3095–105.
2. Carney CE, Segal ZV, Edinger JD, Krystal AD. A comparison of rates of residual insomnia symptoms following pharmacotherapy or cognitive-behavioral therapy for major depressive disorder. *J Clin Psychiatry* 2007;**68**:254–60.
3. Buysse DJ, Angst J, Gamma A, et al. Prevalence, course, and comorbidity of insomnia and depression in young adults. *Sleep* 2008;**31**:473–80.
4. Ford DE, Kamerow DB. Epidemiologic study of sleep disturbances and psychiatric disorders. An opportunity for prevention? *JAMA* 1989;**262**:1479–84.
5. Tsuno N, Besset A, Ritchie K. Sleep and depression. *J Clin Psychiatry* 2005;**66**:1254–69.
6. Morin CM, Kowatch RA, O'Shanick G. Sleep restriction for the inpatient treatment of insomnia. *Sleep* 1990;**13**:183–6.
7. Taylor DJ, Lichstein KL, Weinstock J, Sanford S, Temple JR. A pilot study of cognitive-behavioral therapy of insomnia in people with mild depression. *Behav Ther* 2007;**38**:49–57.
8. Manber R, Edinger JD, Gress JL, et al. Cognitive behavioral therapy for insomnia enhances depression outcome in patients with comorbid major depressive disorder and insomnia. *Sleep* 2008;**31**:489–95.

29

Overlooking insomnia in a patient with alcohol abuse or dependence can increase risk of relapse

Deirdre A. Conroy

Insomnia is a common sleep complaint among patients who are actively drinking alcohol, and also among patients who have stopped drinking. When alcohol is consumed close to bedtime, it shortens time to fall asleep, prolongs latency to the onset of rapid eye movement sleep, and increases slow-wave sleep in the first half of the night. However, sleep quality is often worsened in the second half of the night. With chronic alcohol use, tolerance may develop to the sedating side effects but the alcohol may continue to have disruptive effects on sleep.[1] The DSM-IV lists insomnia among its list of symptoms that can occur within several hours to a few days after cessation of alcohol use. Among alcohol-dependent patients undergoing treatment, the average rate of self-reported insomnia ranges from 36 to 91%,[2] substantially higher than rates of insomnia among the general population.

Insomnia and alcoholism can have a reciprocal relationship.[1] In an epidemiologic study, the incidence of alcohol abuse or dependence during a 1-year follow-up period was twice as high in individuals with persistent complaints of insomnia as it was in individuals without insomnia complaints, after controlling for baseline psychiatric disorders.[3] Both polysomnographic and subjective findings of disturbed sleep among alcohol dependent patients have been associated with higher rates of relapse. These individuals with insomnia may be more likely to turn to alcohol or other sedating medications as a way to self-medicate the insomnia. Therefore, failing to identify and address sleep complaints in a patient with a history of alcohol abuse or dependence may increase the patient's risk of relapse.

Case

A 61-year-old man with a past medical history of diabetes type 2, and psychiatric history of depression and alcohol dependence was referred to the University of Michigan Behavioral Sleep Medicine (BSM) Clinic from Addiction Treatment Services. The patient's alcohol dependence had been in remission for more than 20 years, and he had been attending regular individual therapy at Addiction Treatment Services and at Alcoholics Anonymous.

The patient reported that his insomnia had been present since his teen years. He reported self-medicating his insomnia using drugs and alcohol throughout much of his adult life. Several years after achieving sobriety, the patient gradually developed both anxiety and a return of insomnia. He was prescribed quetiapine and then alprazolam at unknown doses for both disorders. Over the years, he elevated his dosages, became tolerant to the sedating effects, and then discontinued the medications. He had difficulty maintaining sleep and reported early terminal awakenings, at 3:00 or 4:00 AM, at which point he felt quite alert. He was prescribed eszopiclone 3 mg at bedtime. He also began going to bed earlier to ensure that he would get "enough sleep." When his difficulty maintaining sleep persisted, his eszopiclone dose was

Common Pitfalls in Sleep Medicine, ed. Ronald D. Chervin. Published by Cambridge University Press. © Cambridge University Press 2014.

increased to 6 mg by his prescriber. The patient also would occasionally take an additional eszopiclone 3 mg during the night for a total of up to 9 mg per day.

When the patient presented at the BSM Clinic, he was still having difficulty maintaining sleep despite his use of at least 6 mg of eszopiclone each night. Questionnaires revealed that the patient described his insomnia as severe, his depression as moderate, and his anxiety as moderate. The patient did not have a bed partner and therefore there was no one to comment on snoring or motor activity during the night. He was referred to a sleep physician for an evaluation and consideration for a nocturnal diagnostic polysomnogram (PSG).

The patient began to monitor his sleep patterns with a sleep diary. The diaries revealed a nightly pattern of 8 hours in bed but only 5 hours of sleep. The patient's routine was to go to bed early in the evening (~8:00 PM) to avoid marital conflict and to "escape" his low mood. Treatment interventions over the next five sessions focused on behavioral sleep strategies (avoiding spending excessive time in bed, getting out of bed when not sleeping), use of evening bright light to address possible underlying circadian dysregulation (advanced sleep phase), cognitive therapy for insomnia (addressing his rationale for using the bed for reasons other than to sleep as well as his excessive focus on possible consequences of not getting "enough sleep"), and a subsequent gradual taper of eszopiclone. He did not undergo a PSG as it was determined that there was low suspicion for a primary sleep disorder. Over the course of therapy, the patient was able to improve his sleep and decrease his dose of eszopiclone back to 3 mg. At a 1-year follow-up, the patient had maintained sobriety from alcohol.

What factors could be contributing to the patient's difficulty maintaining sleep?

Sleep-disordered breathing

Sleep-disordered breathing is common among alcohol-dependent patients, particularly in older males.[4] Snoring, upper airway resistance syndrome, or frank obstructive sleep apnea can contribute to frequent arousals or awakenings that can be reported by the patient as insomnia. In this case, the patient did not endorse snoring or excessive daytime sleepiness. He did have a body habitus that could raise risk for sleep apnea (6 feet, 5 inches [196 cm] in height and 273 pounds [124 kg] in weight) and he did not share a bedroom with his spouse, so he may not have been aware of the presence or absence of snoring. If snoring or daytime sleepiness were present in this patient, a diagnostic PSG may well have been appropriate.

Insomnia related to mood disorder

Early morning awakenings can sometimes reflect an underlying mood disorder. Given the patient's history of mood disorder, moderate level of depression (on a Patient Health Questionnaire-9), and his desire to socially isolate, insomnia comorbid with a mood disorder must be considered. When insomnia is related to an unstable psychiatric disorder, effective treatment of that disorder may improve sleep. This patient was encouraged to attend his weekly supportive psychotherapy. Other patients may benefit from antidepressants or mood stabilizers as appropriate for their diagnoses.

Advanced sleep-phase syndrome

The patient's report of falling asleep early in the evening and awakening at 3:00 or 4:00 AM feeling alert may have reflected advanced sleep-phase syndrome (ASPS). To address this, the patient was advised to use bright light therapy in the evening to suppress melatonin secretion and delay the endogenous circadian sleep phase.

Medication tolerance and withdrawal

The patient's use of a high dose of sleep medication was suggestive of tolerance as the recommended dose of eszopiclone is up to 3 mg. Sleep medications with relatively short or variable half-lives (3.8–7.3 hours for eszopiclone) can, when taken early in the evening, lead to increased wakefulness later in the desired sleep period, after the drug has been metabolized.

What other pharmacologic options for alcohol-dependent patients with insomnia could have been considered?

Caution is necessary when considering pharmacologic options for insomnia in addicted patients as they are at risk to abuse them, drink hazardously while taking them, or overdose on them. This patient was prescribed alprazolam, but soon began taking high doses and was hospitalized for medication withdrawal. This behavior appeared to begin to be repeated with eszopiclone. Medications with lower risk of abuse may have been alternative options.[5]

Gabapentin

At doses of 300–1800 mg at bedtime, gabapentin is useful in treating insomnia in abstinent alcohol-dependent outpatients and appears to be more effective than trazodone.[6] However, a small pilot study found that administration of gabapentin as compared to placebo during early abstinence did not improve sleep, though it did delay the onset of heavy drinking.[7]

Trazodone

The National Institutes of Health State-of-the-Science Conference on Insomnia in 2005 concluded that in short-term use, trazodone improves several sleep measures, but initial effects may not last beyond 2 weeks. A postal survey by the American Society of Addiction Medicine found that practitioners preferred using trazodone to manage sleep problems in patients recovering from alcoholism, as this medication is thought to have less abuse potential than benzodiazepines. Better sleep outcomes were found with trazodone versus placebo over 12 weeks of treatment in alcohol-dependent patients, but heavy drinking was higher in the trazodone-treated group.[8] Nevertheless, a retrospective study of trazodone-treated patients found no association with relapse to drinking at 6 months.[9]

Ramelteon

The melatonin receptor agonist ramelteon is an option for treating insomnia in recovering alcoholics, though controlled trials are lacking; only one case series to date has tried ramelteon in recovering alcoholics. Four weeks of 8 mg nightly in five alcoholic patients resulted in a reduction of scores on an insomnia questionnaire, a reduction in latency to sleep, and an additional hour of total sleep time.[10]

Discussion

Sleep problems may predispose an individual to development of an alcohol-use disorder, or to relapse to drinking alcohol once abstinent. Given the sedating properties of alcohol, adults with sleep problems may be more likely to turn to alcohol as a way to self-medicate. Pharmacologic or behavioral treatments for insomnia may reduce the rate of relapse.

In the case presented above, the patient presented with persistent sleep disturbance despite medication with eszopiclone. A common pitfall might have been to recommend additional or alternative pharmacologic options despite the patient's known history of alcoholism as well as his history of escalating medication dose (e.g. alprazolam and eszopiclone). A better understanding of the perpetuating factors underlying the insomnia – spending excessive time in bed, going to bed to avoid social contact rather than when sleepy, inappropriate medication dosing, and possible circadian influences – may have helped to reduce the patient's risk of relapse.

Main points

Addressing insomnia in recovering alcoholics is important as it can potentially reduce the risk of relapse. Pharmacologic options exist, and some are better choices than others depending on each individual's circumstances, but non-pharmacologic approaches also can be effective.

FURTHER READING

Arnedt J, Conroy D, Armitage R, Brower K. Cognitive-behavioral therapy for insomnia in alcohol dependent patients: A randomized controlled pilot trial. *Behav Res Ther* 2011;**49**:227–33.

REFERENCES

1. Brower K. Insomnia, alcoholism and relapse. [Clinical Review.] *Sleep Med Rev* 2003;**7**:523–39.

2. Cohn TJ, Foster JH, Peters TJ. Sequential studies of sleep disturbance and quality of life in abstaining alcoholics. *Addict Biol* 2003;**8**:455–62.

3. Weissman MM, Greenwald S, Niño-Nurcia G, Dement WC. The morbidity of insomnia uncomplicated by psychiatric disorders. *Gen Hosp Psychiatry* 1997;**19**: 245–50.

4. Aldrich MS, Brower KJ, Hall JM. Sleep-disordered breathing in alcoholics. *Alcohol Clin Exp Res* 1999;**23**: 134–40.

5. Kolla BP, Mansukhani MP, Schneekloth T. Pharmacological treatment of insomnia in alcohol recovery: a systematic review. *Alcohol Alcohol* 2011;**46**:578–85.

6. Karam-Hage M, Brower KJ. Open pilot study of gabapentin versus trazodone to treat insomnia in alcoholic patients. *Psychiatry Clin Neurosci* 2003;**57**:542–4.

7. Brower KJ, Myra KH, Strobbe S, et al. A randomized double-blind pilot trial of gabapentin versus placebo to treat alcohol dependence and comorbid insomnia. *Alcohol Clin Exp Res* 2008;**32**:1–10.

8. Friedmann PD, Rose JS, Swift R, et al. Trazodone for sleep disturbance after alcohol detoxification: a double-blind, placebo-controlled trial. *Alcohol Clin Exp Res* 2008;**32**:1652–60.

9. Kolla BP, Schneekloth TD, Biernacka JM, et al. Trazodone and alcohol relapse: a retrospective study following residential treatment. *Am J Addict* 2011;**20**:525–9.

10. Brower KJ, Conroy DA, Kurth ME, et al. Ramelteon and improved insomnia in alcohol-dependent patients: a case series. *J Clin Sleep Med* 2011;**7**:274–5.

30

The option of cognitive behavioral therapy should not be ignored simply because a patient has medical reasons for insomnia

Philip Cheng and J. Todd Arnedt

Introduction

Insomnia is a common co-occurrence in medical conditions[1] and can often exacerbate symptoms or impair the patient's ability to cope with subsequent stressors (see Table 30.1 for a list of common co-occurring medical conditions). For example, patients with chronic pain also commonly report insomnia symptoms, such as difficulty initiating sleep, frequent night awakenings, or non-restorative sleep. These patients also often subsequently report both increased pain and decreased tolerance of pain.

Even though the insomnia in these cases can be explained by medical symptoms, cognitive behavioral treatment for insomnia (CBT-I) should still be considered as a treatment option for a number of reasons. While the sleep disturbances may have been initially triggered by the illness, coping behaviors that develop over time may lead to a progression from initial sleep disturbance to full-blown insomnia. To continue with the previous example, patients with chronic pain may begin napping during the day to compensate for poor quality sleep, but the napping in turn could exacerbate early insomnia. This may then lead to further frustration and rumination in bed, which could result in conditioned arousal. What began as a reaction to pain is now an independent illness, even though the patient may continue to attribute it to the initial medical illness.

Other reasons exist for why CBT-I should be considered even when insomnia occurs in the context of other medical illnesses. Research shows that alleviation of sleep disturbances alone can result in some symptom improvement, in addition to enhanced hope and a sense of control. Pain patients, for instance, commonly report reduced pain with improved sleep. Finally, sleep difficulties can often reduce treatment response for co-occurring illnesses, and untreated insomnia may elevate risk for future episodes. As a relatively brief intervention, CBT-I can be easily integrated into a comprehensive treatment regimen, either sequentially or simultaneously. Together, these reasons strongly suggest that CBT-I should be considered as a treatment option even when the sleep difficulties can be attributed to co-occurring medical conditions.

The following example illustrates a case where multiple treatment modalities were integrated into a treatment regimen for co-occurring medical conditions.

Table 30.1 Examples of medical conditions that are often accompanied by insomnia

Obstructive sleep apnea
Congestive heart failure
Chronic pain
Hypertension
Chronic obstructive pulmonary disease
Gastroesophageal reflux disease
Prostatic hypertrophy (frequent nocturia)
Diabetes
Cancer

Case 1: considerations for multiple treatment modalities

Pamela was a 20-year-old college student diagnosed with fibromyalgia who presented to the Behavioral Sleep Medicine Clinic with complaints of fatigue and poor sleep. Additionally, Pamela was recently diagnosed with obstructive sleep apnea (OSA), and was experiencing difficulty with continuous positive airway pressure (CPAP) adherence. Her sleep difficulties resulted in exacerbated depressed mood and impaired school functioning. Pamela was at risk of dropping out of school, which incited some anxiety because her living expenses were paid for by financial aid awarded to her by the university.

Pamela stated that although her fibromyalgia was being medically treated, she continued to experience pain, which worsened during the night. Her pain contributed to difficulties falling asleep with frequent night awakenings. She stated that her night awakenings were sometimes due to pain, but there were also times when she only noticed the pain after being awake. She sometimes had difficulty returning to sleep, even after her pain had responded to medication. As her depression worsened, she also began to experience early morning awakenings.

Following an assessment period, Pamela agreed to work briefly on CPAP adherence, followed by a course of CBT-I if residual sleep difficulties arose. Three sessions of motivational interviewing were used to explore ambivalence and other barriers to CPAP adherence. Pamela responded well to these sessions, and demonstrated regular use of her CPAP machine. Although the increased use of CPAP did not significantly reduce her sleep onset latency and her wake-after-sleep-onset periods, she noted improved sleep quality when she did sleep. Additionally, she reported some improvement in her pain associated with the improved sleep.

Following a subsequent course of CBT-I, Pamela was able to reduce her sleep onset latency from approximately 1 hour to around 30 minutes, with reduced frequency and duration of her wake-after-sleep-onset periods. She continued to report spikes in night awakenings during flare-ups of her fibromyalgia, but these periods were shorter in duration. She experienced continued improvement in her pain as her sleep difficulties lessened. Her mood also drastically improved with her sleep, and her morning awakenings subsided.

Discussion

Although CBT-I is often effective despite the co-occurrence of medical conditions that may contribute to the reported sleep difficulties, treatment considerations should take into account how multiple modalities may be incorporated. In Pamela's case, it was notable that both her sleep quality and her pain improved with increased CPAP adherence, despite minimal improvement in other sleep complaints.

Continuous positive airway pressure adherence was chosen as an initial focus for various reasons. One main reason is that OSA may impede treatment response to CBT-I, as patients are likely to continue experiencing poor quality sleep even with improved sleep efficiency. As apneic events result in less restorative and more fragmented sleep, the process of sleep consolidation from sleep restriction may be impaired, potentially leaving patients feeling even more fatigued with limited treatment gains. Finally, even slight symptom relief from increased CPAP adherence may be extremely motivating for patients, which may enhance treatment adherence for CBT-I. This was the case with Pamela, who approached CBT-I with more enthusiasm and adherence once her initial improvement provided her with assurance and hope that sleep treatment could be effective.

Notably, CBT-I continued to be effective in addressing her sleep difficulties despite her pain. In fact, she reported some alleviation of pain as a result of both CPAP and CBT-I. It is important to note that at the end of treatment, Pamela continued to experience some sleep disturbances that exacerbated during her fibromyalgia flare-ups. However, these disturbances were less severe and less disruptive. This outcome is consistent with research showing that sleep quality can play a significant role in pain perception and management, and contribute to overall quality of life.[2]

Assessment of co-occurring medical conditions

Treatment planning for patients with insomnia and co-occurring medical conditions is often based on information gathered during the initial assessment. Ideally, a thorough assessment includes an evaluation of relevant factors under Spielman and colleagues' behavioral or "3-P model" of insomnia.[3] In this model, **predisposing factors** such as a family history of sleep disturbances are inherent characteristics or traits that increase individual susceptibility to insomnia; **precipitating factors** such as stressful life events contribute to the initial development of insomnia; and **perpetuating factors** such as behavioral practices (e.g. irregular sleep schedules) and cognitive conditions (e.g. worry about inability to sleep) maintain insomnia over time. Questions during an initial evaluation should also identify any use of medications and their contributions to the insomnia. Example questions to assist in the assessment are shown in Table 30.2.

Patient responses to the initial evaluation can often indicate appropriateness of CBT-I. For example, when asked to describe their sleep difficulties if their comorbid illness were hypothetically cured, patients who predict continued sleep difficulties are often more likely to benefit from CBT-I. Additionally, reports of significant anxiety regarding the loss of sleep may also indicate that a portion of sleep difficulties may be addressed through CBT-I. Individuals who report a longer history of

Table 30.2 Examples of questions that can be helpful in assessment of insomnia complaints of a patient with an inter-related medical condition

---

- When did your sleep difficulties begin relative to the dizziness?
- How was your sleep prior to developing fibromyalgia?
- What would your sleep be like if I could give you a magic pill to cure your chronic pain?
- What percentage of your insomnia from 0 to 100% do you believe is due to arthritis?
- When you wake up in the middle of the night, do you awaken from the pain, or do you notice the pain afterwards?
- Once you are awake, how much difficulty would you have returning to sleep if you had less pain?

---

frequent and transient sleep disturbances but do not describe significant insomnia until onset of medical conditions may also benefit from CBT-I.

Once it has been determined that the patient is a good candidate for CBT-I, treatment decisions concern the sequencing of interventions. When barriers to sleep can be quickly or easily addressed by other medical treatments, such as adjustment of pain medications prior to bed, it may be more beneficial to complete CBT-I after the medical intervention. In situations where the initial evaluation suggests that the comorbid medical condition is causally related to insomnia, it is also preferable to proceed initially with treatment of the medical condition, reassess insomnia symptoms following treatment, and initiate CBT-I as appropriate. This clinical scenario is well exemplified when a patient complaining of frequent but brief nighttime arousals also present symptoms suggestive of OSA, which can also explain the sleep maintenance complaints. Accordingly, proceeding with a diagnostic sleep study and, if appropriate, OSA treatment could substantially improve or even entirely alleviate the insomnia complaints.

On the other hand, if the co-occurring medical condition appears to affect sleep independently from other perpetuating factors, CBT-I and appropriate medical interventions may be administered simultaneously. This frequently occurs in patients with co-occurring insomnia and OSA, as sleep fragmentation from apneic events can occur independently from other contributing factors, such as poor sleep hygiene. Patients with comorbid insomnia and OSA may complain about difficulties with sleep initiation (i.e. from conditioned arousal), in addition to sleep maintenance problems related to the OSA. Patients with both insomnia and OSA may also present with frequent night awakenings that are longer than usual. While night awakenings may be initially caused by apneic events, the typical OSA patient is excessively sleepy and does not remain awake very long; difficulty re-initiating sleep may suggest additional perpetuating factors of insomnia.

One final consideration that can help to plan the sequencing of interventions is to bear in mind that patients sometimes lack resources – time, financial, physical, or emotional – to invest in multiple simultaneous treatment regimens. This was the case with Pamela, whose anxiety, depression, and academic commitments precluded the possibility of simultaneous interventions. Thus, the initial evaluation is critical for determining the relative contribution of medical conditions to the presenting insomnia complaint.

This next case illustrates that CBT-I can sometimes improve symptoms of a co-occurring medical condition, even when the medical condition appears to cause the insomnia.

Case 2: CBT-I improves co-occurring medical symptoms

Ann was a 62-year-old retired executive with medical history significant for cervicalgia, migraine headaches, dizziness, and depression who presented to the Behavioral Sleep Medicine Clinic with chief complaints of difficulties primarily in initiation of sleep. The patient attributed the onset of her sleep difficulties 4 years ago to the acute onset of chronic dizziness, which she described as "constantly being at sea." The dizziness symptoms were particularly prominent when she closed her eyes and tried to fall asleep. She had recently been diagnosed with "chronic subjective dizziness" at another academic center, with no significant treatment options. She rated the likelihood that her insomnia symptoms would disappear as 100% if the dizziness symptoms were effectively treated. She indicated that the only time her sleep quality improved was when her dizziness symptoms were less intense. Nevertheless, she reported being distressed about her sleep difficulties and their effects on her medical symptoms.

On evaluation, Ann described her sleep difficulties as being restricted to falling asleep. She was using trazodone 150 mg for sleep and clonazepam for dizziness. She estimated an average sleep latency of 2 hours with a typical bedtime at 9:00–9:30 PM and a typical rise time at 4:00–5:00 AM and minimal wakefulness in between. She attributed fatigue, cognitive difficulties, and worsening migraines to her sleep problems. When unable to sleep, the patient reported significant dizziness and mind racing about life stressors, but she denied sleep-focused worry. She endorsed clock watching and marginal frustration at her sleep problems. Sleep hygiene evaluation revealed minimal caffeine and alcohol intake, a good bedroom environment, and regular exercise. She reported that napping was not possible due to dizziness. She had a past negative overnight diagnostic polysomnogram and reported no current symptoms consistent with other sleep disorders. She described her mood as "OK" and "stable," and she was actively engaged in depression treatment.

Current medications included clonazepam 1.5 mg twice daily, gabapentin 600 mg three times per day, tramadol 50 mg as needed, Fiorecet (butalbital 50 mg, acetaminophen 325 mg, and caffeine 40 mg) as needed, citalopram 40 mg daily, and trazodone 150 mg daily.

Given the close correspondence between the dizziness symptoms and sleep disturbances, the initial diagnostic consideration was Insomnia Due to a Medical Condition (dizziness). In light of the few effective treatments available for dizziness, her stated distress with sleep, and absence of benefit from hypnotic medication, Ann agreed to undergo a trial of CBT-I to improve her sleep quality. It was made clear to her that she should continue to focus attention on dizziness management and that success with CBT-I may be limited if the dizziness did not improve.

Ann participated in a 10-session CBT-I protocol, the results of which are summarized in Figure 30.1. Despite the initial conceptualization that the sleep problems were largely due to dizziness symptoms, the patient showed an excellent response to CBT-I, increasing her sleep efficiency by > 30% from baseline, and increasing her estimated total sleep time by > 3 hours. In addition, she reported significant amelioration in her dizziness symptoms by the end of treatment, although the symptoms did persist, and a reduction in the frequency and severity of migraine headaches (from twice weekly to twice per month). As a result of her sleep quality improvements, Ann was also weaned off trazodone by the prescribing physician, and she was able to maintain good sleep quality without it.

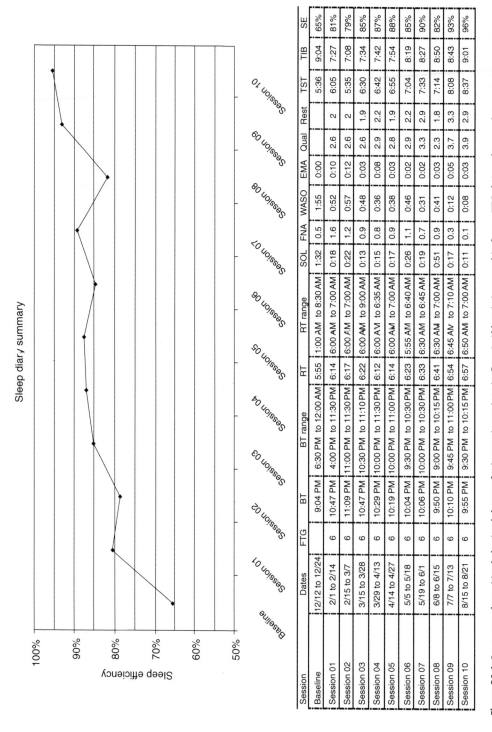

Session	Dates	FTG	BT	BT range	RT	RT range	SOL	FNA	WASO	EMA	Qual	Rest	TST	TIB	SE
Baseline	12/12 to 12/24		9:04 PM	6:30 PM to 12:00 AM	5:55	1:00 AM to 8:30 AM	1:32	0.5	1:55	0:00			5:36	9:04	65%
Session 01	2/1 to 2/14	6	10:47 PM	4:00 PM to 11:30 PM	6:14	6:00 AM to 7:00 AM	0:18	1.6	0:52	0:10	2.6	2	6:05	7:27	81%
Session 02	2/15 to 3/7	6	11:09 PM	11:00 PM to 11:30 PM	6:17	6:00 AM to 7:00 AM	0:22	1.2	0:57	0:12	2.6	2	5:35	7:08	79%
Session 03	3/15 to 3/28	6	10:47 PM	10:30 PM to 11:10 PM	6:22	6:00 AM to 9:00 AM	0:13	0.9	0:48	0:03	2.6	1.9	6:30	7:34	85%
Session 04	3/29 to 4/13	6	10:29 PM	10:00 PM to 11:30 PM	6:12	6:00 AM to 6:35 AM	0:15	0.8	0:36	0:08	2.9	2.2	6:42	7:42	87%
Session 05	4/14 to 4/27	6	10:19 PM	10:00 PM to 11:00 PM	6:14	6:00 AM to 7:00 AM	0:17	0.9	0:38	0:03	2.8	1.9	6:55	7:54	88%
Session 06	5/5 to 5/18	6	10:04 PM	9:30 PM to 10:30 PM	6:23	5:55 AM to 6:40 AM	0:26	1.1	0:46	0:02	2.9	2.2	7:04	8:19	85%
Session 07	5/19 to 6/1	6	10:06 PM	10:00 PM to 10:30 PM	6:33	6:30 AM to 6:45 AM	0:19	0.7	0:31	0:02	3.3	2.9	7:33	8:27	90%
Session 08	6/8 to 6/15	6	9:50 PM	9:00 PM to 10:15 PM	6:41	6:30 AM to 7:00 AM	0:51	0.9	0:41	0:03	2.3	1.8	7:14	8:50	82%
Session 09	7/7 to 7/13	6	10:10 PM	9:45 PM to 11:00 PM	6:54	6:45 AM to 7:10 AM	0:17	0.3	0:12	0:05	3.7	3.3	8:08	8:43	93%
Session 10	8/15 to 8/21	6	9:55 PM	9:30 PM to 10:15 PM	6:57	6:50 AM to 7:00 AM	0:11	0.1	0:08	0:03	3.9	2.9	8:37	9:01	96%

Figure 30.1 Summary of cognitive behavioral therapy for insomnia sessions in Case 2. Abbreviations used in figure: FTG, fatigue (1 = no fatigue to 10 = maximum fatigue); BT, bed time; RT, rise time; SOL, sleep onset latency; FNA, frequency of nocturnal awakenings; WASO, wake after sleep onset; EMA, early morning awakening; Qual, quality (1 = very poor to 5 = very good); Rest, restedness (1 = not at all rested to 5 = very rested); TST, total sleep time; TIB, time in bed; SE, sleep efficiency.

Discussion

The above case example nicely illustrates the potential advantages of CBT-I beyond improving sleep in patients with co-occurring medical conditions. Ann experienced clear improvements in her salient medical symptoms as her sleep quality improved. The amelioration of her dizziness, in particular, was somewhat surprising given that the original conceptualization was that the dizziness symptoms caused the insomnia complaints. Ann's experience suggests that, as in many cases of chronic insomnia, sleep difficulties often become uncoupled from the original causal agent and deserve independent treatment. As noted in the last case example, the 3-P model of insomnia can be particularly useful to help determine what sleep-specific thoughts and behaviors may be contributing to the current clinical picture and to provide guidance on how to sequence treatments. The specific mechanisms contributing to improved medical symptoms in these cases are unclear, but symptomatic improvement may be directly related to sleep quality improvements or the relationship may be indirect through sleep-related improvements in daytime functioning, such as improved coping with medical symptoms.

In cases like the example above where the initial clinical presentation suggests a close association between insomnia symptoms and the co-occurring medical condition, it is important to set patient expectations appropriately with regard to insomnia-focused treatment. In the initial consultation, Ann was encouraged to continue to focus attention on treatment of the dizziness and it was emphasized that progress with insomnia treatment may be mitigated by lack of improvement in the primary medical condition. Nevertheless, CBT-I is a low-risk empirically based treatment that can be initiated even when it appears likely that the sleep problems are directly due to a medical condition.

Main points

Overall, the evidence suggests that CBT-I should be considered as part of the treatment regimen, even in patients for whom the sleep complaints can be explained, at least in part, by co-occurring medical conditions:

- Cognitive behavioral therapy for insomnia can be effective even when sleep disturbances co-occur with medical conditions.
- Treatment regimens (including CBT-I) can be modified to account for comorbid conditions.
- Improved sleep through CBT-I may alleviate symptoms of the co-occurring conditions.
- Improved sleep through CBT-I may help individuals cope with environmental or medical stressors.

REFERENCES

1. Taylor DJ, Mallory LJ, Lichstein KL, et al. Comorbidity of chronic insomnia with medical problems. *Sleep* 2007;**30**:213–18.
2. Roehrs T, Roth T. Sleep and pain: interaction of two vital functions. *Semin Neurol* 2005;**25**:106–16.
3. Spielman AJ, Caruso LS, Glovinsky PB. A behavioral perspective on insomnia treatment. *Psychiatr Clin North Am* 1987;**10**:541–53.

Restless legs syndrome and periodic leg movements

Like so many other sleep disorders, restless legs syndrome (RLS) and periodic limb movement disorder (PLMD) – a sensorimotor and movement disorder, respectively – appear to affect many individuals for years or decades before they are diagnosed and treated. Their pathophysiologies remain incompletely understood, though they are believed to involve deficits in dopaminergic transmission, at least in part. Fortunately, several different therapeutic options are available and often effective.

Potential pitfalls arise for several different reasons. Many physicians fail to appreciate the intense impact on health and well-being that RLS can have on affected patients. The diagnosis of RLS is based entirely on the patient's history. Initial therapies sometimes fail, leading in some cases to doubt about the diagnosis rather than redoubled efforts to secure effective control of symptoms. Underlying conditions – such as certain medications or low-normal total iron stores in particular – that can provoke RLS may be missed or ignored for years or decades. Many physicians and sometimes even sleep specialists may forget that periodic leg movements can be responsible for insomnia.

The following cases in this section illustrate some of these common pitfalls when it comes to recognition, evaluation, and treatment of patients with RLS and PLMD. As with other sleep disorders, these conditions could suddenly appear to permeate the reader's clinical practice, after reading this section, to an extent that could prove quite rewarding because RLS and PLMD are in most cases readily controlled.

31

Misdiagnosis can delay appropriate and effective treatment for many years

Charles R. Davies

A 36-year-old man reported leg discomfort for the past 10 years. He described aching in his legs, and the problem was most notable at night when sitting or lying down. These symptoms were associated with an urge to move the legs. The sensations subsided upon leg movement. Initially, these symptoms were present 1–2 nights per week. He tried an over-the-counter soporific, which helped nominally. He had no history of snoring or witnessed apneas. His Epworth Sleepiness Scale score was 5 (on a scale of 0–24). Routine habits included smoking, 2–4 cups of coffee per day, and late night alcohol on the weekends. On physical exam his body mass index was 25 kg/m² and his oropharyngeal inlet was relatively open with a Mallampati Class II score. The leg strength, sensation, and reflexes were normal.

During the next few years, urges to move his legs worsened considerably. The symptoms began occurring nightly with involvement of his arms in addition to his legs. He sought help from his primary care provider, who suspected restless legs syndrome (RLS) and prescribed pramipexole with a titration up to 0.625 mg at bedtime. The patient experienced no relief, and no side effects. Ropinirole was then tried and titrated up to 0.5 mg. This caused excessive sedation but did not improve his symptoms. He began having nights of little or no sleep due to leg discomfort. To address increasing anxiety, he was prescribed over time a succession of psychotropic medications including alprazolam, diazepam, and doxepin. Each one calmed him to a degree, but did not improve the urges to move his arms and legs. Symptoms spread temporally to the point that they occurred any time of the day or night. Gabapentin and trazodone were also tried without success.

During a particularly bad period, with no sleep for 2 days, he presented to the emergency department. Laboratory testing that included complete blood count, comprehensive electrolytes, and thyroid-stimulating hormone showed normal results.

What additional tests should be performed?

Restless legs symptoms can be associated with low-normal iron stores. Iron is a cofactor for tyrosine hydroxylase, an enzyme that catalyzes a rate-limiting step in the formation of dopamine. Dopamine deficiency is a putative mechanism for RLS. A ferritin level was checked and found to be within normal limits at 155 ng/ml. This suggests normal body iron stores, though one must keep in mind that ferritin is an acute phase reactant, and can be elevated in the setting of generalized inflammation from infection, chronic disease, or obesity. A C-reactive protein can be checked to assess the inflammatory status. If the C-reactive protein is normal, no further tests are necessary. If the C-reactive protein is elevated, iron studies should be checked including the absolute iron level and iron saturation of transferrin. These values represent the true iron status and are not influenced by inflammatory status.

What is the next step in treatment?

Although a dopamine agonist such as pramipexole or ropinirole is often the first line of treatment for RLS, it is not effective in all instances. Furthermore, in cases of severe and refractory RLS such as this, opioids can be the most powerful option for treatment. This patient eventually was begun on tramadol 50 mg, taking 2 tablets up to 3 times per day. He was also advised to stop smoking, taper off caffeine, and eliminate late night alcohol. With this treatment, his symptoms improved dramatically. He was able resume his usual routine, going to bed at 9:00 PM, falling asleep within 15 minutes, and waking at 4:30 AM.

Discussion

This case illustrates the importance of following through with a complete treatment algorithm when confronted with severe RLS. The initial suspicion for this diagnosis was correct, and the diagnosis is made based on symptoms: an unpleasant urge to move the legs, worst at night, worse when lying in bed or sitting still, and relieved by movement. In the patient described above, however, after two dopamine agonists failed to provide relief as the first line of treatment, a strategy inconsistent with the correct diagnosis was pursued. Medications for anxiety and insomnia only addressed the consequences of this patient's RLS, rather than his primary diagnosis. Had this patient been started on an opioid in the first year of symptoms, after the dopamine agonists, 9 years of severe disease impact could have been avoided.

Diagnosis and differential diagnosis of RLS

Restless legs syndrome, aka Willis–Ekbom disease, is a condition that can vex patients and physicians alike. The diagnosis is made by history, which can sometimes lead to ambiguity and delays in proper treatment. While periodic leg movements during sleep (PLMS) represent a quantifiable, frequent accompaniment to restless legs symptoms, they remain a distinct phenomenon. Up to 90% of persons with RLS have PLMS, while

roughly 30% of persons with PLMS are found to have RLS. Furthermore, PLMS may represent a benign phenomenon. This is especially true in older individuals, as PLMS tend to increase in prevalence and frequency with age. Establishing a diagnosis of RLS therefore rests on the presence of four key elements of the history: uncomfortable urges to move the legs, which are worse at night, worse at rest, and relieved with leg movement.[1] In situations involving nocturnal work, the circadian predominance can be reversed. Although the criteria are straightforward, the diagnosis can be confounded by a number of other conditions, so-called mimics that can share all of these features.[2] Furthermore, if RLS is longstanding, symptoms may diffuse to the arms and other times of the day with muting of the circadian predominance. Sleep studies are not needed to evaluate symptoms of RLS, although documentation on polysomnography of PLMS can occasionally help to confirm an ambiguous diagnosis of RLS.

The predominance of familial patterns for RLS supports the idea that genetic factors shape the pathophysiology of RLS. Allelic polymorphisms found to be common in RLS include BTBD9, MEIS1, and MAP2K5.[3] In one study, more than half the risk of RLS was related to the combined impact of these variants.

Common mimics of RLS include nocturnal leg cramps, peripheral neuropathy, osteoarthritis, and akathisia. In most instances, as long as the physician demonstrates cognizance of these conditions through the history, review of systems, and physical portion of the exam, confusion can be avoided. Nocturnal leg cramps typically develop at rest and meet two of the four criteria for RLS. Cramps often provoke movement as a first impulse for relief, and movement of the legs (i.e. stretching) is usually effective. A key difference between nocturnal leg cramps and RLS is the visible muscle contraction and pain that accompanies the former. It is critical to inquire about leg cramps at night and whether stretching, especially isometric stretching has been helpful. A history of improvement by sustained foot dorsiflexion or knee extension essentially rules out RLS, which requires repetitive *movement* for relief.

Physical exam features, on the other hand, are necessary to distinguish RLS from peripheral neuropathy. Given the physiology of integration and filtering of

Table 31.1 Features of restless legs syndrome and common mimics*

Predominant features	Restless legs syndrome	Akathisia	Osteo-arthritis	Peripheral neuropathy	Nocturnal leg cramps
Urge to move	X	X			
Worse at night	X			X	X
Worse at rest	X				X
Improved by moving	X				X
Possible involvement of upper limbs	X	X	X	X	
Associated with psychotropic medication	~	X			
Pain	~		X	X	X
Abnormal sensory exam	~			X	
Palpable muscle spasm					X

* ~Indicates moderate or variable association.

sensory information, dysesthesias in patients with peripheral neuropathy are typically more noticeable at night, and at rest, when the brain is not occupied with higher order functions. Indeed, this may contribute to the circadian nature of RLS as well. Peripheral neuropathy can involve discomfort, or outright pain that is rarely attributed to RLS. Improvement with movement can be noted in both conditions. On exam, a stocking distribution sensory loss with absent ankle reflexes is consistent with peripheral neuropathy. An association between RLS and peripheral neuropathy has been discussed but not clearly established. Although some studies have shown an increased prevalence of neuropathy in RLS subjects, others have found no increase in RLS prevalence among persons diagnosed with polyneuropathy, as compared with the general population.

Osteoarthritis typically involves pain and stiffness. Early in the disease process, symptoms are brought on by activity. With progression, symptoms can occur at rest and at night. In some instances patients may report moving their legs as a reflexive attempt to find some relief. The critical distinction from RLS is the absence in osteoarthritis of any improvement in symptoms with movement.

Akathisia can be seen as a component of certain psychiatric conditions, as a side effect of medications such as levodopa, or even during withdrawal of medications such as benzodiazepines. In later stages of RLS, when all limbs are involved, the two conditions may be difficult to distinguish. The absence of a circadian pattern, presence of a psychiatric condition, or use of a medication known to cause akathisia should lead to the consideration of akathisia rather than RLS.

Symptoms of RLS may be the result of another condition and therefore represent secondary RLS (Table 31.1). As discussed below, RLS can be precipitated by low normal iron stores. Other triggers can include pregnancy, renal failure, and certain medications, such as selective serotonin reuptake inhibitor antidepressants (SSRIs), dopamine antagonists, and sedating antihistamines.

Treatment of RLS

The International RLS Study Group recently published an updated clinical practice guideline for the treatment of RLS.[4] The use of dopamine agonists such as pramipexole or ropinirole continues to be the standard first-line treatment for RLS. High level evidence supports this practice. In light of this evidence, the US Food and Drug Administration (FDA) has approved both of these medications for this indication. The recent FDA re-approval of the dopamine agonist, rotigotine, occurred after submission of the above AASM recommendations. In a limited number of trials thus far,[4] this medication, administered by a once-daily transdermal patch, has been shown to significantly improve RLS symptoms with few side effects. In addition, high level evidence supports a guideline to use of carbidopa/levodopa for RLS. However, potential harms can balance the benefits as carbidopa/levodopa is associated with a significant risk for medication tolerance and "augmentation" among many patients. After weeks or months on carbidopa/levodopa, dose requirements can increase, the timespan for benefit can decrease so that doses must be administered at shorter intervals, and underlying symptoms can worsen and spread to new parts of the circadian cycle (augmentation). Some patients start to require treatment around the clock. In this patient's case, it was reasonable to avoid carbidopa/levodopa given the risk for augmentation.

Although low level evidence supports the guideline to use opioids for the treatment of RLS, the potential for improved symptoms sometimes outweighs the potential for harm and low risk for augmentation. Opioids represent an off-label option for RLS and may be abused. In addition, opioid use may increase sleep-disordered breathing. The rationale for using the relatively weak opioid agonist tramadol in the above patient includes a low clinical suspicion for sleep-disordered breathing and a generally lower potential for abuse. The merit of this approach was highlighted by the immediate and favorable clinical outcome.

Other guidelines for treatment of RLS include the use of gabapentin enacarbil. Despite its recent FDA approval for this indication, the evidence was not completely certain regarding the balance between benefits and harms.[4] The off-label use of gabapentin, pregabalin, carbamazepine, and clonidine is optional as indicated by the AASM recommendations. The patient in this case would have benefited greatly from proper implementation of this algorithm. Prior to pursuing such a treatment algorithm, a correct diagnosis is imperative.

Iron status has long been noted to influence RLS.[5] The dopaminergic, diencephalo-spinal tract (all neurons) has been proposed as a site of pathology that contributes to RLS symptoms.[6] Given that iron is involved in the synthesis of dopamine, low iron stores may reduce dopamine tone and exacerbate restless legs symptoms. Iron supplementation may mitigate the dopamine deficiency and improve symptoms.

Ferritin represents a storage form of iron that can be measured in serum. Treatment in a patient with RLS is indicated for low-normal ferritin levels below 45–50 ng/ml,[7] even though this is above levels that most laboratories flag as deficient. Oral supplementation using ferrous sulfate 325 mg tablets may be taken with 200 mg of vitamin C twice a day. Vitamin C is necessary to lower gastric pH, which favors the absorption of iron. Side effects of oral iron can include severe constipation and stomach upset. In such cases, iron infusions may be an option under the guidance of a hematologist to minimize the morbidity associated with parenteral iron. It may take 6–12 months for iron stores to improve with oral supplementation. Ferritin and iron studies should be checked every 3 months to monitor the patient's response and avoid risk for iron overload. Supplemental iron may be discontinued once ferritin levels reach 75 ng/ml or iron saturation reaches 50%.

Other interventions to consider in the treatment of RLS include curtailment of late night alcohol, caffeine intake, and nicotine. These can exacerbate RLS and should be minimized or eliminated to achieve maximal control of restless legs symptoms.

In addition to follow-up with their physicians, patients may find support groups such as the Willis–Ekbom Disease Foundation (www.rls.org) to be valuable sources of information on RLS.

Main points

If all criteria for RLS are met, and mimics have been excluded, all options in the treatment algorithm should be considered. Although dopamine agonists are often first-line options, other medications or possibly iron replacement should be considered in a progressive manner based on the patient's findings, conditions, tolerance, and responses.

REFERENCES

1. Allen RP, Picchietti D, Hening WA, et al. Restless legs syndrome diagnosis and epidemiology workshop at the

National Institutes of Health; International Restless Legs Syndrome Study Group. *Sleep Med* 2003;**4**:101–19.

2. Hening WA, Allen RP, Washburn M, Lesage SR, Earley CJ. The four diagnostic criteria for restless legs syndrome are unable to exclude confounding conditions ("mimics"). *Sleep Med* 2009;**10**:976–81.

3. Winkelmann J, Schormair B, Lichtner P, et al. Genome-wide association study of restless legs syndrome identifies common variants in three genomic regions. *Nat Genetics* 2007;**39**:1000–6.

4. Garcia-Borreguero D, Kohnen R, Silber MH, et al. The long-term treatment of restless legs syndrome/Willis–Ekbom disease: evidence-based guidelines and clinical consensus best practice guidance: a report from the International Restless Legs Syndrome Study Group. *Sleep Med* 2013;**14**:675–84.

5. Ekbom KA. Restless legs syndrome. *Neurology* 1960;**10**:868–73.

6. Qu S, Ondo WG, Zhang X, et al. Projection of diencephalic dopamine neurons into the spinal cord in mice. *Exp Brain Research* 2006;**168**:152–6.

7. Montplaisir J, Allen RP, Walters AS, Ferini-Strambi, L. Restless legs syndrome and periodic leg movements in sleep. In Kryger M, Roth T, Dement W, eds. *Principles and Practice of Sleep Medicine*, Fourth Edition. St Louis, MO: Elsevier;2005: p. 848.

32

Periodic leg movements should not be overlooked as a possible cause of insomnia, and perhaps rarely, excessive daytime sleepiness

Lizabeth Binns

Case 1

A 56-year-old veterinarian sought a second opinion for excessive daytime sleepiness, and for what the patient referred to as "restless body syndrome." He fell asleep driving, leading to a motor vehicle crash that precipitated his initial evaluation. Leg movements were his main complaint and had been a life-long issue. He recalled wearing out the bottom of his sheets in college. His wife reported that the movements were large and often included his arms. Restless leg symptoms, reported as an urge to move his legs, were rare and only present if he hadn't slept in 24–36 hours. Leg movements typically started just before bedtime, during sedentary activities. He did not have a history of parasomnias. His Epworth Sleepiness Scale score was 21 (on a scale of 0–24), indicating severe subjective sleepiness. His excessive daytime sleepiness symptoms, in addition to drowsiness while driving, consisted of falling asleep during business meetings, meals, and conversation, and while standing up.

What are the criteria for diagnosis of periodic limb movement disorder?

Periodic limb movement disorder (PLMD) is defined by periodic limb movements along with otherwise unexplained clinical sleep disturbance or complaint of daytime fatigue.[1] Other potential diagnoses, such as those in Table 32.1, must be ruled out first. This

Table 32.1 Differential diagnoses to periodic limb movement disorder

Sleep-related epilepsy
Propriospinal myoclonus
Rapid eye movement sleep behavior disorder
Rhythmic movement disorder
Nocturnal paroxysmal dystonia

patient denied any symptoms that would suggest parasomnias, sleep paralysis, hypnogogic hallucinations, or cataplexy, making rapid eye movement (REM) sleep behavior disorder unlikely and narcolepsy less likely.

What tests can be performed to evaluate periodic limb movements during sleep?

The primary objective test for periodic limb movements of sleep (PLMS) is a polysomnogram (PSG). A diagnostic polysomnogram includes surface electromyography (EMG) electrodes that are placed on the anterior tibialis muscles of both legs. These muscles almost always participate in the movements. Respiratory monitoring of airflow, nasal pressure, and thoracic and abdominal effort is also necessary, as arousals and associated movements caused by sleep-related breathing disorders cannot be distinguished from periodic limb movements based on EMG alone.[2]

Common Pitfalls in Sleep Medicine, ed. Ronald D. Chervin. Published by Cambridge University Press. © Cambridge University Press 2014.

Table 32.2 Diagnostic criteria for periodic limb movement disorder

Patient complaint of clinical sleep disturbance
Sleep maintenance insomnia
Daytime sleepiness or fatigue
Periodic leg movements during sleep and sleep disturbance
    are not explained by other medical, neurologic, or
    psychiatric disorders

Actigraphy has occasionally been considered as an objective test for PLMS. A small accelerometer with central processing and memory detects movement and stores recorded data.[3] The actigraph is placed on the ankle or foot. Actigraphy is much less costly than a PSG but provides less information. An actigraph estimates but does not determine definitively whether a patient is asleep, and cannot indicate whether movements are associated with arousals. Therefore use of actigraphy to evaluate patients for PLMS has been limited.[4]

The baseline polysomnogram for Patient 1 demonstrated 219 total PLMS, with a periodic leg movement index (PLMI) of 44 per hour of sleep. Thirty-five of the 219 movements were associated with arousals. Also present were 25 obstructive apneas and 167 hypopneas yielding an apnea/hypopnea index (AHI, events per hour of sleep) of 39. The minimum oxygen saturation was 89%.

Clinically, the patient had hypersomnolence along with insomnia. His reported sleep latency was < 5 minutes. After being asleep for < 30 minutes, he would awaken and take 1–2 hours to return to sleep. He would have hourly awakenings after his initial sleep period.

Despite the substantial amount of sleep apnea on his PSG, the patient refused a continuous positive airway pressure (CPAP) trial. He was treated for the PLMS, initially with gabapentin 300 mg, 2 hours before bedtime. He saw a significant improvement after the first night of treatment. He participated in a boring meeting the following day and found that he was much more alert than usual. At follow-up several weeks later, his Epworth Sleepiness Scale score on gabapentin was 3 out of 24, with only a slight chance of dozing riding as a passenger in a car, lying down to rest in the afternoon, and sitting quietly after lunch. Naps were no longer necessary and drowsiness while driving resolved.

The dramatic resolution of the patient's symptoms was short lived, however, ending after 5 months. The gabapentin was increased to 1200 mg before he developed tolerance even to this dose. He then had trials of pregabalin 150–300 mg, zaleplon 5 mg, trazodone, clonazepam, and cyclobenzaprine, but each agent either failed to improve his symptoms, or caused undesired side effects, or lost efficacy. The last medication trial was then pramipexole, which increased his insomnia. He still did not accept treatment for his obstructive sleep apnea (OSA), a medical disorder that could well have been contributing to his persistent excessive daytime sleepiness (Table 32.2).

Case 2

A 51-year-old auto-mechanic was diagnosed with OSA 2 years prior to his current presentation. The baseline polysomnogram 2 years ago demonstrated an AHI of 36. The PLMI was 18 per hour with rare associated arousals. He was initially anxious about using CPAP for treatment. He was evaluated by otolaryngology and by oral and maxillofacial surgery for surgical alternatives, and he underwent an uvulopalatopharyngoplasty. A diagnostic polysomnogram after the surgery demonstrated continued OSA with an AHI score of 30, a PLMI score of 21, with rare associated arousals. A CPAP titration study was completed because of the unresolved OSA. The titration study demonstrated that 16 cm of water provided effective control of the OSA, but also showed an increase in PLMS to 33 per hour of sleep, still with rare associated arousals.

After using CPAP for several years, he developed insomnia with frequent awakenings. It was at this time that the patient and his wife became aware of frequent periodic limb movements that disturbed him and his wife. He denied any excessive daytime sleepiness.

What would indicate that the diagnosis is PLMD?

A diagnosis of PLMD can only be made if one of two additional criteria is present. Periodic leg movements

Table 32.3 Periodic leg movements during sleep scoring criteria from the American Academy of Sleep Medicine Review 2012[8]

Repetitive muscle contractions of the extremities

Dorsiflexion of toes and ankle, partial flexion of the knee and hip lasting 0.5–10.0 seconds

Movements occurring in a series of at least 4 and a periodicity of 5–90 seconds

Amplitude > 8 μV above baseline electromyogram

---

during sleep must be accompanied by either insomnia or unexplained excessive daytime sleepiness. The patient was compliant using CPAP at 16 cm H_2O. He did not have excessive daytime sleepiness. He reported insomnia that consisted of disturbed sleep with frequent awakenings. He had eliminated the 64 ounces (1.81 kg) of caffeinated diet cola that had been a part of his daily diet. No other sources of insomnia could be determined.

Treatment of his PLMD was initiated with a dopamine agonist, pramipexole 0.125 mg, 45 minutes before bedtime. He was advised to increase by 1 tablet every 5 days up to a maximum of 0.375 mg. Determination for increasing the dose was to be based on continued awakenings or his wife noting leg movements during his sleep.

The patient contacted the author within 48 hours, complaining of adverse effects. He had taken one dose of pramipexole 0.125 mg as directed and had significant excessive daytime sleepiness the following day. He had fallen asleep at a red light driving to work, and could not stay awake on the shuttle bus into work. He left work early due to his excessive daytime sleepiness. He stopped the medication and had resolution of his excessive daytime sleepiness the following day.

Discussion

These two cases illustrate the complexity of diagnosing and treating a symptom/disorder that has been considered controversial since its discovery.

Periodic limb movements have been thought to be the cause of insomnia and excessive daytime sleepiness. Early data noted PLMS to be observed in 13.3% of insomnia patients and 6.9% of patients evaluated for excessive daytime sleepiness.[5] The prevalence of PLMS in the general population has been estimated to be 5.9% based on telephone interviews of 18 980 subjects.[6] The treatment of PLMD has been controversial and currently no recommendations by the American Academy of Sleep Medicine (AASM) are given.[7]

Both patients met the criteria for PLMS, as outlined in Table 32.3.[8] Patient 1 had an abnormal PLMI at 44 events per hour of sleep, and a PLM arousal index (PLMI-A) of 8. The patient reported rare instances of restless leg syndrome. Patient 2 had PLMIs of 18 and 21, with rare associated arousals, on two PSG studies and had no reports of restless legs.

The PLMS that occur in patients with otherwise unexplained insomnia or excessive daytime sleepiness may qualify a patient for a diagnosis of PLMD. Diagnosis requires PSG confirmation of at least 15 PLMS per hour of sleep, and exclusion of other causes of the sleep disturbance.

Periodic limb movements of sleep occur most often in patients with restless legs syndrome. In a study of 133 cases of restless leg syndrome, a PLMI > 5 was found in 80% of patients.[9] Above, only Patient 1 had complaints of rare restless leg syndrome that occurred after an extended period of time without sleep. Patient 2 had no history of restless leg symptoms.

PLMS are common in obstructive sleep apnea syndrome (OSAS). The movements may be closely associated with the apneas or independent.[10] The relevance of PLMS in OSAS is not yet known. Most clinicians treat OSAS before determining whether PLMS are clinically significant. Patient 1 had significant untreated OSA, leaving the cause of his excessive daytime sleepiness unclear. Patient 2 was compliant with PAP treatment of OSA and denied excessive sleepiness, though he complained of insomnia.

A number of studies of PLMS have been undertaken. In 1996, Mendelson[11] examined 67 patients with PLMS. He found no significant correlation between the PLMI-A and subjective sleepiness or mean sleep latency on Multiple Sleep Latency Tests. Haba-Rubio et al.[12] had results that were similar to Mendelson's. A group of 57 patients were examined retrospectively to assess the

Table 32.4 Comments on treatments for periodic limb movement disorder from the American Academy of Sleep Medicine Review 2012[8]

Medication	Focus of study	Results
Clonazepam	Periodic limb movement disorder	Increase in sleep efficiency and subjective sleep quality, no decrease in leg movements
Dopaminergic drugs	Restless legs syndrome; periodic leg movements of sleep	Statistically significant reductions in periodic leg movements
Gabapentin/ pregabalin	Restless legs syndrome	Decrease in periodic leg movements
Melatonin	Leg movements	Decrease in leg movements, subjective improvement in well-being
Valproate	Periodic limb movement disorder	No change in periodic leg movements, subjective improvement in daytime alertness

possibility that PLMS could play a role in sleepiness associated with OSAS before treatment. They also evaluated whether PLMS play a role in residual sleepiness among OSAS patients successfully treated with CPAP. A follow-up CPAP titration was done after 1 year. "Sleepiness was not substantially different between the two groups (PLMS > 5 or PLMS < 5), but the group with the PLMS showed a tendency to be less somnolent."[12] The conclusion of the group was that the presence of the PLMS is not associated with increased sleepiness measured with the Multiple Sleep Latency Test and the Epworth Sleepiness Scale. The electroencephalography (EEG) arousals were not scored and therefore a PLMI-A was not calculated. Chervin[13] tested for an association between the PLMI and excessive daytime sleepiness in a clinical series of 1124 patients with suspected or confirmed sleep-disordered breathing. The conclusion was that PLMI, and especially PLMI-A scored in a subsample of 321 patients, predicted less (to a small extent) rather than more objective daytime sleepiness on the Multiple Sleep Latency Test. The author speculated that patients who are less sleepy than others may be more likely to arouse, in association with a periodic leg movement, than patients who are more sleepy. Rates of periodic leg movements did not predict subjective sleepiness measures in subsets of the sample who provided this information.

The AASM has published three treatment reviews and two practice parameter papers on restless leg

syndrome and PLMD since 1999. The focus has been mainly on restless leg syndrome. The 2012 review on PLMD therapy was basically unchanged from previous reviews. Guidance on treatment of PLMD is based on incidental findings during studies of restless legs syndrome and its treatment. The 2012 review concluded that there was insufficient evidence to comment on the use of pharmacologic therapy in PLMD.[7]

The 2012 review commented on the treatments for PLMD as outlined in Table 32.4.[8]

Clinical studies looking at the relationship between subjective sleep complaints and PLMS are contradictory. Guilleminault et al.[14] and Coleman[15] reported early on that PLMS were important causes of insomnia. In another study, Coleman came to the conclusion that in patients with primary complaints of insomnia and PLMS, there was no correlation between leg movements, arousals, and excessive daytime sleepiness.[16] Saskin early noted that PLMS patients with insomnia have more leg movements, longer delay to sleep onset, and less total sleep time than those with excessive daytime sleepiness.[17] In Mendelson's study,[11] 73%, reported difficulty sleeping. Overall there is stronger evidence that PLMS may contribute to insomnia than to excessive daytime sleepiness.[14]

Patient 1 was treated with seven medications for PLMS. Based on restless leg syndrome treatment recommendations, which most PLMD treatment has been modeled after, initial treatment should have been a dopamine agonist. Pramipexole and ropinirole, dopamine agonists, have considerable evidence of effectiveness in treatment of restless legs syndrome. Gabapentin and pregabalin, the patient's two initial treatments, are listed as options with less supportive evidence.[7] Patient 1 was also treated with zaleplon, trazodone, and cyclobenzaprine, which have not been studied. Clonazepam was used by the patient and was not effective. The conclusion of a recent review was that clonazepam has therapeutic effect on insomnia but not leg movements.[7] The patient's initial significant improvement of excessive daytime sleepiness and insomnia could be due to a decrease in leg movements on the gabapentin. Over a period of time, however, the gabapentin lost its efficacy.

Patient 2 was compliant with treatment of OSA and had eliminated other potential causes of his insomnia. The patient did not have the other related sleep disorders, restless leg syndrome, narcolepsy, or REM sleep behavior disorder. This suggests that PLMD was the primary cause of his insomnia. He refused further treatment, which may have resolved his sleep maintenance insomnia. Prominent sleepiness and sleep attacks in particular – episodes of irresistible sleep, or episodes of abrupt, inadvertent sleep during a wake period – are serious potential side effects of dopaminergic agonists.[18]

Main points

Periodic leg movements are common, especially among patients with restless legs syndrome, and can be documented on laboratory-based PSG.

Most patients are initially treated for OSA and other causes of insomnia and excessive daytime sleepiness before treatment of PLMD is considered.

Periodic leg movements during sleep are sometimes associated with arousals, but this association has little demonstrated clinical meaning because leg movements associated with arousals, as opposed to those without arousals, do not predict more daytime sleepiness.

Periodic limb movement disorder should not be overlooked, because it can be a treatable cause of insomnia; whether PLMD is also a rare cause of excessive daytime sleepiness is debated.

FURTHER READING

Aurora RN, Kristo DA, Bista SR, et al. The treatment of restless legs syndrome and periodic limb movement disorder in adults – an update for 2012: practice parameters with an evidence-based systematic review and meta-analyses. *Sleep* 2012;**35**:1039–62.

Hornyak M, Feige B, Riemann D, Voderholzer U. Periodic leg movements in sleep and periodic limb movement disorder: prevalence, clinical significance and treatment. *Sleep Med Rev* 2006;**10**:169–77.

Hornyak M, Riemann D, Voderholzer U. Do periodic leg movements influence patients' perception of sleep quality? *Sleep Med* 2004;**5**:597–600.

REFERENCES

1. American Academy of Sleep Medicine. *International Classification of Sleep Disorders. Diagnostic and Coding Manual*, Second Edition. Westchester, IL: American Academy of Sleep Medicine;2005.
2. Atlas Task Force of the American Sleep Disorders Association. Recording and scoring leg movements. *Sleep* 1993;**16**:748–59.
3. Henig W. The clinical neurophysiology of the restless legs syndrome and periodic limb movements. Part I: diagnosis, assessment and characterization. *Clin Neurophysiol* 2004;**115**:1965–74.
4. Littner M, Kushida CA, Anderson WM, et al. Practice parameters for the role of actigraphy in the study of sleep and circadian rhythms: an update for 2002. *Sleep* 2003;**26**:337–41.
5. Coleman RM, Bliwise DL, Sabjen N, et al. Natural history, epidemiology and long term evaluation. In Guilleminault C, Lugaras E, eds. *Sleep Wake Disorders*. New York, NY: Raven Press;1983, pp. 217–29.
6. Ohayon M, Roth T. Prevalence of restless legs syndrome and periodic limb movement disorder in the general population. *J Psychosom Res* 2002;**53**:547–54.
7. Aurora RN, Kristo DA, Bista SR, et al. The treatment of restless legs syndrome and periodic limb movement disorder in adults – an update for 2012: practice parameters with an evidence-based systemic and meta-analyses. *Sleep* 2012;**35**:1039–62.

8. Berry RB, Brooks R, Gamaldo CE, et al. *The AASM Manual for the Scoring of Sleep and Associated Events: Rules, Terminology and Technical Specifications, Version 2.0.* www.aasmnet.org, Darien, IL: American Academy of Sleep Medicine;2012.

9. Montplaisir J, Boucher S, Poirier G, et al. Clinical, polysomographic, and genetic characteristics of restless legs syndrome: a study of 133 patients diagnoses with new standard criteria. *Mov Disord* 1997;**12**:61–5.

10. Baran AS, Richert AC, Douglass AB, et al. Change in periodic limb movement index during treatment of obstructive sleep apnea with continuous positive airway pressure. *Sleep* 2003;**26**:717–20.

11. Mendelson WB. Are periodic leg movements associated with clinical sleep disturbance. *Sleep* 1996;**19**:219–23.

12. Haba-Rubio J, Staner L, Krieger J, Macher J. Periodic limb movements and sleepiness in obstructive sleep apnea patients. *Sleep Med* 2005;**6**:225–9.

13. Chervin RD. Periodic leg movements and sleepiness in patients evaluated for sleep-disturbed breathing. *Am J Respir Crit Care Med* 2001;**164**:1454–8.

14. Guilleminault C, Raynal D, Weitzman ED, Dement WC. Sleep related periodic myoclonus in patients complaining of insomnia. *Trans Am Neur Assoc* 1975;**100**:19–21.

15. Coleman RM. Periodic movements in sleep (nocturnal myoclonus) and restless legs syndrome. In Guilleminault C, ed. *Sleeping and Waking Disorders.* Menlo Park, CA: Addison-Wesley;1982, pp. 265–95.

16. Coleman RM, Niwise DL, Sajben N. Daytime sleepiness in patients with periodic movements in sleep. *Sleep* 1982;**5**:191–202.

17. Saskin P, Moldofsky HA, Lue F. Periodic movements in sleep and sleep-wake complaint. *Sleep* 1985;**8**:319–24.

18. Paus S, Brecht HM, Koster J, et al. Sleep attacks, daytime sleepiness, and dopamine agonists in Parkinson's disease. *Mov Disord* 2003;**18**:659–67.

33

Oral iron supplementation can help ameliorate symptoms of restless legs syndrome but may not suffice to improve low iron stores

Shelley Hershner

A 32-year-old woman, with a past medical history of obesity treated with bariatric surgery, presented with a 2-year history of insomnia. The patient describes an uncomfortable sensation in both legs which starts in the early evening and is worse at her bedtime of 9:00 PM. It occurs 5–6 nights a week. The leg symptoms are bothersome enough that on some nights she gets out of bed and paces. Movement temporarily improves her symptoms, but they return when she lies back down. Most nights she tosses and turns in bed for 2–3 hours before she can fall asleep. The patient denies experiencing these sensations during the day, but they have occurred on long car and airplane rides. She feels sleepy and fatigued during the day and has an Epworth Sleepiness Scale score of 11 on a scale that ranges from 0 to 24.

The patient was diagnosed with restless legs syndrome (RLS). A serum ferritin was checked and was low-normal at 29 ng/ml. She was started on ferrous sulfate extended release 325 mg at breakfast. A check-up at 6 months showed minimal improvement in her RLS symptoms and marginal improvement in serum ferritin, to 37 ng/ml.

Why has the patient's ferritin not improved despite treatment with oral iron?

There are several common possibilities to consider when a patient does not respond adequately to oral iron supplementation (Table 33.1):

Table 33.1 Factors that often increase or decrease iron absorption

Increases iron absorption	Decreases iron absorption
Heme sources (meat, fish)	Enteric-coated or delayed release tablets
Acidic environment-use of vitamin C	Non-heme sources (vegetables, grains etc.)
Higher amount of elemental iron	Antacids
An empty stomach	Phytatea (dietary fiber)
	Polyphenols (tea and coffee)
	Some antibiotics (quinolones, tetracycline)

1. Non-compliance
2. Inadequate absorption
3. Blood loss.

To understand a patient's iron status and response to supplementation it is necessary to understand the factors involved in iron regulation. Iron regulation depends on three different factors:

1. Iron stores
2. Iron absorption
3. Iron loss.

Iron is stored primarily in the liver, spleen, and bone marrow; most men have approximately 1 g of iron stores and women often significantly less. The largest storage of iron is located in hemoglobin, with a smaller amount in iron-containing proteins such as myoglobin, while the rest is stored either in ferritin or hemosiderin. Several available serum laboratory tests provide a snapshot of a patient's iron status. Commonly used tests are serum: ferritin, iron, and total iron binding capacity (TIBC). Ferritin, the intracellular storage protein for iron, is a good marker for whole body iron storage. The TIBC is a calculated value and represents the capacity of blood to bind iron with transferrin. Transferrin is the major transporter of iron through the blood. Both TIBC and ferritin are low in iron deficiency states. Total iron stores are the net result of iron absorption minus iron loss.

Medication non-compliance is always a possible reason for an inadequate response to oral iron. In this case, after assurance that the patient has been taking her medications, other potential causes such as inadequate iron absorption or excess iron loss need to be investigated. Iron absorption is poor under the best of circumstances. Iron is absorbed in the jejunum and duodenum, which can be compromised by disorders that affect the intestine, including inflammatory bowel disease and bariatric surgery. Some bariatric surgeries may bypass part or all of the duodenum and the jejunum (Roux-en-Y gastric bypass); after gastric bypass surgery 47–100% of patients will have a low serum ferritin. Other gastrointestinal diseases associated with decreased oral iron absorption include celiac disease, autoimmune gastritis and *Helicobacter pylori*. Iron absorption is also dependent on the source of iron. Approximately 30% of heme dietary sources are absorbed; these include fish, poultry, and other meats. Only about 10% of non heme sources are absorbed. Non-heme sources include vegetable and grains.

In this case, the patient has had a non-specific bariatric surgery likely contributing to inadequate iron absorption.

Iron stores are influenced by iron loss, which can be divided into normal, expected loss, such as the iron lost in sweat, shed skin cells, pregnancy, or lactation, and abnormal loss, usually in the form of blood loss, typically from the gastrointestinal tract or menses. Premenopausal women have lower iron stores due in part to blood loss from menses. Menses can result in 1–2 mg of loss per day. Menorrhagia can result in iron deficiency. Restless legs syndrome symptoms have

been shown to worsen by 29% during menses; however, this does not mean that the blood loss is the sole cause. Although heavy menses are associated with iron deficiency, studies investigating heavy menses and RLS are not available. Restless legs syndrome is also more common among frequent blood donors. Upon further questioning, the patient above reports heavy menstrual periods lasting for 6 days.

When evaluating blood loss as a cause of low ferritin levels, it is important to categorize blood loss as normal (expected) or abnormal. The most concerning source of abnormal or occult blood loss would be malignancy or other gastrointestinal sources. Men and postmenopausal women with iron deficiency (with or without anemia) are at an increased risk for gastrointestinal malignancy. In men and postmenopausal women, a low ferritin with no other source of potential blood loss should prompt consideration for further evaluation for occult blood loss.

Discussion

Restless legs syndrome is a sensorimotor disorder that is often divided into primary and secondary forms. Primary RLS is defined when there is no other contributing disorder while secondary RLS is associated with an underlying causative disorder; the most common etiology of secondary RLS is an abnormality in iron metabolism as represented by a low ferritin.

Restless legs syndrome has been associated with ferritin levels < 45–50 ng/ml. The normal lower limit for ferritin is often cited at 11–30 ng/ml; therefore the ferritin levels associated with RLS often are normal by lab standards. Treatment with oral iron for levels < 50 ng/ml often improves ferritin levels and may reduce severity of RLS symptoms.[1]

In a patient with RLS and a low ferritin, what is the best iron treatment?

Several factors commonly aid or hinder iron absorption. As iron is absorbed in the jejunum and duodenum, delayed release and enteric-coated tablets reduce absorption, as does high dietary fiber, calcium, antacids and some antibiotics. This patient was taking a delayed release iron formulation, which further compromises her iron absorption. If an iron formulation with a high amount of elemental iron is taken with an empty stomach and the addition of vitamin C at the same time, absorption can be enhanced. Unfortunately many people cannot tolerate oral iron due to diarrhea, constipation, and black tarry stools. Iron supplements that engender less gastrointestinal upset have decreased side effects because the amount of iron absorbed is diminished. For example, enteric-coated tablets delay iron release past the area of absorption in the jejunum and duodenum, hence resulting in less gastrointestinal upset. Products with an overall lower amount of elemental iron have fewer side effects because less iron is absorbed.

What oral iron formulations are commonly available?

There are multitudes of over-the counter iron supplements available in the market; many have additional agents to enhance absorption or minimize gastrointestinal side effects. Due to the variability of iron-containing products, recommendations should be based on the amount of elemental iron in each product, which can be found on the product label. Below are some commonly available products in the United States:

1. Ferrous or sodium sulfate: this has 65 mg elemental iron per 325 mg tablet
2. Ferrous fumarate: this has 106 mg elemental iron per tablet
3. Ferrous gluconate: this ranges from 27 to 36 mg elemental iron per tablet depending on the tablet.

Although the American Academy of Sleep Medicine practice parameters reviews supplemental oral iron, no specific target dose is suggested. For mild to moderate iron deficiency, a typical recommended dose is 2–3 mg/kg per day of elemental iron divided into 1–2 doses, or for a 165 pound (75 kg) person a total dose of 150–200 mg elemental iron. Clinically, ferrous

sulfate 325 mg (65 mg of elemental iron) is the most widely available formulation and is often prescribed once or twice a day as tolerated. Repeat iron studies should be done in 3–6 months after treatment starts, to assure adequate treatment and absence of iron overload.

What if the patient's ferritin does not respond to oral iron supplementation?

In those cases, for patients with significant RLS and persistently low ferritin, intravenous (IV) iron can be considered. Iron dextran, especially the high-molecular-weight formulation, has been associated with anaphylaxis; a 25 mg test dose and a 1-hour observation should be performed prior to administration. However, anaphylactic and hypersensitivity reactions have occurred even in patients who tolerated the test dose. There is a greater risk of a reaction in patients with a history of drug allergies and concomitant use of an angiotensin-converting enzyme (ACE) inhibitor. Intravenous low-molecular-weight formulation of iron dextran, iron sucrose, ferric gluconate, and ferumoxytol may have a lower rate of anaphylaxis.

What IV iron formulations are available?

1. Iron dextran
   (a) High-molecular-weight iron dextran: elemental iron 50 mg/ml
   (b) Low-molecular-weight iron dextran: elemental iron 50 mg/ml
2. Iron sucrose: elemental iron 20 mg/ml
3. Ferric gluconate: elemental iron 12.5 mg/ml
4. Ferumoxytol: elemental iron 30 mg/ml.

The medical literature suggests mixed benefit of IV iron in RLS. Iron sucrose versus placebo showed no significant difference at Week 11 on the International Restless Legs Study Group Rating Scale (IRLS).[1,2] At baseline, study subjects had an average ferritin of 20 µg/l.[2] The treatment protocol was 200 mg of IV iron sucrose administered on 5 occasions over a 3-week period. Although this study did not find a superior response to IV iron sucrose, other secondary outcome measures did favor IV iron: these included a lower dropout rate for iron users, and a higher percentage of treatment responders (> 50% reduction in the IRLS) among iron users versus placebo (65% vs. 35% $P = 0.02$). At an interim study analysis for a small randomized, double-blind, placebo-controlled study among subjects with normal ferritin levels, 1000 mg of IV iron sucrose produced only marginal improvement in the global rating scale for RLS symptoms at 2 weeks, despite a small change in cerebrospinal fluid (CSF) ferritin and a marked change in serum ferritin.[3] Periodic leg movements also did not change, and the study was terminated early.

Iron dextran may have more benefit, but few studies are available. Treatment with 1000 mg of IV iron dextran resulted in remission of RLS symptoms in 60% of subjects for 3–36 months, a decrease in periodic limb movements, and an increase in total sleep time.[4] These results appeared irrespective of baseline ferritin levels, and subjects had an average ferritin of 85 µg/l ± 64. An evaluation of the effect of low-molecular-weight iron dextran – 4 weekly infusions of 250 mg – showed 68% of subjects had improvement in RLS symptoms, and adverse side effects including anaphylaxis did not occur. Improvement in symptoms was not related to baseline ferritin levels (mean 39 ± 36) and no pretreatment biologic markers including CSF and serum ferritin, or iron variables predicted a positive response to IV iron dextran.[5]

The American Academy of Sleep Medicine Clinical Practice Guidelines make these optional recommendations for oral and IV iron:[6]

4.2.5 Iron supplementation has not been shown to be effective in the treatment of RLS, except perhaps in patients with iron deficiency or refractory RLS (level of evidence: Very Low).
4.2.5a Clinicians may use supplemental iron to treat RLS patients with low ferritin levels.

If the patient's RLS symptoms are significant, iron may be indicated as an adjunct treatment, (when ferritin is low) but without more evidence of benefit, iron should not be relied on as the sole treatment.[7] In this case described above, the patient had frequent symptoms of RLS (5–6 days a week) that resulted in insomnia

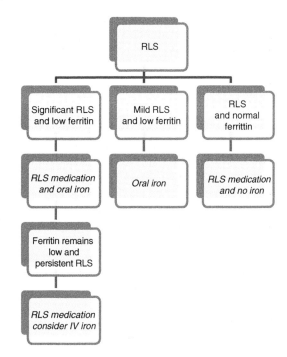

Figure 33.1 Treatment with concomitant restless legs syndrome (RLS) medications in addition to iron should be decided based on the severity and frequency of the patient's RLS symptoms.

(2–3 hour sleep latency). When treating a patient with significant RLS and low ferritin there are several treatment and management considerations as outlined in Figure 33.1.

This patient was treated with a single dose of 500 mg of IV iron dextran. Two weeks after the infusion, her ferritin had improved to168 ng/ml. Although her RLS symptoms decreased in severity and frequency, clinically significant symptoms persisted 3 nights per week. Pramipexole 0.125 mg 1–2 pills at symptom onset resulted in adequate control. Despite poor oral iron absorption she continued on ferrous fumerate 106 mg elemental iron taken once daily, on an empty stomach with some orange juice. She increased her consumption of meats and iron-containing foods (kale, spinach, beans, and meat). She has scheduled an appointment with her primary care physician to discuss whether oral contraceptive pills are indicated to decrease menorrhagia. Further treatment with IV iron will be considered in the future based on her ferritin and clinical symptoms.

Main points

Restless legs syndrome has been associated with serum ferritin levels < 45–50 ng/ml. Oral iron treatment is often offered to patients with serum ferritin levels below 50 ng/ml. Based on clinical circumstances, patients with low ferritin levels – men and postmenopausal women in particular – should be evaluated for occult blood loss. If a patient's ferritin level does not improve after an adequate oral iron trial (3–6 months), IV iron may be an option, though this therapy carries its own risks. Evaluation of patients who have failed oral iron therapy, in particular, for causes of inadequate iron absorption or excessive iron loss, should be considered. Patients with RLS are often treated concomitantly with medications to control RLS symptoms, whether or not iron is administered, depending on the severity and frequency of the RLS symptoms. After treatment with oral or IV iron, repeat iron studies are indicated to assure adequate response and absence of iron overload.

REFERENCES

1. Wang J, O'Reilly B, Venkataraman R, Mysliwiec V, Mysliwiec A. Efficacy of oral iron in patients with restless legs syndrome and a low-normal ferritin: a randomized, double-blind, placebo-controlled study. *Sleep Med* 2009;**10**:973–5.
2. Grote L, Leissner L, Hedner J, Ulfberg J. A randomized, double-blind, placebo controlled, multi-center study of intravenous iron sucrose and placebo in the treatment of restless legs syndrome. *Mov Disord* 2009;**24**:1445–52.
3. Earley CJ, Horska A, Mohamed MA, et al. A randomized, double-blind, placebo-controlled trial of intravenous iron sucrose in restless legs syndrome. *Sleep Med* 2009;**10**: 206–11.
4. Earley CJ, Heckler D, Allen RP. The treatment of restless legs syndrome with intravenous iron dextran. *Sleep Med* 2004;**5**:231–5.
5. Cho Y, Allen R, Earley CJ. Lower molecular weight intravenous iron dextran for restless legs syndrome. *Sleep Med* 2013;**14**:380–1.
6. Aurora RN, Kristo DA, Bista SR, et al. The treatment of restless legs syndrome and periodic limb movement disorder in adults an update for 2012: practice parameters with an evidence-based systematic review and meta-analyses. *Sleep* 2012;**35**:1039–62.
7. Silber MH, Ehrenberg BL, Allen RP, et al. An algorithm for the management of restless legs syndrome *Mayo Clin Proc* 2004;**79**:916–22.

Parasomnias

Parasomnias, broadly defined as unwanted behaviors during the normal sleep period, include some of the most common and intrinsically fascinating sleep disorders. Parasomnias can occur throughout the lifespan, from early childhood throughout old age, though the types of parasomnias likely to present during each period of development can be quite different. Whereas some parasomnias are so common as to be considered part of normal development under some circumstances, others carry substantial risks to health and well-being, or serve as a signal that other serious medical or mental health challenges could be developing.

The following cases, described by a psychologist, two neurologists, an internist, and a pulmonologist, illustrate several common pitfalls that can arise in the assessment, diagnosis, and treatment of individuals with parasomnias. Beyond the inherent scientific interest engendered by elaborate and sometimes consequential behavior that arises during the unconscious state imposed by sleep, clinicians must also be aware of how parasomnias can arise from seemingly unrelated sleep, medical, or psychological conditions, which also merit investigation, diagnosis, and treatment to achieve optimal outcomes for affected patients. Several types of parasomnias, for example, represent partial arousal from the normal sleep state by another primary sleep disorder or sleep fragmenting condition. In the short term, patients with parasomnias and their families often deserve counseling about safety precautions while the behaviors are still occurring, but in the long term, effective efforts to diagnose and eliminate underlying causes, or use of appropriate pharmacologic intervention, can often reduce or eliminate the problem.

34

Diagnosis of a non-REM parasomnia without consideration of a patient's psychological makeup and its possible contribution can leave key issues unaddressed

Alan S. Eiser

The delineation of the varieties of complex behavior that arise out of sleep has been one of the most fascinating developments in clinical sleep medicine. With respect to the non-REM (NREM) parasomnias, three major categories of behavior that have been described are sleep-related violence, eating, and sexual activity. Understanding these entities as sleep disorders has permitted diagnostic specification, etiologic clarification, and development of effective treatments. Earlier tendencies to view them strictly through the lens of psychiatric disorders have been rightly superseded. However, much evidence also supports the idea that psychological elements often play a significant role in determining the nature and occurrence of episodes of complex behavior arising out of sleep, in interaction with the underlying physiological substrate and other factors that comprise the sleep-related basis for the NREM parasomnias. Neglect of these psychological elements will lead in such cases to an incomplete understanding and treatment approach to the patients' clinical disorders. The cases below illustrate these points. Some details have been altered to protect patient confidentiality.

Case 1

A 35-year-old, married woman presented to the Sleep Disorders Clinic for a longstanding history of sleep-related eating. The disorder had begun about 7 years earlier, and episodes had become more frequent over

time, reaching a peak of 3 times per night. During the episodes, she typically would walk to the kitchen and eat. Sometimes, she would awaken but feel compelled to continue eating, while at other times she learned she had eaten only from evidence found in the morning. The eating behavior was the source of a tremendous amount of shame, as well as sleep disruption and fatigue. There was a prominent childhood history of sleep terrors and sleepwalking, which had resolved spontaneously at around puberty.

What tests might you perform to assist in diagnosing these phenomena?

Among patients with NREM parasomnias, a nocturnal polysomnogram can sometimes permit observation of partial awakenings during NREM sleep, or, more rarely, actual episodes of complex behavior arising out of sleep. A finding of preservation of muscle atonia during REM sleep can contribute to ruling out REM sleep behavior disorder. This patient also reported occasional snoring. In view of the fact that episodes of complex behavior can be triggered by disorders that cause arousals during sleep, assessment for obstructive sleep apnea and periodic limb movements of sleep was warranted. A polysomnogram was performed and did not show evidence of obstructive sleep apnea or periodic limb movements during sleep. There were no episodes of complex behavior arising out of sleep. REM sleep muscle atonia was preserved.

Treatment with clonazepam resulted in a reduction in the number of episodes of eating to about one per night. (At the present time, topiramate is often tried as a first-line treatment for sleep-related eating.)

The treating clinicians had the impression that psychological issues might be playing a role in the symptomatology, and the patient was referred for in-depth psychological evaluation. This revealed a very difficult and chaotic childhood environment marked particularly by the severe psychiatric illness and disturbed, at times violent, behavior of the patient's mother. The mother's behavior was also a source of intense shame for the patient. A very profound sense of aloneness was evident, both during childhood and in the patient's present life. There were some significant losses in her later development. An event happening many years prior to referral had created a lasting sense of alienation from her husband, as well as a painful sense of shame about remaining in the marriage. A period of excessive substance use and eating of unhealthy foods was followed by the patient's imposing on herself a very strict regimen of dieting and exercise, likely due in part to anxiety about falling into the chaotic behavior patterns of people who had played significant roles in her early childhood. It was in this context that the sleep-related eating emerged. It appeared to function as a means of obtaining some gratification in the context of intense loneliness and the ascetic deprivation she had imposed on herself. Anxieties about abandonment, impoverishment, loss of control, and her low self-esteem constrained adaptive possibilities and led to a feeling of being stuck in her situation. A recommendation for exploratory psychotherapy, in conjunction with medications for the sleep-related eating, was made.

Case 2

A 26-year-old, divorced woman, mother of one child, presented to the Sleep Disorders Clinic for evaluation of frequent episodes of eating during her sleep. Her level of awareness during these episodes, which often included walking to the kitchen, varied widely from little or no awareness to almost full alertness.

Frequently she would know she had eaten only from evidence she found in the morning, in the bed or in the kitchen. She estimated having five such episodes per night. The sleep eating had begun more than a decade earlier, and had become much more frequent over time. It developed that in addition she had other behavior, including masturbation, in her sleep. A family history of sleep-related eating was reported. The patient was concerned about weight gain from the eating, as well as disrupted sleep and tiredness during the day. These clinical findings were strongly suggestive of sleep-related eating and sexual behavior.

The patient reported rare snoring, and had gained weight in recent years. A nocturnal polysomnogram with parasomnia montage was performed and did not show significant obstructive sleep apnea or periodic limb movements. Behaviorally, there was an episode in which the patient sat up during sleep and appeared to want to get out of bed. REM sleep muscle atonia was preserved. Ultimately, in view of the frequency of her behavioral events, a repeat polysomnogram with esophageal manometry was performed to assess for more subtle forms of obstructive sleep apnea. The study was negative for obstructive sleep apnea or increased resistance of the upper airway.

Treatment with clonazepam resulted in a reduction, but not elimination, of the behaviors during sleep. As the patient also reported intermittent restless legs symptoms, pramipexole was added, but did not result in any further beneficial effect.

The history gathered in the Sleep Disorders Clinic suggested that psychological issues might be involved, and the patient was referred for in-depth evaluation. A complex set of difficult childhood circumstances that continued to be influential in adulthood was uncovered. The patient was raised in a very strict family in which all forms of pleasure-seeking were forbidden. Rules were enforced by harsh, at times physically injurious discipline, as well as the threat of emotional exclusion. At the same time, aspects of parental relatedness as well as discipline were overstimulating and had a quality of out-of-control physicality; the patient was thus exposed to covert stimulation in instinctual realms that was overtly denied. Also highly important, there was a powerful sense of emotional deprivation. She felt there was no one she could turn to for help or support, and needed to rely emotionally on herself from an early age.

Both the sleep-related eating and the sexual behavior were found to be linked to earlier, wakeful childhood precursors. There had been a pattern of secretly eating at night to counter a sense of deprivation and prohibition of gratification. Masturbation had had special importance as a realm in which pleasure could be obtained under the patient's full control, without need to rely on others who would be depriving or forbidding.

The expression of eating and sexual behavior in sleep, when agency can be denied, may be seen as a continuation of the family mode of covert expression of officially prohibited pleasure-seeking behavior. The eating also provided relief from a sense of bleak emotional deprivation at the hands of an unsupportive, harshly critical world.

These same issues affected wide-ranging areas of the patient's life, including her relationships with others, comfort with herself, and parenting. A recommendation was made for exploratory psychotherapy in conjunction with medication treatment of the sleep-related behaviors.

Discussion

As sleep clinicians began to develop knowledge of the frequency and variety of complex behaviors that arise out of sleep, there was a tendency to exclusively emphasize their dimensions as sleep disorders and overlook or deny the possibility of additional, psychological contributions. In part, this was understandable as a means of ensuring that newly won, essential understanding of the integral relationship of these disorders (and their proper diagnosis and effective treatment) to sleep would be maintained in the face of earlier, widespread, incorrect assumptions that these puzzling behaviors must be reflections of psychiatric disorders or comprehensible entirely in psychological terms. However, in the author's experience it is not uncommon clinically to find that psychological factors play an important role, in

interaction with the underlying sleep disorder, in determining the occurrence and nature of significant complex behavior arising out of sleep. Indeed, evidence to support this can be found in some of the earliest work in this area. In an important study of sleep-related injurious (to self and others) behavior, Schenck et al.[1] found that of the 54 patients in their group with sleepwalking/sleep terrors, 48.1% had a current or past history of an Axis I psychiatric disorder. Two-thirds of these patients completed usable Minnesota Multiphasic Personality Inventory (MMPI) profiles, of which 64% were abnormal and a third indicated the presence of personality disorders. These findings indicate a great deal of psychopathology in these patients with injurious NREM parasomnias, and strongly suggest an association between the two. In a carefully studied clinical series of patients with sexual behavior arising out of sleep, Guilleminault et al.[2] found potentially relevant psychological factors, in addition to aspects related to sleep disorders, in a number of their cases. Schenck has noted that some of his cases of sleep-related eating were precipitated by "separation anxiety," suggesting that emotional hunger may come into play in the sleep-related symptoms. The involvement of psychological factors may be made more readily comprehensible if it is recalled that the behaviors are understood to occur in a hybrid state of partial sleep and partial wakefulness.

The occurrence of pleasure-seeking or instinctual behavior in a state in which self-awareness and conscience are diminished suggests a relationship to the dissociative disorders. This possibility was explored, and found to be present, in six of twenty-two patients with NREM parasomnias studied by Hartman et al.[3] It may be that sleep-related dissociative disorders are currently conceived too categorically, and that psychological mechanisms very similar to what are seen in dissociative disorders may come into play in some longstanding cases of complex behavior arising out of NREM sleep. The fact that the behaviors can afford gratification is helpful in understanding why some patients may be reluctant to relinquish their symptoms. This can be viewed as an instance of primary rather than secondary gain, in the sense that the gratification is a contributing factor in the original formation of the symptom.

Main points

Psychological factors, in addition to more commonly-described physiological triggers, can be a significant determinant of sleep-related episodes of behavior in the NREM parasomnias. Attention to the possible presence of these factors is essential in many cases for a thorough understanding and comprehensive treatment approach to the patient's clinical disorders.

FURTHER READING

Schenck CH, Mahowald MW. Review of nocturnal sleep-related eating disorders. *Int J Eat Disord* 1994;**15**:343–56.

REFERENCES

1. Schenck CH, Milner DM, Hurwitz TD, et al. A polysomnographic and clinical report on sleep-related injury in 100 adult patients. *Am J Psychiatry* 1989;**146**:1166–73.
2. Guilleminault C, Moscovitch A, Yuen K, et al. Atypical sexual behavior during sleep. *Psychosom Med* 2002;**64**: 328–36.
3. Hartman D, Crisp AH, Sedgwick P, et al. Is there a dissociative process in sleepwalking and night terrors? *Postgrad Med J* 2001;**77**:244–9.

35

History and polysomnographic findings are both critical to distinguish different parasomnias

Alon Y. Avidan

Description of cases

The following six cases are derived from patients who visited the sleep disorders clinic. The reader is presented with the key clinical and polysomnographic data to formulate presumptive clinical diagnoses. An answer key is provided on page 214.

Case 1

A 5-year-old boy is observed by his parents to experience episodes of screaming about an hour after falling asleep. The frequency of these are about two to three per week, but occurred nightly when he had the flu a week ago prompting a visit to the pediatrician. The parents are concerned, as he is very agitated during these episodes and appears diaphoretic. His mother is particularly worried as he opposes her and becomes more anxious and aggressive when she tries to comfort him. He finally falls asleep after these episodes and upon waking up in the morning does not remember anything that happened. The episodes never last more than a few minutes. His twin brother also had these episodes at age 4, and they lasted for a few months, but then disappeared completely. The patient obtains about 8 hours of sleep each night, does not snore, and does not have any underlying neurologic or medical disorders.

Case 2

A 5-year-old boy has episodes of screaming that arise out of sleep in the latter part of the night.

He vividly describes a pink hand appearing out of the darkness and peaking at him. When he wakes up he appears anxious, and is reaching out to his parents. The frequency of these episodes is about two to three per month, and they appear more likely to occur after snacking on chocolate ice cream before going to sleep.

Case 3

A 26-year-old firefighter complains that he wakes up disoriented at the sound of an alarm in the firehouse. His bed partner reports that she hears him snoring, but she's not sure if he stops breathing at night. On exam, his Mallampati score is between Class II and III. His coworkers, who describe his episodes of disorientation as the "flare-ups," note that immediately following the sound of the fire alarm, the patient is confused, speaks in incomprehensible sentences, and finally gets out of the bed without recalling anything. Per his wife, the episodes never occur at home or when he gets a "good night of continuous sleep." Figure 35.1 depicts a 60-second epoch, during stage N3 sleep, from a recent polysomnogram. The electrographic data follow a night of sleep deprivation and the spell that is captured is typical. The sleep technologists documented a sudden arousal during which he yelled, "Where are the keys?" and was searching under the bed telling the technologist that he is in a hurry. After a period of about 20 seconds, he quickly

Common Pitfalls in Sleep Medicine, ed. Ronald D. Chervin. Published by Cambridge University Press. © Cambridge University Press 2014.

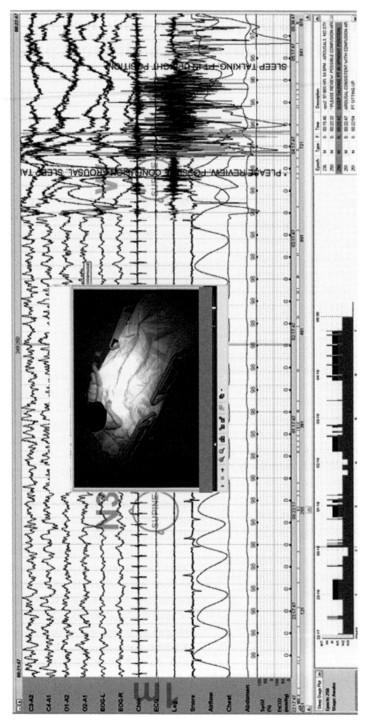

Figure 35.1 A 60-second epoch, during stage N3 sleep, from a recent polysomnogram. See text for figure abbreviations.

returned to baseline and stated that he was just trying to "get comfortable." He was oriented to person, place, and time and did not have any recollection about the episode.

Case 4

A 62-year-old man is bothered by episodes of injurious behaviors during sleep, occurring weekly leading to wrist injury. The episodes began about 3 years ago and were initially mild, consisting of yelling as he was dreaming that he was arguing with someone. Over the past 7 months he has had more "action filled" events where he is fighting and trying to hit something. Last week, he experienced a significant fall while dreaming that he was attempting to confront someone; he lacerated his scalp on the glass nightstand. The most violent episode occurred a month earlier when he tried to punch his wife during sleep, screaming, "Move away from my property." Luckily she moved away in time, but he hit the wall leading to a fracture of his wrist. Both the wife and husband are extremely concerned about the emergence of these severe spells and the injury associated with them. The patient is an executive at a toy factory and is never an aggressive person during the daytime. Upon further questioning by the sleep physician, it is learned that he began to experience the gradual onset of a tremor at rest about 6 months ago. The patient presented for a diagnostic polysomnogram that revealed occasional snoring episodes and occasional hypopneas. Figure 35.2, from REM sleep recorded during his nocturnal polysomnogram (60-second epoch), shows an event in which he moved his hands and legs as if he were running.

Case 5

A 31-year-old second-year obstetrics and gynecology physician resident presented with nightly episodes of suspicious eating episodes after work shifts in which he had obtained very little sleep. He kept a careful diary of these episodes, which confirm that the episodes are most likely to follow a stressful call night in which he has had no sleep. He lives alone and sometimes awakens to find partially eaten food items left on the counter. He became increasingly alarmed after he found cuts on his fingers in the morning. He proceeded to place a motion-activated video camera in the kitchen. The device captured him preparing a turkey sandwich with peanut butter and cutting pickles with a sharp knife. He recently gained 25 pounds (11 kg), and his fiancé reports that he recently began to snore, which was not an issue before starting residency, 2 years ago. Figure 35.3 demonstrates a 30-second epoch from a recent polysomnogram during which the recording sleep technologist was instructed to purposefully leave food items by the bedside. The left panel depicts the corresponding video demonstrating an episode of eating popcorn ("patient chewing food item"). This episode arose from stage N2 sleep.

Case 6

A 66-year-old gentleman presented with the new onset of finding bruises on his extremities upon awakening in the morning. He has a history of restless legs syndrome but has achieved reasonable control of his symptoms with ropinirole and brisk walking exercise in the evening time. Recently, following the loss of his business due to defaulting on several bank loans, he began to experience sleep-onset insomnia. His primary care physician placed him on a hypnotic agent to help him fall asleep. This medication has indeed helped improve his sleep onset. However, his wife often finds him sleeping in other areas of the house after initially going to sleep in their bedroom. He has no recollection of ever leaving the bedroom. His wife remarks that his bruising episodes began following initiation of the treatment for insomnia and wonders if there could be an association. Figure 35.4 demonstrates a photograph, taken during a recent clinic visit with the author, highlighting right arm ecchymosis following a night in which he experienced a typical episode. His wife found him sleeping in his car, parked on the sidewalk with the engine on.

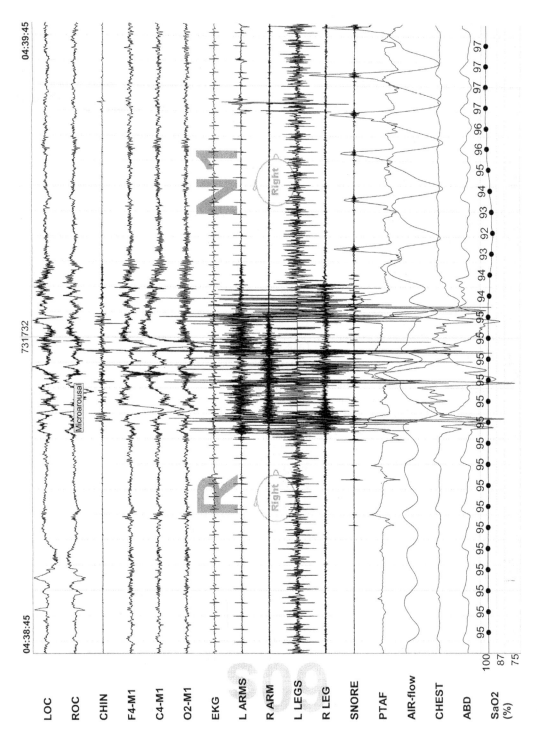

Figure 35.2 Rapid eye movement sleep recorded during nocturnal polysomnogram (60-second epoch). See text for figure abbreviations.

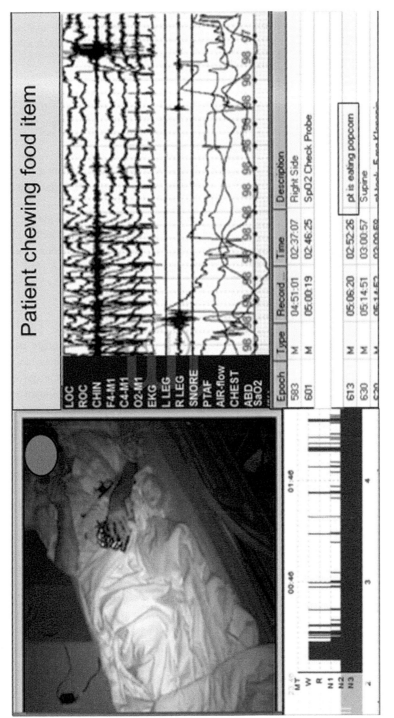

Figure 35.3 Patient chewing a food item. See text for figure abbreviations.

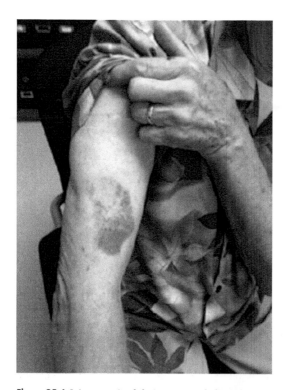

Figure 35.4 Injury sustained during somnambulism. See text for figure abbreviations.

Key for the most likely diagnosis

Case 1: Sleep terrors

Case 2: Nightmares

Case 3: Confusional arousals (Figure 35.1)

Case 4: Rapid eye movement sleep behavior disorder (RBD) (Figure 35.2).

Case 5: Sleep-related eating disorder (SRED) (Figure 35.3)

Case 6: Sleepwalking (Figure 35.4).

Key channels in figures

Electrooculogram (left: LOC-A2, right: ROC-A1) = LOC and ROC left and respectively right outer cantus electrooculography (EOG) electrodes

Electroencephalogram (EEG) =

M1: Left mastoid electrode location

M2: Right mastoid electrode location

C3 and O1, left central and respectively: occipital EEG electrodes

C4 and O2, right central and respectively: occipital EEG electrodes

Chin electromyogram (EMG) = (Chin 1–Chin 2)

Limb EMG (L = left leg, R = right leg) = LAT1–LAT2

EKG = Electrocardiogram

SNORE = Snore sensor sound

ORAL/N/O AIR-flow = Nasal–oral airflow

THOR/CHEST and ABD = chest and abdominal walls motion effort

EtCO2 = End tidal carbon dioxide

(*PTAF*) = Pressure transducer airflow

SpO2 = Percent oxygen saturation by pulse oximetry (finger probe).

Introduction

The cases presented above highlight the wide range and complex nature of parasomnias, but also highlight how clinical history, semiology, the age of the patients, predisposing factors, and accompanying symptoms may help the sleep healthcare provider arrive at the correct diagnosis.

Sleep specialists are often consulted to help identify, evaluate, and manage a spectrum of active behavior – parasomnias – during the night that range from phenomena as benign as sleep talking to others that could be the first harbinger of a progressive neurodegenerative disorder. Disorders of partial arousal from deep non-rapid eye movement (NREM) sleep, such as sleepwalking, sleep terrors, and confusional arousals, represent states of incomplete awakening. The REM Sleep Behavior Disorder (RBD), the most common parasomnia in older adults, arises from REM sleep with abnormal augmentation of electromyographic activity and enactment of dream experiences.

Parasomnias are defined as undesirable and sometimes abnormal behaviors that occur during transition from wakefulness into sleep or arise during awakenings or partial awakenings from sleep. The episodes are not a unitary phenomenon, but rather are the

Table 35.1 Summary of the key differences between sleep terrors and nightmares

Characteristic	Sleep terror	Nightmare
Alternative name	Pavor nocturnus	Anxiety dream
Time of night	First third	Last third
Stage of sleep	Slow-wave sleep	Rapid eye movement sleep
Movements	Common	Rare
Severity	Severe	Mild
Vocalizations	Screaming common	Rare
Autonomic discharge	Severe and intense	Mild
Recall	Fragmented	Good
State on waking	Confused/ disoriented	Function well
Injuries	Can occur	Rare
Violence	Can occur	Rare
Displacement from bed	Can occur	Very rare

manifestation of a wide variety of different conditions, many of which are readily identified and managed. Parasomnias are hypothesized to be due to changes in brain organization across multiple states of being and are particularly apt to occur during the incomplete transition or oscillation from one sleep state to another.

The American Academy of Sleep Medicine's International Classification of Sleep Disorders (ICSD-2)[1] classifies parasomnias as: (a) "Disorders of arousals from non-rapid eye movement sleep (NREM);" (b) "Parasomnias usually associated with rapid eye movement (REM) sleep;" and (c) "Other parasomnias." The next section presents a description of each of the parasomnias reflected in the above cases.

Case 1: sleep terrors

Sleep terrors are characterized by a sudden arousal from deep slow-wave sleep, often with an intense scream, overwhelming fear, extreme panic, confusion, and heightened sympathetic discharge (tachycardia, tachypnea, diaphoresis, mydriasis, and increased muscle tone).

The autonomic reaction is a unique feature that often differentiates sleep terrors from other parasomnias. After an episode, the patient often returns to sleep, generally with no memory of the event by the next day. The episodes can be accompanied by prominent motor activity and displacement, sometimes leading to bodily injury.

Case 1 described a patient whose sleep terror episodes may have been worsened by an illness – the flu. The case also highlights the underlying genetic predilection in first-degree relatives. In fact, many of the NREM parasomnias have an autosomal dominant pattern of inheritance.

Polysomnographic features consist of a sudden arousal during slow-wave sleep aligned with autonomic (sympathetic) hyperactivation. Differentiation from nightmares, as depicted in Case 2, is most important. Unlike nightmares, which occur during REM sleep, for which vivid recollection is present, patients with sleep terrors have universal amnesia for the event. Differentiating sleep terrors from sleep-related epilepsy is occasionally difficult, and polysomnography with an expanded electroencephalographic montage may be helpful for patients in whom the episodes are atypical for sleep terrors – frequent (several episodes per night), repetitive, stereotypical in semiology, with poor response to management.

Treatment is often unnecessary when episodes are infrequent, or in young children as in this age group sleep terrors are so common that they are not necessarily considered abnormal. However, treatment may be necessary in an adult, especially when the events are frequent, intense, or disruptive to the patient's sleep. Suggested therapy includes a low dose, short-acting benzodiazepine (clonazepam, diazepam) at bedtime.[2] For adults, psychotherapy and stress reduction may be implemented in the setting of psychiatric disorders (anxiety, stress).[3,4] Finally, in patients with chronic NREM disorders of arousal, a careful search for a primary sleep disorder that fragments sleep – and obstructive sleep apnea in particular – sometimes reveals a treatable underlying cause for the parasomnia. A chronic NREM parasomnia usually resolves when comorbid obstructive sleep apnea is treated.

Table 35.1 lists the differences between sleep terrors and nightmares.

Case 2: nightmares

Nightmares probably affect 10% to 50% of children and up to 75% of the population can remember at least one or a few nightmares in the course of their childhood. Half of all adults admit to having an occasional nightmare, while 1% report more than a single nightmare a week. Nightmares present as a vivid and prolonged dream that tends to become progressively more complicated and frightening before terminating in an awakening and recall. Episodes may increase during times of stress, and can be related to use of pharmacologic agents such as L-dopa or β-adrenergic blockers. Nightmares may be induced following abrupt withdrawal of REM-suppressant medications.

Case 3: confusional arousals

Confusional arousals consist of confusion and disorientation during and following abrupt, partial awakenings from slow-wave sleep (deep NREM sleep). Patients experience confusion and disorientation and may have errors of logic. Typical episodes last a few minutes and are typically terminated with amnesia for the event, but quick recovery to baseline. The underlying etiology may be related to recovery from sleep deprivation; circadian rhythm sleep disorders (shift work, as in the firefighter, in Case 3) or use of central nervous system depressants. Polysomnographic recordings during the episode, as in Figure 35.1, depict an arousal pattern out of deep slow-wave sleep associated with error of logic ("Where are the keys?"), disorientation, unintelligent speech pattern, and rapid return to baseline. Confusional arousals may be managed conservatively by avoidance of the precipitating factors such as sleep deprivation, preventing irregular sleep/wake schedule patterns, and evaluating and managing coexisting sleep disorders. The firefighter in Case 3 had complete remission of his spells after he switched to a different work setting with more regular work hours. Typically, patients with confusion arousals do not need to undergo formal polysomnography unless one suspects underlying sleep-disordered breathing or an alternative

diagnosis of nocturnal seizures. Given his crowded upper airway and history of snoring, an evaluation for sleep apnea was appropriate. In his case, this did not reveal treatable obstructive sleep apnea. Pharmacologic management is often not necessary as episodes are self-limiting, but confusional arousals may be managed with tricyclic antidepressants or benzodiazepines when they are refractory to conservative therapy.

Case 4: REM sleep behavior disorder

The prevalence of RBD is estimated to be about 0.5% in the general population.[5] Up to 47% of patients with Parkinson's disease experience sleep disturbances.[6,7] The disorder has an increased predilection to affect men, about 90%, and has a higher prevalence in patients older than age 50 years.

Rapid eye movement sleep behavior disorder is one of the most fascinating parasomnias seen by sleep clinicians, and is currently the only one that requires formal evaluation by polysomnography. The episodes are characterized by abnormal augmentation of chin or limb surface EMG tone during REM sleep and by recalled dream mentation. Patients exhibit a wide variety of abnormal behaviors, ranging from simple talking or singing to more dramatic yelling, shouting, and screaming. Complex movements, such as running, walking, jumping, punching, kicking, and violent agitated behaviors should prompt swift and effective therapy. In contrast to patients who have sleepwalking episodes, eyes usually remain closed. In addition to absence or reduction of normal atonia during REM sleep, patients with RBD also appear to have distinctive dream content. The typical dream involves being chased or attacked and having to defend oneself against an assailant. As many sleep physicians can attest, the injury that is often associated with the severe spells – injury to the patient or to the bed partner – can be the key trigger that first brings the patient to medical attention.

Polysomnographic findings in RBD reveal abnormal augmentation of muscle activity during REM sleep: either tonic background activity of the surface EMG

Table 35.2 The key similarities and differentiating features between non-rapid eye movement (REM) and rapid eye movement parasomnias

	Confusional arousals	Sleep terrors	Sleepwalking	Nightmares	REM sleep behavior disorder
Timing in night	Early	Early	Early/mid	Late	Late
Sleep stage	N3	N3	N3	REM	REM
Electroencephalographic discharges	–	–	–	–	–
Scream	–	++++	–	++	+
Central nervous system activation	+	++++	+	+	+
Motor activity	–	+	+++	+	++++
Awakens	–	–	–	+	+
Typical duration (min)	0.5–10.0	1–10	2–30	3–20	1–10
Post-event confusion	+	+	+	–	–
Typical age	Child	Child	Child	Child/ Adult	Older adult
Genetics	+	+	+	–	–
Organic brain lesion	–	–	–	–	++

Abbreviations: N3, Stage N3 sleep; Min, time in minutes;–indicates absence of, whereas +, ++, ++++ indicates increased likelihood/presence of encountering in the various parasomnias.

can be increased, or phasic twitches in the chin or limbs can be excessive (Figure 35.2). The result of the neurologic evaluation may indicate the need for other neurologic testing, including neurologic imaging when structural or underlying neurodegenerative processes are suspected. Imaging may be more important to consider if the episodes follow a neurologic insult or occur in younger patients or women.[8–10]

The differential diagnosis of RBD includes nocturnal frontal lobe seizures, confusional arousals, sleepwalking, sleep terrors, post-traumatic stress disorder, and nightmares (Table 35.2). Patients with RBD are often differentiated from patients with other REM and NREM parasomnias based on the complex nature of their behavioral episodes, timing later in the night when REM sleep is most prominent, and older age that is characteristic for RBD.

Treatment includes safety measures such as covering or securing windows, and sleeping on the ground floor in a sleeping bag until the episodes are fully managed.[11] Every patient with suspected RBD should be assessed carefully with meticulous attention to risk for potential harm. Pharmacotherapy for RBD may be in the form of clonazepam (0.25 mg to 2.0 mg

po QHS), which achieves improvement in the majority (90%) of patients with little evidence of tolerance or abuse.[12–14] A second option for pharmacologic treatment includes melatonin, which restores REM-sleep atonia and is effective in 87% of patients taking 3–12 mg at bedtime.[15,16] The reader is reminded that in the United States, melatonin is considered a dietary supplement, is not approved by the US Food and Drug Administration, has a poor track record with respect to pharmacologic preparation, and could have side effects that have not been carefully studied. Recent data show that a customized, motion-activated bed alarm may also offer an elegant non-pharmacologic therapy for RBD.[17]

Case 5: sleep-related eating disorder

Sleep-related eating disorder (SRED) consists of recurrent episodes of involuntary eating that occur during the main sleep period. The episodes typically involve eating peculiar forms or combinations of food (as in Case 5 in which the patient ate a peanut butter, turkey, and pickles sandwich), or unusual, inedible, or toxic substances (frozen food, dog food, dish soap).

As in other forms of arousal disorders, most patients do not have full recall of the event. Other sleep disorders may also trigger SRED including obstructive sleep apnea, restless legs syndrome, periodic leg movement disorder, and circadian rhythm disorders. Use of hypnotics[18] along with cessation of smoking or alcohol have also been reported as triggers.[19] Sleep-related eating disorder should be differentiated from the night eating syndrome (NES), which is characterized by full awareness of the abnormal eating and the absence of bizarre or toxic ingestion.

Treatment includes management of any underlying sleep disorder (such as OSA). If the patient suffers from other disorders of arousal, recommended treatments for these conditions, for example with benzodiazepines or tricyclic antidepressants (TCAs), can help reduce SRED. Dopamine agonists, selective serotonin reuptake inhibitors, and topiramate have all been reported to help improve symptoms, although lack of support from large trials is a limitation as in the other parasomnia categories.[20,21] Interestingly, SRED is shown to be more common in patients with restless legs syndrome, probably because these individuals are often treated with hypnotics to help address the sleep-onset insomnia in this condition, which induced SRED.

The patient in Case 5 was managed with topiramate and improving his sleep while on call by providing time for rest and power naps. His episodes improved dramatically, and his weight stabilized to his normal premorbid state.

Case 6: sleepwalking (somnambulism)

Sleepwalking is common in children between the ages of 4 and 8 years but can occur as soon as a child is able to walk. Typical episodes arise from deep NREM sleep and can involve minor movements, simple walking around the bed, or more rarely, "escape" and prolonged behaviors when extreme. The episodes end with the patient awakening confused, disoriented, and amnestic for the events. Somnambulism may occasionally result in falls and injuries (Figure 35.4) following displacement, during attempts to "escape," or when walking down stairs or into windows or glass doors. In adults, precipitating factors include the use of hypnotic agents, acute sleep deprivation, and primary sleep disorders. Underlying sleep disorders such as sleep apnea or extrinsic stimuli (noise) may produce sleep disruption, which can predispose patients to exhibit ambulation in sleep. Treatment includes the avoidance of the precipitating factors and establishing a safe living environment (removing sharp objects from bedroom, covering windows, sleeping on the ground floor). The use of medications such as TCAs or benzodiazepines may be indicated when the episodes are refractory, severe, or dangerous.

The concern with the patient in Case 6 was his risk for injury, the fact that he had already sustained injury, and his risk of injuring others (i.e. through sleep driving). Upon discontinuation of the hypnotic agent, the episodes improved dramatically, and he was placed on more aggressive therapy to manage the restless leg symptoms.

Main points

The NREM parasomnias generally involve partial arousal from deep NREM sleep in the first half of the night; examples include sleep terrors, sleepwalking, and confusional arousals.

The NREM parasomnias, and also sleep-related eating disorder and REM sleep behavior disorder, can arise from sleep fragmentation induced by another primary sleep disorder, most commonly obstructive sleep apnea.

The REM sleep parasomnias include RBD and nightmares, which can be distinguished by the considerable observable behavior associated with the former.

When necessary, parasomnias can often be controlled with appropriate medication, though precautions may also be necessary in the home to reduce the chance of injury for the patient or bed partner.

REFERENCES

1. American Academy of Sleep Medicine. *International Classification of Sleep Disorders. Diagnostic and Coding Manual*, Second Edition. Westchester, IL: American Academy of Sleep Medicine;2005, p. 293.

2. Nino-Murcia G, Dement WC. Psychophysiological and pharmacological aspects of somnambulism and night terrors in children. In Meltzer HY, ed. *Psychopharmacology: The Third Generation of Progress*. New York, NY: Raven Press;1987, pp. 873–9.

3. Mahowald MW. *Overview of Parasomnias. National Sleep Medicine Course*. Westchester, IL: American Academy of Sleep Medicine;1999.

4. Mahowald MW, Schenck CH. NREM sleep parasomnias. *Neurol Clin* 1996;**14**:675–96.

5. Ohayon MM, Caulet M, Priest RG. Violent behavior during sleep. *J Clin Psychiatry* 1997;**58**:369–76; quiz 77.

6. Comella CL, Nardine TM, Diederich NJ, Stebbins GT. Sleep-related violence, injury, and REM sleep behavior disorder in Parkinson's disease. *Neurology* 1998;**51**:526–9.

7. Eisehsehr I, Parrino L, Noachtar S, Smerieri A, Terzano, MG. Sleep in Lennox-Gastaut syndrome: the role of the cyclic alternating pattern (CAP) in the gate control of clinical seizures and generalized polyspikes. *Epilepsy Res* 2001;**46**:241–50.

8. Bonakis A, Howard RS, Ebrahim IO, Merritt S, Williams A. REM sleep behaviour disorder (RBD) and its associations in young patients. *Sleep Med* 2009;**10**:641–5.

9. Stores G. Rapid eye movement sleep behaviour disorder in children and adolescents. *Dev Med Child Neurol* 2008;**50**:728–32.

10. Plazzi G, Montagna P. Remitting REM sleep behavior disorder as the initial sign of multiple sclerosis. *Sleep Med* 2002;**3**:437–9.

11. Aurora RN, Zak RS, Maganti RK, et al. Best practice guide for the treatment of REM sleep behavior disorder (RBD). *J Clin Sleep Med* 2010;**6**:85–95.

12. Schenck CH, Mahowald MW. Polysomnographic, neurologic, psychiatric, and clinical outcome report on 70 consecutive cases with REM sleep behavior disorder (RBD): sustained clonazepam efficacy in 89.5% of 57 treated patients. *Cleve Clin J Med* 1990;**57** (Suppl): S9–23.

13. Mahowald MW, Schenck CH. REM sleep behavior disorder. In Kryger MH, Dement W, Roth T, eds. *Principles and Practice of Sleep Medicine*, Second Edition. Philadelphia, PA: WB Saunders;1994, pp. 574–88.

14. Mahowald MW, Ettinger MG. Things that go bump in the night: the parasomnias revisited. *J Clin Neurophysiol* 1990;**7**:119–43.

15. Takeuchi N, Uchimura N, Hashizume Y, et al. Melatonin therapy for REM sleep behavior disorder. *Psychiatry Clin Neurosci* 2001;**55**:267–9.

16. Boeve B. Melatonin for treatment of REM sleep behavior disorder: response in eight patients. *Sleep* 2001;**24** (Suppl):A35.

17. Howell MJ, Arneson PA, Schenck CH. A novel therapy for REM sleep behavior disorder (RBD). *J Clin Sleep Med* 2011;**7**:639–44A.

18. Chiang A, Krystal A. Report of two cases where sleep related eating behavior occurred with the extended-release formulation but not the immediate-release formulation of a sedative-hypnotic agent. *J Clin Sleep Med* 2008;**4**:155–6.

19. Morgenthaler TI, Silber MH. Amnestic sleep-related eating disorder associated with zolpidem. *Sleep Med* 2002;**3**:323–7.

20. Miyaoka T, Yasukawa R, Tsubouchi K, et al. Successful treatment of nocturnal eating/drinking syndrome with selective serotonin reuptake inhibitors. *Int Clin Psychopharmacol* 2003;**18**:175–7.

21. Howell MJ, Schenck CH. Treatment of nocturnal eating disorders. *Curr Treat Options Neurol* 2009;**11**:333–9.

36

Diagnosis and counseling for rapid eye movement sleep behavior disorder: a potential window into an uncertain neurologic future

James D. Geyer and Paul R. Carney

Introduction

Normal rapid eye movement (REM) sleep in humans is accompanied by generalized muscle atonia. Muscle atonia arises from intrinsic regulation within pontine nuclei near the locus ceruleus. This occurs by hyperpolarization of the alpha-motoneurons, resulting in subsequent muscle atonia. The mechanism was initially described in cats, after specific pontine lesions were observed to cause a reproducible loss of REM sleep-induced atonia. This model was subsequently extrapolated to humans to explain naturally occurring but abnormal behaviors during sleep.

Rapid eye movement sleep behavior disorder (RBD) occurs when there is a loss of subcortical regulation of REM sleep atonia and generally involves skeletal muscle activity. Basically, the loss of normal REM atonia allows the patient to "act out" his or her dreams. Behaviors such as punching, yelling, swearing, kicking, screaming, grabbing, talking, running, crawling, and jumping out of bed are commonly described. Injuries to both the patient and a bed partner are not uncommon. This phenomenon arises only from REM sleep, making this behavior more common in the latter half of the night.

Case

Chief complaint: The patient's wife stated, "He fights in his sleep."

History of present illness: A 62-year-old man presented with his wife. The man stated he did not believe any of his wife's reports concerning his nocturnal behavior until he recently fractured his hand in the middle of the night. The man's wife reported that for the last 3–4 years he would begin yelling and then punch and kick in his sleep like he was fighting. He usually went to bed around 11:00 PM. He struck her on one occasion as she tried to check on him, resulting in a black eye. Most recently he punched the nightstand, fracturing several bones in his hand. The patient told his wife he was dreaming that he was back in the military. She became afraid to sleep in the same room with him.

Past medical history: Hypertension.

Medications: Hydrochlorothiazide and aspirin.

Social history: Retired farmer. He served in the military years ago with several tours of duty in combat. He stopped smoking 26 years ago. He drinks an occasional beer.

Family history: Father had hypertension and died after having a myocardial infarction. Mother died from cancer. There is no one in family with a history of seizures.

Review of systems: Unremarkable except for some headaches. Specifically the patient denied any resting tremors. He denied any falls.

Exam: Well-dressed gentleman with the right arm in a cast. The cranial nerve examination was

Common Pitfalls in Sleep Medicine, ed. Ronald D. Chervin. Published by Cambridge University Press. © Cambridge University Press 2014.

unremarkable. There were no identified tremors or abnormal movements. The motor examination did not show increased muscle tone or bradykinesia. There may have been a very mildly decreased arm swing with ambulation.

Polysomnogram: Sleep onset latency 22 minutes. Sleep efficiency 78%. Increase in slow-wave sleep and REM sleep. The periodic limb movement index (PLM index, number of limb movements per hour of sleep) was 17. The apnea/hypopnea index (AHI, events per hour of sleep) was 2.1 and minimum oxygen saturation was 89%. The surface electromyogram (EMG) showed an increase in muscle activity in stage R sleep. Once during the night while in stage R sleep, the patient began yelling and punching violently for several seconds (Figure 36.1[1]).

Diagnosis

Rapid eye movement sleep behavior disorder is characterized by abnormal behaviors that occur during REM sleep and threaten or cause injury or sleep disruption. The patient physically acts out a dream. This can lead to a variety of movements and actions, which may be violent in nature. Patients can break bones, strike bed partners, and knock items off bedside tables. Episodes can be and often are violent. The patients may report that the dreams are extremely vivid. Furthermore, dream content recall is typically much more detailed following an event with violent acting out of dreams.

Rapid eye movement sleep behavior disorder is more common in men than in women. It may be idiopathic but has been associated with a variety of progressive neurologic disorders including α-synucleinopathies that can cause parkinsonism and associated dementia. Although RBD can be seen at any age, it is most prevalent in the sixth and seventh decades.

The polysomnogram shows episodes of sustained increased muscle tone or increased transient phasic muscle activity during stage R sleep, instead of the decreased tone normally seen at this time. The sleep study may also show an increase in non-REM (NREM)

periodic limb movements and REM density. The polysomnogram should be performed with continuous time-locked video. The video may show that movements including punching and guttural utterances occur during REM sleep. If carefully awakened during an episode, the patient can often recall the content of the dream, and relate a reason for the movements. However, attempting to awaken someone with RBD from the dream can lead to physical injury as the person may fight or grab. This has been referred to as "getting inside the envelope."

Differential diagnosis

A careful general medical and neurologic history is necessary. Certain medications such as tricyclic antidepressants and other anticholinergic medications may lead to RBD symptoms. There are also reports of transient RBD symptoms following hypnotic or alcohol withdrawal (Table 36.1).

The differential diagnosis includes nocturnal seizures. Concomitant expanded 16-channel scalp electroencephalography (EEG) recording, during the polysomnogram, can be useful. Nocturnal seizures are often highly stereotyped, from one episode to the next, whereas RBD usually exhibits more variability, depending on the particulars of the dream episode involved. Nightmares, another REM sleep-related parasomnia, is sometimes confused with RBD. A nightmare is a frightening dream that often awakens the sleeper. Rarely, striking out can be part of a nightmare but usually does not occur during the stage R phase itself. In comparision, RBD patients tend to be more explosive and usually do not awaken with the frightening aspect, as may commonly occur in a true nightmare. The differential diagnosis also includes other NREM parasomnias, specifically sleepwalking, confusional arousals, and sleep terrors.

A clinical diagnosis of RBD can be strongly suspected by history alone if an individual has a classic description that is often observed by a bed partner. Confirmation of the diagnosis requires a polysomnogram, which can also help to rule out other potential

222

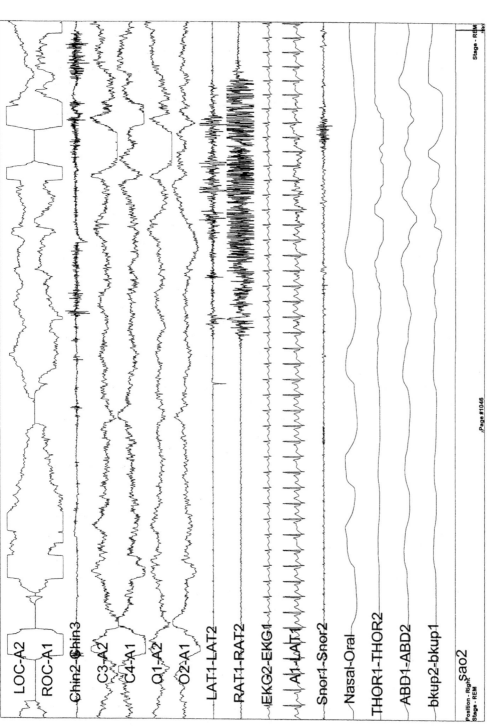

Figure 36.1 In rapid eye movement sleep behavior disorder (RBD), elevated muscle tone can appear during rapid eye movement sleep, in a continuous manner or in bursts of activity often accompanied by stereotyped movements that can be violent in nature. The 30-second epoch shown here, from a polysomnogram, reveals rapid eye movements in the eye movement channels (LOC and ROC) and low muscle tone initially in the chin electromyogram (EMG) channel, typical of REM sleep. However, a sudden increase in muscle tone then occurs, with movement artifact, despite continued REM sleep, consistent with RBD. Abbreviations used in figure: LOC-A2, left eye movement; ROC-A1, right eye movement; Chin2-Chin3, chin EMG; C3-A2, left central electroencephalogram (EEG); C4-A1, right central EEG; O1-A2, left occipital EEG; O2-A1, right occipital EEG; LAT1-LAT2, left anterior tibialis EMG; RAT1-RAT2, right anterior tibialis EMG; EKG2-EKG1, electrocardiogram (EKG); A1-LAT1, secondary EKG; Snor1-Snor2, snore vibration sensor; Nasal-Oral, airflow thermistor; THOR1-THOR2, thoracic effort monitor; ABD1-ABD2, abdominal effort monitor; bkup2-bkup1, secondary effort monitor; SaO2, oxygen saturation. Reprinted with permission from Geyer J, Payne T, Carney P.[1]

Table 36.1 Differential diagnosis for acting out dreams or fighting during sleep

Rapid eye movement sleep behavior disorder
  Nightmares
  Sleep talking
  Sleepwalking
  Confusional arousals
  Sleep terrors
  Seizures

differential diagnoses of RBD. The polysomnogram can also sometimes identify a primary cause for sleep disruption – most commonly obstructive sleep apnea – that causes what amounts to partial arousal from REM sleep. In such cases, the partial arousals are believed to precipitate the behavioral episodes.

Treatment

This patient was treated with low-dose clonazepam at 0.5 mg per night with an excellent clinical result. He also stopped drinking alcohol in the evening. The treatment of RBD includes the use of clonazepam as the medication of choice. The major caveat to the use of long-acting benzodiazepines, such as clonazepam for the treatment of RBD, is that the majority of these patients are older individuals and, as previously suggested, may have other concomitant neurologic issues. The long-term use of benzodiazepines in this population may predispose these elderly patients to worsening cognitive function. Ideally, the lowest therapeutic dose of benzodiazepines that eliminates nocturnal behaviors without daytime sequelae should be used. Medium- and short-acting benzodiazepines might be considered as alternative treatments if any such undesired effects of sedation or impaired cognitive function should occur with clonazepam, but appear to be somewhat less efficacious, in part because a cycle of REM sleep often occurs just prior to awakening in the morning. Other treatment options include carbamazepine, L-dopa, and dopamine agonists, which are typically somewhat less effective than clonazepam. Beyond treatment with medication, patients and bed partners should also hear about safety precautions to take in the sleeping environment to minimize potential for injury. Removal of sharp or dangerous objects from the bedroom; sleeping on the ground floor of the home; and thoughtful approaches to safety with regard to windows and doors are examples of precautions to consider.

Counseling about prognosis

In recent years, studies have demonstrated a significant correlation between idiopathic RBD and neurodegenerative disorders, such as Parkinson's disease, Lewy body dementia, and multiple-system atrophy. These conditions are also termed *synucleinopathies*, since they all contain intracellular inclusion bodies containing alpha-synuclein. Dopaminergic dysfunction in the striatum is often demonstrable in patients with alpha-synucleinopathies and may play a role in RBD. In fact, RBD is often the initial presenting complaint of patients who subsequently develop these neurodegenerative conditions. The appearance of the RBD may precede the onset of parkinsonian syndrome by many years.

Other associations between RBD and preceding events, such as a history of prior neurologic disease, including stroke, dementia, subarachnoid hemorrhage, and Guillain–Barré syndrome, have been noted.

How should counseling be approached for a patient with RBD?

Controversy exists amongst sleep medicine physicians as to the appropriate counseling for a patient who has been diagnosed with idiopathic RBD, meaning that no evidence has emerged to suggest another neurodegenerative disorder. Some physicians avoid the discussion of the possible association between RBD and parkinsonian syndromes: as the development of a parkinsonian syndrome cannot be avoided or delayed by treatment, the patient should be spared this concern. However significant pitfalls can arise from this approach. Foremost amongst these is the likelihood that the patient will discover the association with a simple web search. Unfortunately in this case, the patient will not have been counseled appropriately about potential alternative causes for RBD, such as idiopathic RBD that remains an isolated condition during the patient's lifetime, narcolepsy, use of certain medications, and withdrawal states.

After a full history that includes psychiatric screening for conditions such as post-traumatic stress disorder, medication, and histories of medications that could potentially cause iatrogenic RBD, social history for drug and alcohol use, and a family history for concomitant sleep disorders as well as the degenerative disorders, a counseling approach can be developed. If the patient has an obvious etiology for the RBD such as an acute withdrawal state, this should be stressed as a likely primary cause. In other cases, counseling regarding the differential diagnosis is probably warranted. The patient should be provided with this information in order to appropriately monitor his or her condition so that any parkinsonian symptoms can be addressed at an early stage. Furthermore, this approach helps avoid exposure to erroneous or even correct but unexplained information on the Internet and the undue fear is that this can generate. In some cases, the information could conceivably have impact on important life or family planning decisions. Such an approach is a component of good patient advocacy, full disclosure, and responsibilities for full disclosure that are increasingly assumed in the modern physician–patient relationship.

Main points

- Careful evaluation and diagnosis is vital.
- Institute aggressive management for patient and family safety.
- Counseling is often important, especially for primary cases with no precipitating factors.

FURTHER READING

Iber C, Ancoli-Israel S, Chesson, Am Quan SF. *The AASM Manual for the Scoring of Sleep and Associated Events: Rules, Terminology, and Technical Specifications*, First Edition. Westchester, IL: American Academy of Sleep Medicine;2007.

Olson E. Rapid eye movement sleep behavior disorder: demographic, clinical and laboratory findings in 93 cases. *Brain* 2000;**123**:331–9.

Schenck CH. Managing bizarre sleep-related behavior disorders. *Parasomnias* 2000;**107**:145–56.

Schenk CH, Mahowald MW. A polysomnographic, neurologic, psychiatric, and clinical outcome report on 70 consecutive cases with REM sleep behavior disorder: sustained clonazepam efficacy in 89.5% of 57 treated patients. *Cleveland Clin J Med* 1990;**57**(Suppl):10–24.

Shirakawa S, Takeuchi N, Ucimura N, et al. Study of image findings in rapid eye movement sleep behavioral disorder. *Psych Clin Neurosci* 2004;**56**:291–2.

REFERENCE

1. Geyer J, Payne T, Carney P. Parasomnias. In Geyer T, Payne P, Carney P, eds. *Atlas of Polysomnography*, Second Edition. Philadelphia, PA: J. Lippincott Williams and Wilkins; 2010, p. 223.

37

Obstructive sleep apnea must be ruled out as a potential underlying cause of sleepwalking in a child

Shalini Paruthi

Case

An 8-year-old boy presented to the Pediatric Sleep Disorders Clinic with a 4-year history of sleepwalking. Recently, the child exited the home through the front door while asleep, which clearly alarmed his parents. Sleepwalking episodes occurred between two and seven nights per week, and at least once to twice per night. The first episode of sleepwalking occurred between midnight and 3:00 AM. A second episode often followed within an hour. During sleepwalking episodes, he had urinated in multiple places within the home. Father also noted that when his son is especially tired, the likelihood of sleepwalking greatly increases. Parents report he snores once per month. Parents only hear the snoring when standing next to him. Parents deny pauses in breathing, gasping, choking, mouth breathing, or diaphoresis. However, he is a very restless sleeper, tosses and turns frequently, and falls out of bed. His daily bedtime is 9:30 PM and wake up time is 7:30 AM. Sleep latency is under 10 minutes. Bedtime routine includes: dinner, reading, television time, snack, and then lights out. He sleeps in his own room with a night light on.

He has no past medical or surgical history. Family history reveals that his father snores, but has not undergone formal evaluation. The patient lives with his mother, father, and sister. He is in the second grade and receives "B" grades. He does not get in trouble at school or home. He has no medication allergies. He is on no medications.

The physical exam revealed the following findings on the head and neck exam: normal nasal turbinates, midline septum, Mallampati Class II, 1+ tonsils bilaterally, and a high arched hard palate. It was a narrow airway. Neurologic exam was entirely within normal limits. His height was 4 feet, 9 inches (143.6 cm) and his weight was 88 pounds (40.1 kg), for a body mass index of 19.4 kg/m^2 and body mass index z-score of 1.49. He had an Epworth Sleepiness Scale score of 6.

After the thorough clinical history and physical exam, he was diagnosed with (i) sleepwalking and (ii) snoring, with possible obstructive sleep apnea (OSA).

What treatment options should be considered?

Given the snoring history and dangerous sleepwalking, an in-laboratory diagnostic polysomnogram was ordered. Safety precautions were discussed such as door alarms.

The sleep study showed OSA with an apnea/hypopnea index of 5.3 events per hour of sleep, and a minimum oxygen saturation of 96%. End-tidal carbon dioxide values were > 50 mmHg for 30% of total sleep time.

What is the next best step for treatment?

The boy was then evaluated by an otolaryngologist for adenotonsillectomy. Although he had a narrow airway, he had small tonsils and adenoids, and was not considered an appropriate candidate for surgical intervention. After education regarding continuous positive airway pressure (CPAP) therapy, the parents and child agreed to proceed with a CPAP titration polysomnogram. A CPAP setting of 6 cm H_2O best treated this child's sleep-disordered breathing and was prescribed.

The child acclimated well to CPAP therapy at home. Downloaded adherence reports showed CPAP usage 83% of nights, with > 4 hours usage on 67% of nights. Sleepwalking resolved completely.

Discussion

Sleepwalking is a common childhood disorder, with a prevalence of up to 40% for a single episode of childhood sleepwalking; 2–3% of children have frequent episodes of sleepwalking. The primary goals in treatment include identification of any trigger for sleepwalking and also creation of a safe sleep environment. The focus for this discussion is to review features associated with sleepwalking, the most common precipitating factors, and lastly the evaluation and treatment of OSA in children with sleepwalking.

Many parents describe children with sleepwalking as in a state of sleep, easily redirected to bed, and found in unusual locations in the home in the mornings. Some children will urinate in unusual locations such as a kitchen corner or bedroom closet; others will eat unusual foods. Complex motor activity may be observed; essentially any action may be possible when sleepwalking.

In some children, sleepwalking can become dangerous. Cases have been reported of children who exited the home while asleep, walked into oncoming traffic, became lost in the woods when camping, or even drowned in nearby ponds or lakes. Many parents report the need to stay awake and watch their child sleep. Many parents have also installed additional locks on doors, gates in hallways, or home alarm systems in order to keep their child safe.

Sleepwalking is a non-rapid eye movement (NREM) parasomnia, triggered by any sleep disturbance that causes a partial arousal from sleep, most often stage N3 (deep, slow-wave NREM sleep). Thus sleepwalking is most likely to occur in the early half of the night, and rarely in the second half of the night. A positive family history increases the risk of sleepwalking with one study finding a 60% risk of sleepwalking in a child if both parents were sleepwalkers.

Several clues may help parents better recognize if the child is sleepwalking versus awake and out of bed. Children who sleepwalk will frequently walk without clear purpose, may injure themselves unintentionally, become combative when approached, or guided back to bed easily by verbal command or gentle leading by parent. Furthermore, children who sleepwalk may not interact "appropriately" with their environment, for example when family members ask questions. These children typically cannot recall sleepwalking and may become embarrassed when parents or siblings discuss the episodes.

In many children, sleepwalking appears to spontaneously resolve with increasing age. Common precipitating factors for consideration include sleep deprivation, restless legs syndrome (RLS) and OSA. Other less common but reported causes of sleepwalking include hyperthyroidism, migraines, brain injury, travel, unfamiliar sleep environments, stress, fever, psychotropic medications, and substance use.

Treatment includes providing a quiet, dark, familiar sleep environment with an age-appropriate amount of time in bed and treatment for possible RLS or OSA. Rarely, no cause is identified for sleepwalking, and the treatment plan may include scheduled awakenings (parents gently awaken the child very briefly and quietly, 30 minutes prior to the typical time of the episode) or medications such as clonazepam.

If OSA is suspected, it is best confirmed in children through an in-laboratory diagnostic polysomnogram (Figure 37.1). Children found to have OSA should be evaluated by an otolaryngologist for adenotonsillectomy as first-line treatment. If a child has small adenoids and tonsils and is not considered a candidate for surgery, a conversation directly with the otolaryngologist may be worthwhile. Extraction of tonsils that do not appear enlarged on examination may still have benefit in pediatric OSA, because non-enlarged tonsils

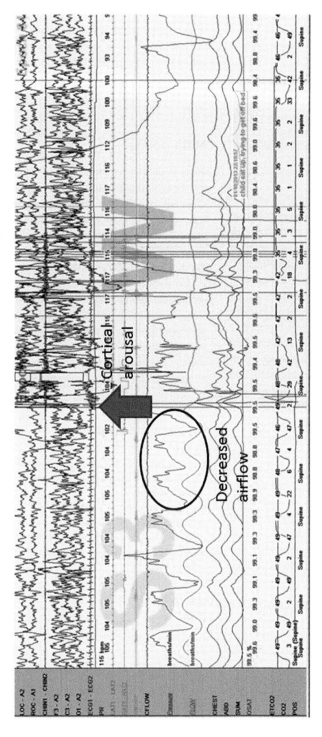

Figure 37.1 A 60-second epoch from the diagnostic polysomnogram of a 7-year-old child who was referred to the pediatric sleep center for evaluation of sleepwalking and was also noted to have snoring on clinical history. A typical episode of sleepwalking is shown as the child sits up and starts to get out of bed. Note the delta wave activity (large slow waves in the electroencephalographic channels) before, during (where legible), and after the cortical arousal that starts at the red arrow and continues through the duration of the child's movement. Channels are as follows: electrooculogram (left, LOC-A2; right, ROC-A1), chin electromyogram (EMG) (CHIN1-CHIN2), electroencephalogram (left frontal, F3-A2; left central, C3-A2; left occipital, O1-A2), electrocardiogram channel, pulse rate (PR), limb EMG (left, LAT-LAT2; right, RAT1-RAT2), snore channel, positive airway pressure signal (CFLOW), nasal pressure airflow (Pressure), nasal–oral airflow (FLOW), respiratory effort by respiratory inductance plethysmography (thoracic [CHEST], abdominal [ABD], sum channel [SUM]), oxygen saturation (OSAT), capnography value (ETCO2), capnography waveform (CO2), and position (POS). See plate section for color version.

227

Table 37.1 Examples of safety recommendations for children who sleepwalk

Child to sleep on a mattress on a floor
Child to sleep on the first floor of the house
Remove/pad sharp corners on furniture
Use safety gates on stairs or in doorways
Consider door alarms on doors which exit the home
Consider window alarms on second-floor windows
Parents to secure any potentially dangerous items out of
    child's reach

can still occupy a substantial proportion of an anatomically narrowed upper airway. If surgery is not an option, the child has had prior adenotonsillectomy, or the family has a strong preference for non-surgical treatment, then discussion should also include CPAP therapy. Through education, incentives, or recognition of symptom improvement, many children show excellent adherence to CPAP therapy. Treatment of OSA with adenotonsillectomy or CPAP therapy will improve or resolve obstructions in the airway, thereby decreasing the event-related cortical arousals during sleep, which may trigger parasomnias, including sleepwalking. The decrease in nighttime arousals also may lead to more restful, consolidated sleep, likely with improvements in daytime sleepiness, concentration, and mood as well.

Additionally, care should be taken to maintain safety of the child at all times (Table 37.1). It is recommended that children who sleepwalk should not sleep on the top bunk of bunk beds. Parents may want to remove furniture with sharp corners or pad sharp corners to avoid injury. Furthermore parents should consider door or window alarms that may be placed on second-floor windows and any doors that exit the home such as front doors, back doors, garage doors, and basement doors. Safety gates at the top of staircases or in doorways could avert potential falls. Sleeping on the first floor may be advisable. Parents should carefully lock up potentially dangerous items such as guns, knives, and car keys when appropriate.

Main points

Many pediatricians and clinicians dismiss sleepwalking as a normal phenomenon of childhood. This is often not true. Through thoughtful and thorough clinical history, clinicians should evaluate for a sleep disorder that may trigger partial cortical arousals from sleep. This includes obtaining history regarding snoring or other symptoms of sleep-disordered breathing. If OSA is suspected or features of the clinical history are unclear, then a polysomnogram may help identify sleep-disordered breathing, or another sleep disorder that can trigger sleepwalking. If OSA is observed, then initial treatment with adenotonsillectomy or CPAP therapy is indicated. Additionally, parents should try to ensure a safe sleeping environment.

FURTHER READING

Guilleminault C, Lee JH, Chan A, et al. Non-REM-sleep instability in recurrent sleepwalking in pre-pubertal children. *Sleep Med* 2005;**6**:515–21.

Guilleminault C, Palombini L, Pelayo R, Chervin RD. Sleepwalking and sleep terrors in prepubertal children: what triggers them? *Pediatrics* 2003;**111**:e17–25.

Hoban TF. Sleep disorders in children. *Ann NY Acad Sci* 2010;**1184**:1–14.

38

An adult parasomnia can sometimes reflect effects of occult obstructive sleep apnea

Naricha Chirakalwasan

Case

A 60-year-old Asian man was referred to our sleep disorder clinic because of history of abnormal behavior during sleep for approximately 10 years. His bed partner reported that she observed the patient to be moving in an aggressive manner including punching, kicking his legs around, and occasionally with vocalization. There were no tongue biting or urinary incontinence associated with the reported abnormal behaviors. These aggressive behaviors almost resulted in injuries to her several times, and appeared to be more frequent in the past 2 years, which caused her to seek medical attention. She reported that these episodes can occur at any time during the night. She had also observed loud snoring and witnessed some apneic episodes. The patient admitted to recall of some unpleasant dreams. He also had frequent nocturia and experienced an average of three awakenings per night, but was able to fall back asleep in < 10 minutes. The patient had developed excessive daytime sleepiness in the last 5 years. His Epworth Sleepiness Scale score was 16 out of 24.

Past medical history was significant for hypertension and hyperlipidemia. His medications included hydrochlorothiazide 25 mg daily and simvastatin 20 mg daily. He denied drinking alcohol and he was a non-smoker.

On physical exam, the patient was a middle age Asian male who was in no distress. The vital signs were normal except for a blood pressure of 150/90 mmHg.

His height was 5 feet, 6 inches (168 cm) and his weight was 138 pounds (63 kg) with a body mass index (BMI) of 22.3 kg/m^2. Oral examination demonstrated a modified Mallampati Class IV and an overjet of 6 mm. The patient was observed to have retrognathia and micrognathia. The neck circumference was 14 inches (36 cm). The nasal exam was normal as was his neurologic examination.

What are the differential diagnoses in this case?

This patient presented with abnormal behavior during sleep, or parasomnia. According to the International Classification of Sleep Disorders (ICSD-2),[1] parasomnia can be divided into three main categories; disorders of arousal (non-rapid eye movement [NREM] parasomnia), parasomnias usually associated with rapid eye movement (REM) sleep, and other parasomnias. Since the reported symptoms are aggressive and the patient reported some unpleasant dreams, REM sleep behavior disorder (RBD), one of the most commonly described parasomnias, is a possible diagnosis. The patient demographic (middle age male) also suits the diagnosis of RBD. However the patient and his bed partner also reported symptoms suggestive of obstructive sleep apnea (OSA), including loud snoring, witnessed apneas, and excessive daytime sleepiness. The patient was not overweight by standards used in Western countries (BMI > 25 kg/m^2), but patients of

Common Pitfalls in Sleep Medicine, ed. Ronald D. Chervin. Published by Cambridge University Press. © Cambridge University Press 2014.

Asian descent have been reported to have a lower BMI. Furthermore, at the same BMI, patients of Asian descent were reported to have more severe OSA with higher apnea/hypopnea indices (AHIs, events per hour of sleep). This patient was observed to have craniofacial structures predisposing to upper airway obstruction, including a modified Mallampati Class IV, retrognatia, micrognatia, and overjet. Association between severe OSA and abnormal sleep behavior suggestive of RBD has been reported in the literature. Pseudo-RBD has been described as a form of confusional arousal observed following obstructive events in patients with severe OSA.[2] In these reported cases, the history suggested RBD, but polysomnography did not support this diagnosis. Since the above patient had the symptoms and clinical characteristics suggestive of RBD and OSA, the most likely diagnoses in this case are pseudo-RBD, or perhaps RBD and OSA (separate disorders).

What is the essential investigation in this patient?

Overnight polysomnography is the recommended investigation in this patient. Even though not all patients who are suspected to have a parasomnia would need polysomnography, to diagnose RBD or pseudo-RBD, polysomnography is warranted. The decision to obtain full 16-lead electroencephalography to exclude the possibility of nocturnal epilepsy would be based on the level of clinical suspicion for seizures. Lack of underlying diseases predisposing to nocturnal epilepsy or the typical presentations such as stereotypic movements, tongue biting, or urinary incontinence made nocturnal epilepsy less likely in this case. Overnight polysomnography with video recording and extra limb leads to record the abnormal movements and behaviors was performed in this patient. This patient's polysomnogram revealed severe OSA with an AHI of 44 events per hour of sleep, a respiratory disturbance index of 56 events per hour, an arousal index of 45 events per hour, and nadir oxygen saturation of 72%. Several episodes of gesturing, kicking, punching, and vocalization were observed following

arousals from obstructive events. These abnormal behaviors were equally distributed between REM and NREM sleep. Normal chin atonia was observed during REM sleep. No epileptiform activity was detected on the electroencephalogram (EEG) (Figure 38.1). These findings are consistent with the diagnosis or pseudo-RBD from OSA.

Discussion

This case demonstrated the importance of polysomnography with video recording in patients who present with abnormal dream enactment. Generally, the observed aggressive dream enacting behaviors occurring during arousals at the end of obstructive events are diagnostic of pseudo-RBD. Polysomnography is also required to exclude other potential diagnoses such as nocturnal epilepsy or idiopathic RBD. A reported case series of 16 patients with pseudo-RBD revealed that OSA was observed to be severe in all patients, with a mean AHI of 68 ± 19 events per hour of sleep. These patients also had frequent arousals with a mean AI of 74 ± 17 events per hour of sleep. The typical abnormal behaviors were observed to be gesturing, kicking, raising the arms, and talking. Abnormal behaviors were observed in 54% of the patients in arousals from both REM and NREM sleep, and in 46% of the subjects only in REM sleep. As mentioned earlier, idiopathic RBD and OSA (separate disorders) are diagnoses that can sometimes give rise to similar clinical presentations. However, increased tonic or phasic electromyographic activity during REM sleep, in the chin or limb muscles, would be expected in idiopathic RBD, and this was not observed in this patient. It is important to separate these two entities (pseudo-RBD and idiopathic RBD) by polysomnography with video recording. Prior studies have shown that 65% of the subjects initially diagnosed as having idiopathic RBD developed parkinsonism and/or dementia following a mean interval of 13 years. If patients are misdiagnosed with idiopathic RBD, they may be subjected to inappropriate investigations, prognoses, and treatment. For example, clonazepam is the most effective treatment for idiopathic RBD, but it can worsen OSA in pseudo-RBD.

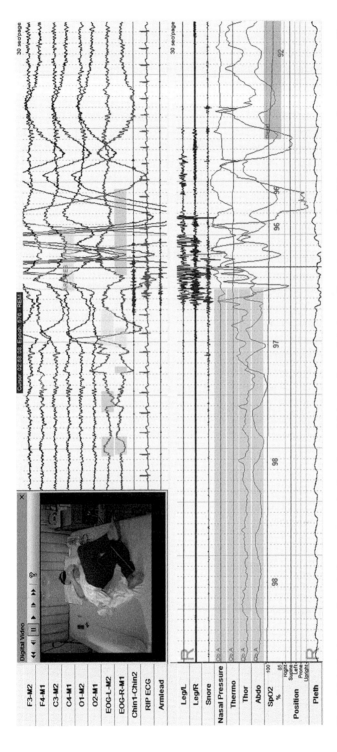

Figure 38.1 This 30-second epoch shows an example of an abnormal behavior observed during rapid eye movement sleep following a long obstructive apnea. The synchronized video recording demonstrates the patient to be aggressively moving his arms and legs during an arousal at the termination of the apnea. During the initial period without an arousal, normal chin atonia is observed. Figure abbreviations: F3-M2, left frontal electroencephalogram (EEG); F4-M1, right frontal EEG; C3-M2, left central EEG; C4-M1, right central EEG; O1-M2, left occipital EEG; O2-M1, right occipital EEG; EOG-L-M2, left eye electrooculography (EOG); EOG-R-M1, right eye electrooculography; Chin1-Chin2, chin electromyogram (EMG); RIP ECG, electrocardiographic leads; Armlead, extensor digitorum profundus surface EMG; Leg/L, left anterior tibialis surface EMG; Leg/R, right anterior tibialis surface EMG; Thermo, oronasal thermocouple; Thor, thoracic excursion; Abdo, abdominal excursion; SpO2, oxyhemoglobin saturation (%); Pleth, pulse waveform from oximeter. See plate section for color version.

231

The observed aggressive dream-enacting behaviors occurring during arousals at the end of obstructive events are diagnostic of pseudo-RBD. However concomitant idiopathic REM sleep behavior disorder cannot be entirely excluded because dream-enacted behavior during REM sleep as well as REM sleep without atonia may not always occur during laboratory sleep studies. Prior studies demonstrated the usefulness of cardiac 123 I-metaiodobenzylguanidine (MIBG) scintigraphic assessment as a supportive diagnostic indicator for concomitant idiopathic RBD.[3] Pseudo-RBD is not the only reported abnormal behavior that occurs during arousals associated with OSA. Movement disorder, specifically sleep-related rhythmic movement disorder, has also previously reported.[4] The rhythmic movements associated with OSA were observed to commence with the onset of each arousal and resolved quickly in synchrony with transition of the EEG back to sleep. In pseudo-RBD, when behavior is observed to occur from arousals related to obstructive events, treatment for OSA generally is effective in ameliorating the abnormal behaviors. Continuous positive airway pressure, the most effective treatment for OSA, was reported to be effective with complete cessation of abnormal sleep behaviors, unpleasant dreams, snoring, and daytime hypersomnolence in patients with pseudo-RBD.

Main point

Abnormal behaviors in the form of RBD by clinical history can be a manifestation of occult OSA called pseudo-RBD. It is important to obtain the medical history and perform a thorough physical examination to uncover the possibility of OSA. Polysomnography with video recording is essential to diagnose pseudo-RBD. Typical findings are abnormal behaviors occurring during arousals that follow obstructive events. Preserved muscle atonia during REM sleep differentiates pseudo-RBD from idiopathic RBD. It is crucial to differentiate the two entities due to different prognosis and treatment modalities. Treatment of OSA has been shown to resolve abnormal behaviors associated with pseudo-RBD.

REFERENCES

1. American Academy of Sleep Medicine. *International Classification of Sleep Disorders. Diagnostic and Coding Manual*, Second Edition. Westchester, IL: American Academy of Sleep Medicine;2005.
2. Iranzo A, Santamaria J. Severe obstructive sleep apnea/hypopnea mimicking REM sleep behavior disorder. *Sleep* 2005;**28**:203–6.
3. Miyamoto T, Miyamoto M, Suzuki K, et al. Comparison of severity of obstructive sleep apnea and degree of accumulation of cardiac 123I-MIBG radioactivity as a diagnostic marker for idiopathic REM sleep behavior disorder. *Sleep Med* 2009;**10**:577–80.
4. Chirakalwasan N, Hassan F, Kaplish N, Fetterolf J, Chervin RD. Near resolution of sleep related rhythmic movement disorder after CPAP for OSA. *Sleep Med* 2009;**10**:497–500.

Circadian rhythm sleep disorders

Roughly 10% of the workforce in the United States engages in shift work. Many individuals experience the effects of abrupt changes in time zones when they travel. Youngest and oldest adults often confront the effects of tendencies to have delayed or advanced sleep phases, if not full-fledged disorders that stem from these physiologic age-related tendencies. These and other circadian rhythm sleep disorders can have enormous impact on health, quality of life, productivity, safety, physical performance, mood, and well-being. The chapters in this section, written by sleep medicine physicians with background in psychiatry and neurology, focus on the assessment and treatment of three key types of circadian rhythm sleep disorders.

In contrast to sleep-related breathing disorders, central hypersomnias, and some parasomnias, polysomnography usually plays no role in the diagnosis of circadian rhythm sleep disorders. Instead, sleep logs and actigraphy over multiple nights at home are often the most useful ancillary investigations, beyond a thorough history during the clinic visit. A variety of treatments can be useful, including behavioral management, bright light therapy, and pharmacologic intervention. Fortunately, clinicians who avoid several potential pitfalls in the recognition and treatment of circadian rhythm disorders will often be rewarded with substantial improvement in patients' symptoms and disease burden.

39

Circadian rhythm sleep disorders can complicate or confuse mental health diagnoses in young persons

Fouad Reda

Case

An 18-year-old female college student presented to a psychiatric emergency center in apparent emotional distress. The patient was evaluated by the on-call psychiatry resident physician. Her chief complaints included increased anxiety, crying spells, and poor sleep over the last 2 days. The patient reported that her symptoms began after she received poor grades for the last academic semester. However, according to the patient, she has been suffering from difficulty with poor sleep/insomnia, low mood, irritability, tiredness, fatigue, daytime sleepiness, and poor concentration since the beginning of the semester. Despite her daytime sleepiness and tiredness, the patient usually feels more alert during the evenings and has difficulty with sleep initiation. She reports having experienced "periods" of such symptoms since her early teens but never sought any medical or psychiatric help. She has no previously diagnosed psychiatric or medical problems. She takes birth control pills, but no other regular medications. The patient's family history is significant for insomnia in her mother, but no history of mood or psychotic disorders. Her review of systems was otherwise unremarkable.

The patient's social history is significant for being the middle child with strong relationships with her parents and siblings. She only has a few friends and describes herself as "shy." She reports that her parents have very high expectations of her. She was very concerned that her parents would be disappointed in her academic performance. The patient is a freshman in college who just completed her first semester. Although she was an excellent student during her high school years, her academic performance has been suffering since she started college. She attributed this to her poor concentration. She also admits to skipping morning classes on multiple occasions. She drinks alcohol socially and denies any other substance abuse.

The patient's physical exam was unremarkable. On Mental Status Examination (MSE) the patient was noted to have a tearful affect. She was, however, able to smile appropriately later on. She was alert and fully oriented, but had a slight decrease in attention span. Otherwise, her MSE was within the expected norm. Blood tests including complete blood count, electrolyte profile, and thyroid-stimulating hormone level were within normal limits.

The resident felt that the patient's most recent symptoms were reactive in nature, and could be attributed to an adjustment disorder with both depressive and anxiety features. However, considering her reported long standing history of neuropsychological symptoms (insomnia, low mood, irritability, tiredness, fatigue, daytime sleepiness, and poor concentration), the resident felt that this acute psychiatric presentation most likely evolved on top of a more chronic process. The resident's differential diagnosis for the chronic mood process included:

1. Dysthymia.
2. Major depressive disorder, recurrent.
3. Bipolar disorder, not otherwise specified.

Common Pitfalls in Sleep Medicine, ed. Ronald D. Chervin. Published by Cambridge University Press. © Cambridge University Press 2014.

The resident's plan was to start the patient on an antidepressant and a hypnotic with consideration to add a mood stabilizer if more evidence for bipolarity was gathered.

What other information should have been considered before reaching the above diagnosis?

At first glance, it is reasonable to consider the existence of a primary psychiatric illness; specifically a primary mood disorder given the above symptoms. However, more information regarding the patient's sleep schedule and its relation to her daytime symptoms turns out to be of key significance. Although the patient did report having difficulty with sleep initiation since her mid-teens, no information regarding any specific patterns for her sleep difficulties was obtained. A more detailed history would have revealed the following:

1. In middle school and high school, the patient encountered difficulty with sleep initiation at night on school days, but not during weekends, holidays, or summertime.
2. Despite her sleeping difficulties, her academic performance in middle school and high school was not affected. The patient attributed that to the fact that she was able to "catch-up" on sleep during the weekends.
3. In her first semester in college, the patient was taking regular classes during weekdays and working at the school library during the weekends, thus reducing her ability to "catch up" on sleep.
4. The patient's preferred bedtime was reported to be around 2:00 AM, at which time she had no difficulty falling asleep. Her preferred wake-up time was at 11:00 AM, at which time she felt most refreshed. She followed this schedule during summertime and school breaks, which resulted in the patient having normal mood and a normal level of energy.
5. Despite her tiredness and sleepiness during the daytime, the patient always felt as if she had a "second wind" in the evening hours.

Discussion

Would the additional information challenge the resident's working diagnosis and treatment plan?

The additional information reveals the existence of delayed sleep-phase disorder (DSPD). According to the International Classification of Sleep Disorders (ICSD-2),[1] a circadian rhythm disorder – delayed sleep-phase type (DSPD), is characterized by sleep onset and wakeup times that are usually delayed by a minimum of 2 hours relative to desired or socially acceptable sleep–wake times. Once sleep initiation is achieved, patients with DSPD do not experience difficulty maintaining sleep. The duration of sleep is typically within the expected age specific norm. The difficulty with sleep initiation that such patients have, when attempting to sleep at a desired earlier bedtime, simulates sleep-onset insomnia. These patients are likely to experience heightened alertness in the evening with the increase in circadian drive.[2] Sleep restriction due to the enforced arousal at socially acceptable wake-up times may result in sleep insufficiency and daytime sleepiness. Delayed sleep-phase disorder is more common in adolescents and young adults compared to the adult population, with an estimated prevalence rate of 7%. However, newer research suggests the prevalence rate in young adults may be less than previous estimates.[3] The cause of DSPD is not fully understood, but both chronobiologic and behavioral mechanisms (ex: circadian and homeostatic drives) likely contribute to its etiology.[2] Around 40% of people with DSPD have a family history of similar sleep-related complaints.[1] (Did you note our patient's family history?)

Delayed sleep-phase disorder has been associated with mental disturbances in adolescents. Association with depressive symptoms and depressive disorders as well as with cluster A and C personality traits has been reported in the literature.[1,4,5] Some notable effects of DSPD specific to adolescents and young adults include irritability, depression, decreased concentration and poor school performance.[2,5] A major driver of such symptoms appears to be the resultant decreased amount of sleep and the related daytime sleepiness. Consequences often mimic or exacerbate neuropsychological symptoms usually found in primary mood disorders, symptoms such as low mood, irritability, and decreased concentration.[5] In addition, the delayed sleep onset in DSPD can be easily attributed mistakenly to other causes of initial insomnia, such as primary insomnia or psychiatric illnesses. The heightened alertness in the evening can be confused with decreased need for sleep. This, coupled with irritability, can raise concern for potential hypomanic or mixed mood symptoms. A recent study suggested that patients with DSPD may show marked anxiety and excess emotional expression in face of perceived stress (note our patient's presenting and most recent symptoms).[6]

Thus in our case, the patient's chronic symptoms could be explained by DSPD coupled with insufficient hours of sleep. Moreover, the clear resolution of the neuropsychological symptoms during summertime and school breaks decreases the likelihood of any primary or comorbid mood illness. The patient's acute episode of increased emotionality (anxiety and crying spells of 2 days duration) is an acute adjustment reaction precipitated by getting bad grades. A simple adjustment reaction does not usually require major psychotropic intervention and can be addressed with counseling and supportive psychotherapy.

Based on the above, it is easy to misdiagnose a circadian rhythm disorder as a primary mood disorder, especially when relying on a fast and shallow history. A misdiagnosis of this type could have a significant impact on the clinical management and the outcome. In this case, starting the patient on an antidepressant most likely would not have improved her chronic daytime symptoms, and may have subjected her to undesirable side effects.[7]

Proper identification and standard treatment of DSPD

The diagnosis of DSPD is usually based on clinical history. Other medical, sleep, and mental disorders and medications or substance use that better explain symptoms should be ruled out. The relationship between daytime symptoms and sleep patterns should be clearly elicited (as in the above case) in order to rule out any primary psychiatric comorbidity. Significant improvement in the neuropsychiatric symptoms when patients are able to follow their natural circadian rhythm drives, for example on weekends or vacations, excludes any primary mood disorder. Utilization of sleep diaries or actigraphy monitoring is recommended for a minimum of 7 days to detect a consistent delay in the timing – sleep onset and offset – of an otherwise normal sleep period. Polysomnography is usually not recommended unless other primary comorbid sleep disorders are suspected, such as obstructive sleep apnea or periodic limb movement disorder. The use of circadian rhythm markers, such as dim light plasma melatonin onset (DLMO) or continuous recording of body temperature, can aid in confirming the diagnosis, but these are not commonly used in clinical settings.[2,8,9]

The aim of treatment of DSPD is to reestablish the alignment between the biologic (circadian) clock and the terrestrial time (24 hour light–dark cycle). Behavioral modifications to promote proper sleep hygiene are important, but not sufficient for treatment. The currently indicated treatments for DSPD include: chronotherapy, light therapy, and timed melatonin administration.[9]

Chronotherapy implements the systematic delaying of bedtime and wake-up time by 3 hours on successive days until the desired bedtime and wake-up time are reached. With this therapy, it usually takes between 5 and 6 days to attain the desired sleep schedule. The use of light therapy has been found to be of benefit given the influence of light on circadian rhythm drive. Exposure to bright light immediately after awakening in the morning leads to the advancement of the phase of circadian rhythm. A light pulse of 2500–10 000 lux is generally administered for about 1–2 hours starting at the socially desired wake-up time. The use of melatonin has also been implemented in the attempt to shift the phase of circadian rhythm. Small doses of melatonin, 0.1–0.5 mg administered in the early evening, are usually sufficient to achieve the phase shifting.[2,9]

Literature suggests that a combination of the above therapies is also implemented and proved effective in clinical settings. The use of hypnotic medications might be helpful, but is not usually recommended and not considered a standard of treatment. This option remains limited by the potential side effects (sedation) and the quick relapse after discontinuation of treatment.[2,8-10]

Main points

Delayed sleep-phase circadian rhythm disorder is common in young adults. By itself it is a benign shift of otherwise normal sleep phase and structure. When coupled with an environmental or social requirement for earlier bedtime and wake-up time, initial insomnia and sleep deprivation ensues. The resultant clinical picture can simulate a primary mood illness. A carefully obtained history about the patient's sleep patterns and subsequent relation to the daytime symptoms can aid in the distinction and can drastically change the management plan.

REFERENCES

1. American Academy of Sleep Medicine. *International Classification of Sleep Disorders. Diagnostic and Coding Manual*, Second Edition. Westchester, IL: American Academy of Sleep Medicine;2005.

2. Kryger M, Roth T, Dement W, eds. *Principles and Practice of Sleep Medicine*, Fifth Edition. St Louis, MO: Elsevier;2010.

3. Hazama GI, Inoue Y, Kojima K, Ueta T, Nakagome K. The prevalence of probable delayed-sleep-phase syndrome in students from junior high school to university in Tottori, Japan. *Tohoku J Exp Med* 2008;**216**:95-8.

4. Turek FW. From circadian rhythms to clock genes in depression. *Int Clin Psychopharmacol* 2007;**22**(Suppl 2): S1-8.

5. Millman RP. Working Group on Sleepiness in Adolescents/Young Adults; AAP Committee on Adolescence. Excessive sleepiness in adolescents and young adults: causes, consequences, and treatment strategies. *Pediatrics* 2005;**115**:1774-86.

6. Shirayama M, Shirayama Y, Iida H, et al. The psychological aspects of patients with delayed sleep phase syndrome (DSPS). *Sleep Med* 2003;4:427-33.

7. Lam RW. Sleep disturbances and depression: a challenge for antidepressants. *Int Clin Psychopharmacol* 2006;**21** (Suppl 1):S25-9.

8. Sack RL, Auckley D, Auger RR, et al. American Academy of Sleep Medicine. *Sleep* 2007;**30**:1484-501.

9. Morgenthaler TI, Lee-Chiong T, Alessi C, et al. Standards of Practice Committee of the American Academy of Sleep Medicine. *Sleep* 2007;30:1445-59.

10. Gradisar M, Dohnt H, Gardner G, et al. A randomized controlled trial of cognitive-behavior therapy plus bright light therapy for adolescent delayed sleep phase disorder. *Sleep* 2011;**34**:1671-80.

40

Advanced sleep phase can cause considerable morbidity in older persons until it is diagnosed and addressed

Cathy A. Goldstein

Case

A 78-year-old female presented to the sleep disorders clinic with 2 years of progressive sleepiness and difficulty staying asleep. She noted feeling particularly sleepy after having dinner around 6:00 PM. She reported napping in a chair inadvertently from around 7:00 PM to 9:00 PM while watching television with her husband. Her sleep schedule is as follows. She retires to the bedroom around 10:00 PM where she sleeps well for approximately 5 hours. She may doze on and off from 3:00 to 4:00 AM at which time she begins to have marked difficulty returning to sleep. She will toss and turn until 5:00 AM when she finally gets out of bed to begin her day, starting with a cup of coffee on her balcony followed by gardening. She feels alert and energetic throughout the morning and early afternoon. Her mood is good with the exception of frustration due to her early morning awakenings and evening sleepiness that has negatively impacted her social life. Her husband denied the presence of snoring, gasping, choking, apneas, excessive body movements, or other abnormal sleep-related behaviors. She reported that after evaluation by her primary physician, a sleep study was ordered which was "normal" and zolpidem prescribed. She sustained a fall and confusion after taking zolpidem. Her only other medication is atorvastatin. Physical exam demonstrates a body mass index of 20.3 kg/m^2, a Class II modified Mallampati score with normal neurologic, cardiovascular, and pulmonary examinations. Overnight polysomnography conducted with lights out at 10:00 PM and lights on at 6:00 AM demonstrated a sleep onset latency of 4 minutes, total sleep time of 281 minutes, sleep efficiency of 58.5%, 12% stage N1 sleep, 59% stage N2 sleep, 8% stage N3 sleep, 21% stage rapid eye movement (REM) sleep, and an arousal index of 20 per hour of sleep. Sleep efficiency was reduced due to increased wake after sleep onset during the second half of the recording. The apnea/hypopnea index was within normal limits at 0.8 per hour of sleep. The oxygen nadir was 93%. In his notes, the sleep technician reported that the patient was asleep when he entered the room for the hook up.

Did this patient need a polysomnogram? What would be more beneficial testing?

Overnight polysomnography was not necessary in this case. The patient described a history suggestive of a disorder of sleep timing (a circadian rhythm sleep disorder). Without more suggestive signs, symptoms, or risk factors, sleep-disordered breathing is not a likely cause of her sleep complaints. In addition, there is no indication that a parasomnia or sleep-related movement disorder exists. Because our suspicion for another primary sleep disorder is very low, overnight polysomnography is not likely to be helpful in this context. Her polysomnogram demonstrated shortened sleep onset latency, and in fact she was nodding off even prior to the application of electroencephalogram

Common Pitfalls in Sleep Medicine, ed. Ronald D. Chervin. Published by Cambridge University Press. © Cambridge University Press 2014.

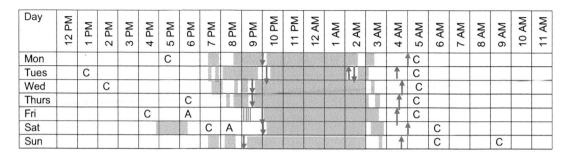

Figure 40.1 Sample sleep log in a patient with advance sleep phase.

leads. The study also showed reduced total sleep time, and decreased sleep efficiency as the recording was performed at a time later than her preferred time for sleep. Sleep logs would be helpful to clarify sleep timing, as would actigraphy, a device that monitors body movement as a surrogate marker for sleep. A 7-day sleep log is shown in Figure 40.1.

Was zolpidem an appropriate treatment?

Zolpidem is a hypnotic medication that is US Food and Drug Administration (FDA) -approved for the treatment of insomnia. Although this patient has difficulty with sleep maintenance, her history suggests that the source of early morning awakenings is a misalignment of her sleep propensity with her desired sleep times. Furthermore, care must be taken with use of zolpidem in older patients, who may be more prone to experience side effects, such as the fall and confusion sustained by our patient. Therefore, zolpidem (or any hypnotic medication) is not an optimal treatment in this case. Treatment to align the patient's sleep propensity with her desired sleep–wake times should be pursued as below.

Discussion

The patient describes a sleep propensity occurring earlier than conventional or desired sleep times. This causes chronic difficulty in maintaining wakefulness up to the desired bedtime and difficulty maintaining sleep up to the desired wake time. This is consistent with the circadian rhythm sleep disorder – advanced sleep phase type (ASPT) as defined by the International Classification of Sleep Disorders (ICSD-2).[1] When sleeping *ad libitum*, sleep duration and quality are not impaired but occur at a stable, advanced phase. Sleep onset typically occurs between 6:00 and 9:00 PM and sleep offset between 2:00 and 5:00 AM. However, when the individual attempts to sleep at clock times later than the circadian preference, evening sleepiness and sleep maintenance insomnia ensue. Even when successful at staying awake later, patients still experience early morning awakening and thus have a shortened sleep period leading to excessive sleepiness.[1]

Although rare, advanced sleep phase becomes more common with advancing age. The condition showed a prevalence of about 1% in a group of middle-aged subjects presenting to a sleep disorders clinic.[2] The disorder is potentially under recognized, as an early sleep–wake schedule does not typically lead to problems in school or work. Familial cases of advanced sleep phase have been described in association with mutations of Per2 and casein kinase 1 delta genes, with an autosomal dominant mode of inheritance.[3,4] Whether advanced sleep phase in aging represents the same condition as advanced sleep phase in younger patients remains unclear.

Advance

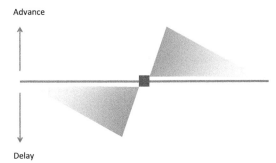

Delay

Figure 40.2 Phase response curve to light. The core body temperature nadir is depicted by the square and occurs roughly 2–3 hours before habitual wake time. Light exposure prior to core body temperature nadir results in a circadian phase delay, which moves biologic rhythms later. Light exposure after the core body temperature minimum has the opposite effect and results in an advance of circadian phase. The largest magnitude of change is produced when light is delivered close to the time of core body temperature nadir.

The pathophysiology of advanced sleep phase is not clearly delineated. Potential mechanisms are based on the current knowledge of circadian biology. Human circadian rhythms usually oscillate with a period of 24.2 hours. Shortening of the circadian period (*tau*) may be implicated in advanced sleep phase. This was demonstrated by a familial ASPT patient whose temperature and sleep–wake rhythm cycled with a period of 23.3 hours when the individual was isolated from temporal cues.[5] Circadian *zeitgebers* (time givers) modulate circadian phase and include light, melatonin, social interaction, feeding, and physical activity. Light is the strongest *zeitgeber*. The direction and degree of phase shift produced by light is defined by the phase response curve to light (Figure 40.2). The human body typically reaches its nadir of core body temperature 2–3 hours prior to habitual wake time. Bright light exposure prior to the core body temperature minimum entrains circadian phase to a later time (delay) whereas exposure to bright light after core body temperature minimum results in a phase shift earlier (advance). Reduced exposure to, or decreased availability of evening light and other *zeitgebers* may advance sleep–wake timing. Alternatively, increased exposure to

morning light may perpetuate the early sleep–wake times seen in ASPT. Patients with ASPT may also have reduced ability to phase delay in response to entraining factors. Abnormalities of the phase response curve to light, such that the delay portion is diminished and the advance portion is enhanced, could theoretically contribute to this disorder as well. Further research is required to fully understand the physiologic causes of this circadian rhythm sleep disorder.

The diagnosis of circadian rhythm sleep disorder, ASPT is made based on the criteria of ICSD-2.[1] A patient's sleep log that records times in and out of bed, estimated sleep duration, caffeine, medication, and alcohol use can provide a useful summary of the relationship of sleep propensity to desired sleep–wake times (Figure 40.1). An actigraph is a device used to monitor movement, and the recorded data provide a surrogate marker for sleep. Derived estimates for total sleep times can show good reliability.[6] The device can provide an objective assessment of sleep–wake patterns during a several day period in the patient's home environment. Both sleep logs (diaries) and actigraphy are recommended by the American Academy of Sleep Medicine at the guideline level in assisting with the evaluation of patients with circadian rhythm sleep disorders. Polysomnography is not suggested in evaluating patients with ASPT unless clinical suspicion for comorbid sleep disorder (such as obstructive sleep apnea) exists.[7] If recorded at the conventional (desired) sleep time, polysomnography may demonstrate a short sleep onset latency, early morning awakening, and increased wake after sleep onset.

The Horne–Ostberg questionnaire is a self assessment of morningness or eveningness. Although patients with advanced sleep phase do score as high or "morning type" on this questionnaire, its use as an isolated diagnostic tool for circadian rhythm sleep disorders remains uncertain.[7] Objective markers of circadian phase, notably melatonin secretion and minimum core body temperature, occur earlier in subjects with ASPT than in other subjects. However, at this time, these assays are not routinely available in the clinical setting.[7] As depression often results in early morning awakenings, evaluation of mood is important to rule out this possibility.

The treatment of ASPT is based on the knowledge of circadian phase shifts in response to *zeitgebers*, and particularly bright light. As discussed above, exposure to bright light in the evening will result in a phase delay. The goal of this shift is to move sleep propensity to a later time so that alertness may be maintained until the desired bedtime and sleep continued until the desired wake time. Light therapy was investigated in a group of subjects with evening sleepiness, early morning awakenings, and early objective markers of circadian phase.[8] Two evenings of bright light therapy at 2500 lux given for 4 hours starting at 8:00 PM resulted in a significant delay of dim light melatonin onset and core body temperature minimum, by approximately 2 hours as compared to controls.[8] Importantly, sleep measures changed significantly after therapy, with wake time occurring > 1 hour later than baseline and total sleep time lengthening similarly.[8] This study was repeated to assess 4-week durability of treatment. Hour-long delays of wake time, 90-minute increases in total sleep time, and 60-minute reductions in wake after sleep onset were seen in the treatment group 1 month after light therapy was delivered. These sleep diary changes were significantly better than baseline, and improvement in total sleep time was also significant in comparison to the control condition.[9] Dim light melatonin onset, although somewhat earlier than it was immediately after treatment, remained significantly later than baseline at the 4-week time point.[9] Another group of investigators found that 12 days of evening bright light exposure (4000 lux for 2 hours at 8:00 PM) delayed core body temperature minimum and bedtime. In addition, time awake after sleep onset was reduced by an hour.[10] Unfortunately, not all studies of evening bright light have had such promising results, particularly in regard to objective sleep parameters. However, this therapy is routinely used due to the scarcity of treatment strategies and low likelihood of side effects. Bright light therapy is recommended by the American Academy of Sleep Medicine as an option for treatment of ASPT (lux and duration of therapy are not specified at this time).[7] Reinforcement of non-light *zeitgebers*, such as exercise, in the evening, could also be beneficial.

Melatonin has a phase response curve demonstrating action in the opposite direction of bright light. Therefore melatonin administration can result in a phase delay when given after the core body temperature minimum. However, it is not routinely used during awakenings in ASPT due to potential for side effects with morning administration. Similarly, hypnotics are not recommended. Chronotherapy, by progressive advancement of sleep–wake times until the desired sleep schedule is achieved, may also be considered, although it has only been described in one case.[7]

Main points

Misalignment of circadian phase and conventional sleep–wake times can result in both excessive sleepiness and insomnia, impairing quality of life. In ASPT, sleep–wake propensity is earlier than expected due to an intrinsic timing abnormality and may be perpetuated by behaviors facilitating a continued phase advance rather than delay. Rigorous clinical evaluation to identify a problem with the timing rather than quality of sleep will help target treatment and avoid unnecessary diagnostic tests. Treatment manipulates the pliable nature of the mammalian internal clock by using *zeitgebers* to delay circadian phase, and avoids the need for hypnotic medications.

REFERENCES

1. American Academy of Sleep Medicine. *International Classification of Sleep Disorders. Diagnostic and Coding Manual*, Second Edition. Westchester, IL: American Academy of Sleep Medicine;2005.
2. Kamei Y, Urata J, Uchiyaya M, et al. Clinical characteristics of circadian rhythm sleep disorders. *Psychiatry Clin Neurosci* 1998;**52**:234–5.
3. Toh KL, Jones CR, He Y, et al. An hPer2 phosphorylation site mutation in familial advanced sleep-phase syndrome. *Science* 2001;**291**:1040–3.
4. Xu Y, Padiath QS, Shapiro RE, et al. Functional consequences of a C K1δ mutation causing familial advanced sleep phase syndrome. *Nature* 2005;**434**:640–4.

5. Jones CR, Campbell SS, Zone SE, et al. Familial advanced sleep-phase syndrome: a short-period circadian rhythm variant in humans. *Nat Med* 1999;**5**:1062–5.

6. Morgenthaler T, Alessi C, Freidman L. Practice parameters for the use of actigraphy in the assessment of sleep and sleep disorders: an update for 2007. *Sleep* 2007;**30**: 519–29.

7. Morgenthaler TI, Lee-Chiong T, Alessi C, et al. Practice parameters for the clinical evaluation and treatment of circadian rhythm sleep disorders. *Sleep* 2007;**30**:1445–9.

8. Lack L, Wright H. The effect of evening bright light in delaying the circadian rhythms and lengthening the sleep of early morning awakening insomniacs. *Sleep* 1993;**16**: 436–43.

9. Lack L, Wright H, Kemp K, Gibbon S. The treatment of early-morning awakening insomnia with two evenings of bright light. *Sleep* 2005;**28**:616–23.

10. Campbel SS, Dawson D, and Anderson MW. Alleviation of sleep maintenance insomnia with timed exposure to bright light. *J Am Geriatr Soc* 1993;**41**:829–36.

41

Shift work disorder is common, consequential, usually unaddressed, but readily treated

Cathy A. Goldstein

Case

A 46-year-old man presented with sleepiness and disrupted sleep. He was feeling well until about 3 months ago when his shift as a police officer was changed from 7:00 AM – 5:00 PM to 11:00 PM – 7:00 AM. He presented to his primary care physician after developing sleepiness to the extent that he was nodding off during his shift and he was chastised at work. A polysomnogram was ordered at that time to determine whether obstructive sleep apnea was a cause of his sleepiness. No sleep-disordered breathing was seen. Subsequently, trazodone was initiated as his somnolence was also accompanied by difficulty initiating and maintaining sleep, resulting in total sleep times of 5–6 hours per day. Trazodone improved his sleep duration slightly but sleepiness worsened to the point that he felt notably drowsy during his commute to and from work. The medication was discontinued. He presented to the sleep disorders clinic for help as he felt his job and safety were at risk.

What important information is missing from the patient's initial evaluation?

A thorough sleep and work schedule, as well as details regarding the work and sleep environment, constitute the most important missing information. Upon further questioning, he explained that he works Monday, Tuesday, Thursday, and Friday nights 11:00 PM to

7:00 AM. His commute is 20 minutes to and from work; he does not wear sunglasses during the drive home. Upon returning from work, he will have breakfast and go on a walk outdoors with his wife and son. He then attempts to sleep around 8:30 AM. His sleep onset latency is estimated at around 20–30 minutes. He sleeps well until around 1:00 PM at which time sleep becomes fragmented and restless, despite the purchase of black-out curtains and ensuring quiet in his bedroom. Typically at 3:00 PM, he will leave the bedroom frustrated and spend the rest of the day with his family. He nods off around 8:00 PM in his son's room after putting him to bed, but is awoken by his wife after an hour to watch their favorite television program and prepare for work. Once at work, he spends most of his time in a dimly lit squad car until he is called for action. On days off he will sleep for 3–4 hours after his shift, but that night retire to bed around 11:00 PM and sleep well through 7:00 AM. He then has difficulty obtaining daytime and afternoon sleep in preparation to resume night shifts. His wife denies witnessed snoring, gasping, choking, apneas, excessive body movements, or other abnormal sleep-related behaviors. Physical exam demonstrates a body mass index of 27.6 kg/m^2, a Class I modified Mallampati score with normal neurologic, cardiovascular, and pulmonary examinations. Overnight polysomnography conducted with lights out at 10:00 PM and lights on at 6:00 AM demonstrated a sleep onset latency of 7 minutes, total sleep time of 412 minutes, sleep efficiency of 85.8%, 7% stage N1 sleep, 48% stage N2 sleep, 27% stage N3

Common Pitfalls in Sleep Medicine, ed. Ronald D. Chervin. Published by Cambridge University Press. © Cambridge University Press 2014.

sleep, 18% stage rapid eye movement (REM) sleep, and an arousal index of 9 per hour of sleep. The apnea/hypopnea index was within normal limits at 1.1 events per hour of sleep. His oxygen saturation nadir was 94%.

Is trazodone the best treatment for his sleep difficulties?

Although trazodone is often used for the treatment of sleep initiation and maintenance insomnia, this patient's difficulty obtaining sleep is due to a misalignment between his natural sleep tendency and the available time for sleep. Therefore, targeted treatment to align internal timing of sleep with the externally imposed sleep opportunity (daytime) is a more effective treatment strategy. Hypnotic agents also carry risk for residual effects that could increase drowsiness during night shift work.

Discussion

This is a case of somnolence during expected wakefulness, and insomnia during the available time for sleep, both in the setting of a non-conventional work schedule (in this case, a night shift). These findings are consistent with Shift Work Disorder. The International Classification of Sleep Disorders (ICSD-2)[1] defines Circadian Rhythm Sleep Disorder, Shift Work Type as at least a month of insomnia or excessive sleepiness in the context of a schedule where the time of work coincides with the typical time for sleep. In our 24-hour, international society, shift work has become commonplace, with at least 15% of the workforce participating in non-traditional shifts worldwide.[2] Most commonly associated with shift work disorder are night and early morning work shifts (start time of 4:00–7:00 AM).[1] The prevalence of shift work disorder in night or rotating shift workers has been estimated at 10%.[3]

The pathophysiology of shift work disorder can be understood within the framework of the two process model of sleep.[4] "Process C" denotes the circadian regulatory component and is mediated by the suprachiasmatic nucleus (SCN) housed in the hypothalamus. This internal clock, controlled by gene transcription and negative feedback loops, promotes sleep during the subjective night through an evening rise in melatonin and reduction in core body temperature, which reaches its lowest value 2–3 hours before waking. "Process S", or the homeostatic sleep drive, reflects the "sleep hunger" that grows with wakefulness and diminishes with sleep. The two processes interact. Homeostatic sleep need begins to increase after awakening, and mounts as the day proceeds. The circadian alerting signal counteracts this sleep pressure as it rises throughout the day to its evening peak, such that wakefulness can be maintained steadily until bedtime. Two hours prior to typical sleep onset, melatonin secretion begins, inhibiting SCN neuronal firing. This phenomenon, in conjunction with the high homeostatic sleep drive, facilitates sleep onset. Although sleep hunger starts to dissipate after sleep ensues, the circadian alerting signal remains low. Thus, sleep is consolidated through morning.

Excessive sleepiness in shift work disorder is due to attempted wakefulness during a time of high sleep propensity (Figure 41.1), and to chronic partial sleep loss. Insomnia – including difficulties with sleep onset, maintenance, and subjective poor sleep quality – is seen in this context because the individual attempts to sleep at a time when the circadian alerting signal is high, during the daytime. Ongoing sleep deprivation then mediates the homeostatic component of somnolence in shift work disorder.

Shift work has been associated with a host of negative effects on health. An increased risk of cancer, metabolic disorders, mood disturbances, reproductive abnormalities, gastrointestinal illnesses, and cardiovascular disease has been associated with shift work.[2] Furthermore, performance may be impaired with resultant occupational consequences and motor vehicle crashes.

A diagnosis of shift work disorder can be made with ICSD-2[1] criteria, which include patient's report of insomnia or excessive sleepiness in the context of a work schedule that coincides with the typical time

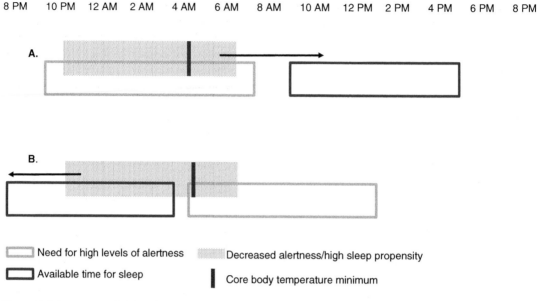

8 PM   10 PM   12 AM   2 AM   4 AM   6 AM   8 AM   10 AM   12 PM   2 PM   4 PM   6 PM   8 PM

A.

B.

☐ Need for high levels of alertness   ▨ Decreased alertness/high sleep propensity

☐ Available time for sleep   ▮ Core body temperature minimum

Figure 41.1 In patients with habitual sleep times of 11:00 PM to 7:00 AM, core body temperature minimum (CBT_{min}) is between 4:00 AM and 5:00 AM. Onset of melatonin secretion is approximately 7 hours before this time (9–10:00 PM) and peaks just prior to CBT_{min}. The time of peak melatonin secretion and CBT_{min} coincides with the nadir of circadian alertness. Label **A**: During a night shift condition, the intrinsic timing of high sleep propensity may result in somnolence during work and insomnia during the day sleep bout. Therapeutic goals include a phase delay (black arrow), such that sleep promoting factors fall within the available rest period rather than the work period. This could potentially be achieved with bright light during the first half of the shift, avoidance of bright light after the shift and on the commute home, and melatonin prior to day sleep. Label **B**: During early rise shift work, the intrinsic timing of high sleep propensity may result in somnolence during the first portion of the work period and insomnia at sleep onset. Therapeutic goals include a phase advance (black arrow), such that sleep promoting factors coincide with the available earlier rest period rather than the work period or morning commute. Use of a bright light box after arriving at work, avoidance of afternoon and evening bright light, and evening melatonin prior to bedtime may be beneficial. See plate section for color version.

for sleep. Symptoms should be present for at least a month. Diagnosis can typically be made by clinical inquiry that includes a detailed sleep and work schedule. Information about caffeine intake, light exposure during the shift and time off, characteristics of the sleep environment, and family and social obligations during time off are helpful in evaluation of this disorder and may provide targets for therapeutic intervention. As with all circadian rhythm sleep disorders, a sleep log or diary is recommended for evaluation. Use of an actigraph – a device worn on the wrist to monitor movement and provide a surrogate measure for sleep patterns – also may provide helpful diagnostic information.[5]

The goal of treatment in shift work disorder is to optimize sleep quality and duration during the allotted time in bed and maximize alertness during the shift. Therapeutic strategies shift circadian phase to move the inherent factors that promote sleep from the externally imposed work time to the available time for sleep. This requires an understanding of the human phase response curves to light and melatonin. Bright light is the strongest circadian *zeitgeber* or "time giver" and is most potent in modulation of circadian timing during the night in individuals with normal phase. Bright light prior to the core body temperature minimum (CBT_{min}) and avoidance of bright light after the CBT_{min} will promote a phase delay, whereas the opposite stimulates phase advance. The hormone melatonin, the body's dark signal, also modifies the internal clock and may be given exogenously. The melatonin phase response curve is reverse that of light. Melatonin administration prior to the CBT_{min} results in a phase advance, melatonin after CBT_{min} promotes a phase delay, and daytime delivery produces the largest magnitude of change. In a night shift worker, a phase delay is beneficial to align circadian phase with a night work/day sleep schedule (see Figure 41.1). In contrast, an early rise shift worker may be assisted by a phase advance (see Figure 41.1). Studies that used bright light of variable intensity and duration during the night shift, or post-shift light avoidance, have shown improvements in mood, performance, and alertness with more uneven effects on objective markers of circadian phase and day sleep quality.[5] Recently, a group of nurses who worked night shifts were exposed to 2000–4000 lux of full spectrum light during the first 6 hours of night shift work as their duties allowed.[6] Additionally, they wore ultraviolet light-emitting goggles for the 2-hour period following their shift including the commute home.[6] Compared to the control group, the intervention group experienced longer sleep duration as reflected by actigraphy, and a delay of melatonin midpoint and core body temperature minimum of almost 5 hours, moving these sleep promoting factors from before to within the day sleep period.[6]

In addition to its phase shifting effects, bright light has direct alerting properties as well, conferring further benefit. Light exposure in the occupational environment and avoidance of morning bright light are recommended by the American Academy of Sleep Medicine (AASM) at the guideline level as a therapeutic intervention for night shift work. Melatonin at doses as low as 0.5 mg has improved the day sleep of night workers with less consistent effects on circadian phase.[5] However, despite improved sleep after melatonin administration, studies have not shown improvements in night shift alertness. Melatonin is suggested by the AASM at the guideline level to enhance day sleep in night shift workers.[5] The melatonin receptor agonist, ramelteon, could also be considered, as objective sleep measures including wake

after sleep onset and sleep duration were significantly improved after its use in a day sleep condition.[7]

Studies of bright light or melatonin to shift circadian phase have not been performed in early rise shift workers. However, in an investigation of workers with shift start times from 4:00 to 7:30 AM, a simple behavioral measure of moving bedtime approximately 1.5 hours earlier increased sleep duration by an hour and improved subjective sleepiness.[8]

In addition to movement of the sleep–wake cycle to correlate with shift work, sleep times and circadian phase on days off may also prove important in the treatment of shift work disorder. A study of simulated night workers delayed CBT_{min} to 10:00 AM with use of appropriately timed bright light exposure and avoidance. Sleep times were scheduled from 8:30 AM to 3:30 PM on work days and 3:00 AM to 12 noon on days off (with a nap from 8:30 AM to 1:30 PM after the last night shift of the week). Subjects shifted to this "compromise position" where the trough in alertness coincides with both the sleep period on work days and days off had significant improvements in fatigue, mood, and performance during the night shift as compared to controls.[9]

Augmenting alertness with napping, caffeine, and stimulant medications has also shown significant benefits in shift work disorder. Scheduled naps prior to or during the first portion of night shift work have improved alertness and performance, and decreased accidents, and therefore are recommended by the AASM as standard therapeutic intervention for night shift workers.[5] Furthermore, in simulated and field studies of night shift work, a combination of preshift napping and caffeine administration (4 mg/kg) significantly improved objective and subjective measures of alertness, and vigilance on performance tests.[10] The combined intervention was superior to placebo or either individual intervention.[10] The wake-promoting agent modafinil and especially its longer acting R isomer, armodafinil, have improved objective alertness during the night shift and both are US Food and Drug Admistration (FDA) -approved for use in this setting.[11,12] Although methamphetamine stimulants have been evaluated as well, the potential for abuse precludes their use.[5] Above all, good sleep hygiene that includes an environment conducive to day sleep and sufficient time in bed must be implemented by shift workers.

Main points

When non-conventional work times are imposed, misalignment of circadian phase and sleep–wake times can result in both excessive sleepiness and insomnia. Safety can be at risk when the commute and work period coincide with the time of high propensity for sleep. Sleep deprivation, a common problem due to insomnia in shift work disorder, further augments somnolence. Careful clinical evaluation of work schedules, sleep timing, and environmental factors may reveal targets for therapeutic intervention to better align the sleep–wake cycle with shift work. Treatment can include manipulation of circadian phase, appropriately timed bright light exposure and avoidance, and use of strategies such as scheduled naps to improve shift alertness.

REFERENCES

1. American Academy of Sleep Medicine. *International Classification of Sleep Disorders. Diagnostic and Coding Manual*, Second Edition. Westchester, IL: American Academy of Sleep Medicine;2005.
2. Wright KP, Bogan RK, Wyatt JK. Shift work and the assessment and management of shift work disorder (SWD). *Sleep Med Rev* 2013;**17**:41–54.
3. Drake C, Roehrs T, Richardson G, Walsh JK, Roth T. Shift work sleep disorder: prevalence and consequences beyond that of symptomatic day workers. *Sleep* 2004;**27**: 1453–62.
4. Daan S, Beesrma DG, Borbely AA. Timing of human sleep: recovery process gated by a circadian pacemaker. *Am J Physiol* 1984;**246**:161–83.
5. Morgentahaler TI, Lee-Chiong T, Alessi C, et al. Practice parameters for the clinical evaluation and treatment of circadian rhythm sleep disorders. *Sleep* 2007;**30**:1445–59.
6. Boivin DB, Bodreau P, James FO, Ng Ying Kin N. Photic resetting in night-shift work: impact on nurses' sleep. *Chronobiol Int* 2012;**29**:619–28.
7. Markwald RR, Lee-Chiong TL, Burke TM, Snider JA, Wright KP. Effects of the melatonin MT-1/MT-2 receptor agonist ramelteon on daytime body temperature and sleep. *Sleep* 2010;**33**:825–31.
8. Yeung J, Sletten TL, Rajaratnam SM. A phase-advanced, extended sleep paradigm to increase sleep duration among early-morning shift workers: a preliminary investigation. *Scand J Work Environ Health* 2011;**37**:62–9.
9. Smith MR, Fogg LF, Eastman CI. A compromise circadian phase position for permanent night work improves mood, fatigue, and performance. *Sleep* 2009;**32**:1481–9.
10. Schweitzer PK, Randazzo AC, Stone K, Erman M, Walsh JK. Laboratory and field studies of naps and caffeine as practical countermeasures for sleep-wake problems associated with night work. *Sleep* 2006;**29**:39–50.
11. Czeisler CA, Walsh JK, Roth T, et al. US modafinil in Shift Work Sleep Disorder Study Group. Modafinil for excessive sleepiness associated with shift-work sleep disorder. *N Engl J Med* 2005;**353**:476–86.
12. Czeisler CA, Walsh JK, Wesnes KA, Arora S, Roth T. Armodafinil for treatment of excessive sleepiness associated with shift work disorder: a randomized controlled study. *Mayo Clin Proc* 2009;**84**:958–72.

Missed diagnoses of obstructive sleep apnea can exacerbate medical and neurologic conditions

Many patients and clinicians have a rather "sleepy" view of sleep disorders: sure, they may be common, and consequential, but they are no emergency. Although many sleep disorders do develop insidiously, to become key concerns only with time and repeated exposure over months or years, sleep-disordered breathing is an exception. Sleep apnea can have acute cardiopulmonary or neurologic impact, with the potential for lethal outcomes.

The cases described in this section highlight the critical roles that obstructive sleep apnea (OSA) can play when it occurs in association with other medical and neurologic conditions. Asthma, for example, is likely to have bi-directional provocative influences in relation to OSA: although asthma is likely to worsen OSA, unaddressed OSA is also likely to impede effective control of asthma. Similarly, untreated OSA also may provoke seizures in patients with poorly

controlled epilepsy. Identification of OSA, and effective treatment for it, in advance of cardioversion or ablation procedures for atrial fibrillation, may have substantial impact on the likelihood that the procedure will provide lasting control of the arrhythmia. Finally, prompt identification and effective treatment of sleep apnea – though challenging over constrained time periods immediately after stroke or before a surgical procedure – could have important impact on health outcomes in these acute settings.

Review of all the medical conditions suspected to show sensitivity to underlying OSA is not possible in this volume. However, the selected examples in this section highlight important, common situations in which clinicians who remember to check for, and control OSA are likely to provide their patients with considerably improved health outcomes, both in the short term and for many years thereafter.

42

Occult obstructive sleep apnea can contribute to chronic persistent asthma

Mihaela Teodorescu and Rahul K. Kakkar

Case

A 56-year-old Caucasian female nurse was first seen in the hospital due to severe asthma exacerbations occurring several times a year, particularly during winter months. She had a history of persistent asthma that required use of rescue inhalers several times each day, in addition to inhaled steroids and oral montelukast. She also had chronic fungal sinusitis, which required surgical intervention and she was also a smoker. She was being treated with intravenous steroids, inhaled albuterol, and ipratropium bromide. She was discharged on a drug regimen of oral and inhaled steroids, long-acting bronchodilators, nasal steroids, and proton pump inhibitors.

However, she continued to have symptoms of asthma, with recurrent cough and wheezing, and also nasal congestion and gastroesophageal acid reflux (GERD). Smoking cessation improved, but did not completely resolve her symptoms. Pulmonary function testing revealed normal spirometry, and allergy testing showed significant allergies to dust mite, dog, cat, birch, and hickory. She was educated about allergen avoidance but refused to part with her dog. During one of the visits, her husband reported a history of loud snoring and the patient admitted waking up tired. The patient was reluctant to go for an attended sleep study. A home sleep test was performed which demonstrated an apnea/hypopnea index of 10 events per hour of recording, and a lowest oxygen saturation of 88%. She was treated with an automatically adjusting continuous positive airway pressure (CPAP) device. Objective data subsequently showed that she was using the CPAP for an average of 6 hours and 9 minutes every night with a 90% pressure of 8.5 cm of water. Within a few weeks she started to feel better, as most of her symptoms including the cough and wheezing improved significantly. In contrast to her recent years, she experienced her first winter without an asthma exacerbation. She continued to use her rescue inhaler, but only about once a week.

Brief overview of uncontrolled asthma and the role of sleep

Asthma and obstructive sleep apnea (OSA) represent problems on different ends of the same airway. While asthma causes intermittent lower airway constriction lasting hours or days, OSA arises from intermittent closure of upper airway during sleep, lasting a few seconds to over a minute, and occurring primarily at the retropalatal or retrolingual level of the pharynx.

Sleep has an adverse effect on the lower airway tract, and therefore on asthma control, which in turn worsens the quality of sleep.[1] Non-asthmatic individuals show an increase in lower airway resistance during sleep, and this increase worsens with sleep duration. It usually has no clinical manifestation in non-asthmatics. However, asthmatics show a more profound increase in lower airway resistance, resulting in worsening of symptoms at night (nocturnal asthma)

Common Pitfalls in Sleep Medicine, ed. Ronald D. Chervin. Published by Cambridge University Press. © Cambridge University Press 2014.

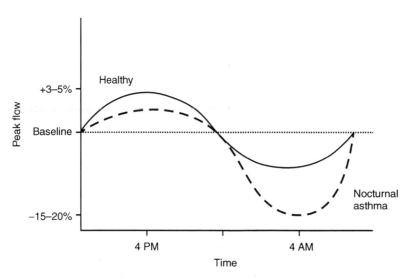

Figure 42.1 Diurnal variation in peak flow in healthy individuals and asthmatics. Reprinted with permission from Sutherland ER.[2]

(Figure 42.1[2]). The reasons for this decline in lung function during sleep are poorly understood. Possible explanations include alterations in autonomic tone, changes in hormonal secretion, circadian rhythm changes in the number of corticosteroid receptors, circadian changes in inflammatory cells and cytokines, and acid reflux. Persistent nocturnal symptoms indicate a lack of adequate control of asthma according to the National Asthma Educations and Prevention Program. In a survey of 7729 people, about 75% of adult patients reported nocturnal symptoms once a week, 64% thrice a week, and 39% every night.[3] According to the 2005 Harris poll, 48% of children suffered from disturbed sleep due to their asthma.[4]

Uncontrolled asthma carries increased morbidity and mortality. Women with asthma are more prone to cardiovascular disease than those without asthma. It has been reported that 53% of asthma deaths occur during sleep and the majority of these patients had nocturnal asthma symptoms. Studies have demonstrated cognitive deficits in asthmatic patients with poor sleep quality, and improvement in cognition with treatment of nocturnal asthma symptoms. Hypoxemia likely contributes at least partly to the impairment in mental faculties of children with nocturnal asthma.

OSA is more common among individuals with asthma

Multiple lines of evidence suggest a bi-directional relationship between asthma and OSA.

First, several cross-sectional studies in general and asthma clinic patient samples have reported a higher frequency of OSA symptoms and of questionnaire-assessed OSA risk among the patients with asthma.[5] In a small study of asthmatics with differing disease severity, Julien et al.[6] found an OSA prevalence of 88% in severe asthmatics, 58% in moderate asthmatics, compared to 31% among normal controls. Furthermore, a prospective cohort study suggested asthma development was a risk factor for incident habitual snoring during 14-year follow-up. What contributes to the increased OSA risk in asthma remains to be studied, but more unique disease related features related to physiologic dynamics between the lower and upper airways during sleep, reflux, and corticosteroid use may contribute, apart from traditional risk factors such as obesity and nasal congestion, more commonly represented in this population. The prevalence of asthma in patients confirmed to have OSA is also not well studied. In a

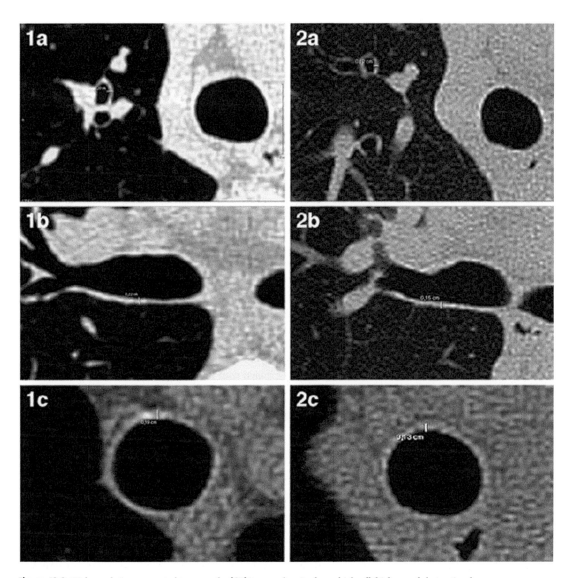

Figure 42.2 High-resolution computed tomography (CT) images showing bronchial wall thickness of obstructive sleep apnea patients (1a, 1b, 1c) and control subjects (2a, 2b, 2c). The thickness of the bronchial walls were 20 mm (1a), 22 mm (1b), 19 mm (1c), 12 mm (2a), 15 mm (2b), and 13 mm (2c). Reprinted with permission from Sariman N, Levent E, Cubuk R, et al.[8]

study of 606 polysomnographically confirmed cases of OSA (67% men), Alharbi et al.[7] found that 35% of patients had asthma. However, the diagnosis of asthma was based upon three-item questionnaires administered to the patients to ask whether a physician had ever diagnosed them with asthma. No spirometry data was available on these patients. Increased bronchial reactivity and bronchial wall thickening has been reported in association with OSA (Figure 42.2[8]).

Role of OSA in asthma control

Once OSA is established in asthma, it is unlikely to be an innocent bystander. Obstructive sleep apnea has recently been identified as a cause of chronic cough, presumably through mechanisms involving the triad of nasal inflammation, loss of lower esophageal sphincter tone, and bronchial inflammation.[9] Cough is both a symptom of asthma as well as a trigger for asthma. Persistent cough can cause reflex bronchospasm and initiate or perpetuate a vicious cycle of cough-asthma-cough. In a study that used the sleep apnea scale of the Sleep Disorders Questionnaire (SA-SDQ) and the Asthma Control Questionnaire (ACQ), Teodorescu et al.[10] found an association of symptom-defined high risk for OSA with poor asthma control, irrespective of other factors known to aggravate asthma. In another study that involved questionnaire-defined OSA risk and historical diagnosis of OSA, each were associated with persistent daytime asthma symptoms, interestingly, to an extent that matched or exceeded associations with nocturnal asthma, suggesting carry-over effects of OSA on asthma during the day. Severity of sleep apnea also correlates with asthma control. In a study of 50 children referred for adenotonsillectomy for OSA, the severity of OSA was related to poor asthma control.[11]

Conversely, OSA treatment appears to improve asthma. In adults, treatment of OSA with CPAP improves asthma symptoms, morning peak expiratory flow rates, and quality of life.[12] In children, the frequency of acute asthma exacerbations requiring Emergency Room visits or systemic steroids; use of rescue inhalers; and frequency of asthma symptoms improve after tonsilladenoectomy (AT). Kheirandish-Gozal et al.[13] prospectively studied 92 children, aged 3–10 years and with poorly controlled asthma, with overnight polysomnography. The prevalence of significant OSA (apnea/hypopnea index > 5 events per hour of sleep) was 63%. After 1 year, information on 35 children was available following AT. Children who had undergone AT demonstrated significant improvement in frequency of acute asthma exacerbations, from 4.1 times a year to 1.4 times a year; in frequency of β2-agonist use; and in an asthma symptom score.

Preliminary research suggests that the forced oscillation technique (FOT) when combined with a Millar catheter can be used to measure both upper and lower airway resistance separately while breathing spontaneously and while using a bi-level positive airway pressure device.[14] This methodology may be especially useful in measurement of treatment outcomes in patients with asthma. Future studies that incorporate such objective measures of upper and lower airway resistance before and after treatment of OSA in asthmatics may shed more light on this topic.

How OSA influences asthma remains to be determined. Obesity may confound the effects of OSA on asthma; however, OSA may be an important mediator in the relationship of obesity with asthma. While prospective studies are needed, evidence available at present has found associations of OSA risk and diagnosis to be independent of obesity, and CPAP use has shown a "protective" effect on daytime asthma, apart from effects of obesity.[10] Although obesity alters lower airway resistance and increases bronchial hyperresponsiveness,[15] both OSA and obesity are associated with increased expression of markers of airway inflammation, including exhaled nitric oxide (eNO), polymorphonuclear cells (PMN), interleukin 6 (IL-6), and 8-isoprotane. Sleep apneic children also have increased expression of leukotrienes and leukotriene receptors in adenotonsillar tissue. Children with asthma exhibit elevated concentrations of leukotrienes and oxidative stress markers in their exhaled breath condensate. Another possible common pathway under investigation is leptin, a 16KDa protein of 167 amino acids, which is a product of the *ob* gene. Obstructive sleep apnea is recognized as a leptin-resistant state, and leptin levels fall after treatment with CPAP therapy.[16] The role of leptin in asthma control seems influenced by gender. Asthmatic children, especially boys, exhibit higher levels of leptin as compared to controls. Leptin levels are also predictive of bronchodilator response as well as asthma in adult males, though not in females. Evidence is accumulating that leptin may play a pro-inflammatory role in the asthmatic airway. Leptin increases O_3-induced airway inflammation, phagocytosis by macrophages, and release of inflammatory cytokines such as tumor necrosis factor-alpha (TNF-α), IL-6, and IL-12. Leptin administration in mice augments airway response to inhaled methacholine following ovalbumin challenge.[16]

Gastroesophageal reflux (GER) and especially nocturnal GER (nGER) is another putative factor in the complex interplay between OSA and asthma. The role of GER as an intermediary in the bi-directional relationship between asthma and OSA is poorly understood. In a study that involved 2640 subjects from Iceland, Belgium, and Sweden over a period of 9 years, Emilsson et al.[17] found that persistent nGER symptoms correlated with the onset of respiratory symptoms of asthma and OSA. However, no correlation of nGER with lung function and bronchial hyperreactivity was demonstrated. Dixon et al.[18] used 24-hour pH probes to accurately assess the relationship between asthma, GER, and OSA. Although limited by lack of objective diagnosis of OSA, the study demonstrated that the risk of poor asthma control as measured by the Juniper Asthma Control Questionnaire was correlated with symptoms of OSA, which in turn was correlated with increasing body mass index (BMI). The majority of the subjects in the study were obese. The symptoms of GER correlated with the BMI but objective measurement of 24-hour pH did not correlate well with asthma control in obese patients.

The 2007 National Asthma Education and Prevention Program and the American Academy of Sleep Medicine recommend clinical evaluation of patients with chronic uncontrolled asthma for symptoms and signs of OSA, and use of polysomnography if indicated. However, clear guidelines based on specific symptoms or severity of symptoms are lacking, due to inadequate research in this area. It is especially important to screen moderate to severe asthmatic individuals, both adults and children, for OSA. The target groups should include ethnic minorities who have a high prevalence of both disorders, the obese, those with nasal diseases, patients with GERD, and higher users of corticosteroid therapies.[19]

Main points

In summary, accumulating evidence suggests that OSA and asthma are likely to exert bi-directional influences on each other. Clinicians should maintain a high index of suspicion for OSA in patients with asthma, and particularly those with moderate to severe disease and other characteristics presented above. In such patients, identification and treatment of OSA may – as in the case of the patient described above – allow substantial improvement in symptoms of persistent asthma.

REFERENCES

1. Ballard RD, Saathoff MC, Patel DK, et al. Effect of bronchoconstriction and ventilator pattern in asthmatics. *J Appl Physiol* 1989;**67**:243–9.
2. Sutherland ER. Nocturnal asthma. *J Allergy Clin Immunol* 2005;**11**:1179–86.
3. Turner-Warwick M. Epidemiology of nocturnal asthma. *Am J Med* 1988;**85**:6–8.
4. Harris poll conducted on behalf of Asthma and Allergy Foundation of America. www.aafa.org.
5. Sharma B, Feinsilver S, Owens RL, et al. Obstructive airway disease and obstructive sleep apnea: effect of pulmonary function. *Lung* 2011;**189**:37–41.
6. Julien JY, Martin JG, Ernst P, et al. Prevalence of obstructive sleep apnea-hypopnea in severe versus moderate asthma. *J Allergy Clin Immunol* 2009;**124**:371–6.
7. Alharbi M, Almutairi A, Alotaibi D, et al. The prevalence of asthma in patients with obstructive sleep apnoea. *Prim Care Resp J* 2009;**18**:328–30.
8. Sariman N, Levent E, Cubuk R, et al. Bronchial hyperreactivity and airway wall thickness in patients with obstructive sleep apnea. *Sleep Breath* 2011;**15**:341–50.
9. Sundar KM, Daly SE. Chronic cough and OSA: a new association? *J Clin Sleep Med* 2011;**7**:669–77.
10. Teodorescu M, Polomis DA, Teodorescu MC, et al. Association of obstructive sleep apnea risk or diagnosis with daytime asthma in adults *J Asthma* 2012;**49**:620–8.
11. Ramgopal M, Mehta A, Roberts AW, et al. Asthma as a predictor of obstructive sleep apnea in urban African-American children. *J Asthma* 2009;**46**:895–9.
12. Alkhalil M. Obstructive sleep apnea syndrome and asthma: the role of continuous positive airway pressure treatment. *Ann Allergy Asthma Immunol* 2008;**101**:350–7.
13. Kheirandish-Gozal L, Dayyat E, Eid N, et al. Obstructive sleep apnea in poorly controlled asthmatic children: effect of adenotonsillectomy. *Pediatr Pulmonol* 2011; **46**:913–18.

14. Campana LM, Owens RL, Suki B, Malhotra A. Measuring upper and lower airway resistance during sleep with forced oscillation technique. *Ann Biomed Eng* 2012;**40**:925–33.

15. Litonjua AA, Sparrow D, Celedon JC, et al. Association of body mass index with the development of methacholine airway hyperresponsiveness in men: the Normative Aging Study. *Thorax* 2002;**57**:581–5.

16. Malli F, Papaionnou, K, Gourgoulianis Z. The role of leptin in the respiratory system: an overview. *Respir Res* 2010;**11**:152–67.

17. Emilsson ÖI, Bengtsson A, Franklin KA, et al. Nocturnal gastro-esophageal reflux, asthma and symptoms of OSA: a longitudinal, general population study. *Eur Respir J* 2013;**41**:1347–54.

18. Dixon AE, Clerisme-Beaty EM, Sugar EA, et al. Effects of obstructive sleep apnea and gastroesophageal reflux disease on asthma control in obesity. *J Asthma* 2011;**48**:707–13.

19. Teodorescu M, Consens FB, Bria WF, et al. Predictors of habitual snoring and obstructive sleep apnea risk in patients with asthma. *Chest* 2009;**135**:1125–32.

43

Occult obstructive sleep apnea can exacerbate an uncontrolled seizure disorder

Beth A. Malow

Neurologists and other medical specialists often enjoy the opportunity to focus on their particular disciplines. While the expertise that develops can enhance patient care, a broad knowledge that includes some other medical areas is often essential for optimal diagnosis and treatment. This case illustrates the value of a sleep history and awareness of the intersection of sleep disorders with one specific medical condition, namely epilepsy. However, sleep and its disorders affect nearly every physiologic system in the human body, and some knowledge of sleep medicine is a valuable asset in most other medical specialties.

Case

A 50-year-old man presented with a worsening of his seizure control. He had been diagnosed with complex partial seizures with secondary generalization in his teens. His seizures had been brought under control with phenytoin 350 mg daily, and he enjoyed seizure freedom for several decades. He presented for reevaluation to our epilepsy clinics after a worsening of seizure control in his late forties. He had complex partial seizures consisting of a blank stare with oral automatisms occurring at least once a week, with occasional secondary generalization. Approximately half of these seizures occurred during sleep. After a phenytoin level was found to be therapeutic (18 μg/ml), he was begun on levetiracetam and titrated up to 1500 mg twice a day. Complex partial seizures continued to occur several times a month. Other than hypertension, his medical history was unremarkable.

What additional information do you want to know?

Fortunately for the patient, the epilepsy fellow who evaluated this patient had just completed a rotation on the sleep medicine service. Therefore, the patient was asked about snoring and sleep habits. His hunting buddies had complained about sharing a cabin with him due to his loud snoring. His wife also complained that he snored loudly, which began bothering her in the last 4–5 years coinciding with a 20-pound (9-kg) weight gain. His sleep was interrupted by night wakings at least 1–2 times a night. He admitted to awakening himself from sleep with snoring on several occasions. In the morning, he had a dry mouth and difficulty getting up for work. Despite getting 8 hours of sleep, he tended to be sleepy after lunch while sitting in front of his computer, or in boring meetings. In the evening, he would fall asleep watching television or reading a book. His Epworth Sleepiness Scale score was 12 (maximum value of 24 with 10 or above indicating sleepiness).[1] Daytime sleepiness was present before the addition of levetiracetam but worsened after addition of this agent.

Family history was unremarkable for seizures but notable for loud snoring in his father and brother.

On examination, his body mass index was 29 kg/m². He had a Friedman palate position of 4 (could not

Common Pitfalls in Sleep Medicine, ed. Ronald D. Chervin. Published by Cambridge University Press. © Cambridge University Press 2014.

visualize any structures other than tongue and hard palate) and a neck circumference of 17 inches (43 cm). Blood pressure was elevated at 150/92 mmHg. His examination was otherwise unremarkable.

What diagnostic testing is indicated? What was the outcome?

To determine whether obstructive sleep apnea (OSA) was present, and also identify any ongoing seizures or interictal epileptiform activity, an overnight polysomnogram was performed with an expanded electroencephalographic (EEG) montage. This study was remarkable for an elevated apnea/hypopnea index (AHI, events per hour of sleep) of 40, with a minimum oxygen saturation of 84%, in the first 2 hours of sleep. No epileptic seizures were recorded, although occasional interictal epileptiform discharges were noted (Figure 43.1). He was treated with continuous positive airway pressure (CPAP) for the remainder of the night. His AHI fell to 3 events per hour on CPAP at a setting of 10 cm of water; he then used CPAP at home thereafter. On CPAP, and without any change in his phenytoin level, he became seizure-free. His snoring resolved, and his level of alertness improved to where he was no longer feeling drowsy or falling asleep during the day. His Epworth Sleepiness Scale score fell to 6.

Discussion

This case illustrates the therapeutic effects of treating OSA on seizure management. The patient most likely developed OSA with increasing age and weight gain. Addition of a second antiepileptic drug increased daytime sleepiness and seizures continued to occur. Upon treatment of the patient's OSA with CPAP, the patient resumed his prior level of seizure freedom and daytime sleepiness improved. While this effect has been documented in numerous case series and prospective trials,[2–6] the mechanisms whereby treatment of sleep apnea improves seizure control remain unclear. Disruption of sleep by obstructive respiratory events, and the accompanying chronic hypoxia, has been postulated to increase neuronal excitability. Nocturnal seizures may improve with CPAP treatment due to stabilization of sleep and reduction of sleep transitions.[4,6] Regardless of the mechanism, considering the diagnosis of OSA in patients with epilepsy and treating OSA once diagnosed is an important clinical pearl. The pitfall in this case was the addition of a second antiepileptic drug to the patient's medication regimen. In a pilot randomized trial of CPAP for OSA in epilepsy, the response of seizures to therapeutic CPAP was comparable to that of a second antiepileptic drug in patients with medically refractory epilepsy.[5] However, whereas antiepileptic drugs are often associated with sedation, CPAP improves daytime sleepiness through the treatment of sleep fragmentation. CPAP adherence is related to improved seizure control in patients with OSA and epilepsy.[6]

How prevalent is OSA in epilepsy, and which patients with epilepsy are at risk? In 130 consecutive adults with epilepsy, assessed with structured interview, questionnaires, and polysomnography, the prevalence of sleep apnea was 30%, with 16% having moderate to severe disease.[7] These rates markedly exceed general population estimates. Predictors of OSA in multivariate models included increasing age, dental problems, and greater antiepileptic drug load, with male gender, older age, higher body mass index, hypertension, and dental problems associated with higher AHI. In older adults with epilepsy, the AHI was higher in patients with late-onset or worsening seizures compared to those who were seizure-free or who had improvement of seizures.[8]

Treatment of OSA may also improve a patient's ability to tolerate antiepileptic drugs and promote adherence to them, in that patients with OSA are often already excessively sleepy and more susceptible to the sedating adverse effects of these agents.

Main points

In summary, OSA should be kept in the forefront of the evaluation of patients with epilepsy, especially those with seizures refractory to medication or who experience an unanticipated deterioration in seizure control. Patients with epilepsy may be particularly vulnerable

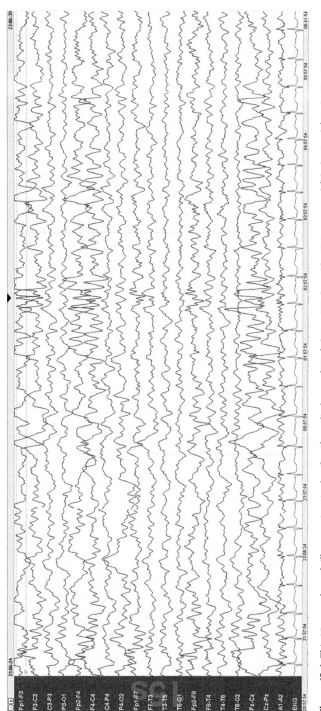

Figure 43.1 This 15-second epoch illustrates interictal epileptiform discharges (IEDs) during N2 sleep. The IEDs are noted (black triangle) in the Fp1-F3, F3-C3, Fp2-F4, and F4-C4 channels with phase reversals at F3 and F4.

to OSA. Furthermore, they have much to gain, as treatment of OSA may improve seizure frequency and occasionally result in seizure freedom, as well as improve daytime sleepiness.

REFERENCES

1. Johns MW. A new method for measuring daytime sleepiness: the Epworth sleepiness scale. *Sleep* 1991;**14**:540-5.
2. Devinsky O, Ehrenberg B, Barthlen GM, Abramson HS, Luciano D. Epilepsy and sleep apnea syndrome. *Neurology* 1994;**44**:2060-4.
3. Vaughn BV, D'Cruz, OF, Beach R, Messenheimer JA. Improvement of epileptic seizure control with treatment of obstructive sleep apnoea. *Seizure* 1996;**5**:73-8.
4. Malow BA, Fromes GA, Aldrich MS. Usefulness of polysomnography in epilepsy patients. *Neurology* 1997;**48**:1389-94.
5. Malow BA, Foldvary-Schaefer N, Vaughn BV, et al. Treating obstructive sleep apnea in adults with epilepsy: a randomized pilot trial. *Neurology* 2008;**71**:572-7.
6. Vendrame M, Auerbach S, Loddenkemper T, Kothare S, Montouris G. Effect of continuous positive airway pressure treatment on seizure control in patients with obstructive sleep apnea and epilepsy. *Epilepsia* 2011;**52**:e168-71.
7. Foldvary-Schaefer N, Andrews ND, Pornsriniyom D, et al. Sleep apnea and epilepsy: who's at risk? *Epilepsy Behav* 2012;**25**:363-7.
8. Chihorek AM, Abou-Khalil B, Malow BA. Obstructive sleep apnea is associated with seizure occurrence in older adults with epilepsy. *Neurology* 2007;**69**:1823-7.

44

Diagnosis and control of sleep apnea may improve the chances of successful treatment for atrial fibrillation

Johnathan Barkham

Case

A 65-year-old man with a history of hypertension presented with complaints of recurrent atrial fibrillation (AF). He was originally diagnosed 15 years ago and has been cardioverted three times since then. A few months ago, he presented to the Emergency Department with palpitations and was found to be in AF with a rapid ventricular rate. He is currently rate controlled on diltiazem and anticoagulated on coumadin. Cardiology is planning on cardioversion again in the next month.

The patient reports snoring loudly all of his life and does not know whether this had become progressively worse. Snoring is improved in the lateral position and worsened in the supine. He denies associated gasping, choking, and snorting arousals. He recalls a sleep study at an outside hospital about a decade ago. He was told he had severe obstructive sleep apnea (OSA) and was given a machine but did not tolerate the noise. He reports unrefreshing sleep and daytime somnolence with an Epworth Sleepiness Scale score of 14, on a scale of 0–24. His physical exam is unremarkable except for a high body mass index of 31 kg/m^2 and an irregular rhythm with a normal rate on cardiovascular examination.

What is the relationship between OSA and AF?

The presence of OSA more than doubles the chance of developing AF (Figure 44.1).[1,2] Although this relationship has been well established and awareness among practitioners is growing, screening tests for OSA should be implemented in standard evaluations at the time of AF diagnosis. Hypercapnia, hypoxemia, increased sympathetic tone, and increased levels of inflammatory marker C-reactive protein are features of OSA that have each been associated with increased risk for AF. These features could potentially play a role in any causative mechanisms by which OSA may facilitate AF. Comorbidities of OSA, such as hypertension and increased body mass index, also are independent risk factors for AF. This patient is at high risk for AF given his history of severe untreated OSA, hypertension, and obesity.

How does OSA cause AF and other arrhythmias?

Arrhythmias are often precipitated by hypoxemia, acidosis, electrolyte abnormalities, structural abnormalities, and conduction system disease. These predisposing abnormalities often occur as the result of OSA. In particular bradyarrhythmias can be triggered by the dive reflex, where hypoxemia during the obstructive event causes bradycardia through vagal activation. Upon termination of the obstructive event there is hyperpnea, which impairs vagal tone and activates the sympathetic nervous system, causing tachycardia. Individual apneic events can trigger AF (Figure 44.2). The consequences of OSA which

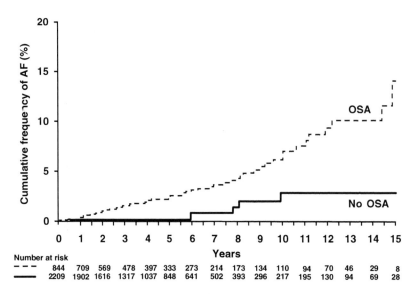

Figure 44.1 Incidence of atrial fibrillation (AF) based on presence or absence of obstructive sleep apnea (OSA). Cumulative frequency curves for incident AF among subjects < 65 years of age with and without OSA during an average 4.7 years of follow-up. $P = 0.002$. Data from Gami AS, Hodge DO, Herges RM, et al.[2]

increase myocardial oxygen demand in the presence of hypoxemia may cause myocardial ischemia in patients with cardiac disease; the result may be an arrhythmogenic substrate for ventricular arrhythmias. This arrhythmogenic potential of OSA was demonstrated in the Sleep Heart Health Study, which showed that specific nocturnal arrhythmias were more common in patients with OSA compared to normal controls, with AF found in 4.8% versus 0.9%, non-sustained ventricular tachycardia found in 5.3% versus 1.2%, and complex ventricular ectopy found in 25% versus 14.5%.[3] Thus, OSA is associated with other arrhythmias in addition to AF.

What are the predictors of AF recurrence after electrical cardioversion or ablation in patients with OSA?

As the severity of OSA increases, the risk for recurrence after cardioversion increases, particularly in patients with an apnea/hypopnea index (AHI) below 15 events per hour of sleep (Figure 44.3).[4] Additionally the recurrence of AF after cardioversion increases dramatically in untreated OSA with lower nocturnal oxygen saturations.[5] Although OSA increases the risk of AF recurrence after cardioversion, evidence suggests that this risk can be reduced by the use of continuous positive airway pressure (CPAP).[5] If ablation for AF is pursued, recurrence is also more likely to occur in patients with untreated OSA, and is reduced if treated with CPAP.[6] This patient's severe untreated OSA increases his risk of AF recurrence after cardioversion and may explain why he has failed cardioversion three times.

How else should this patient be evaluated?

Understanding the pathogenesis of OSA on the cardiovascular system helps one look for clues on history and exam. Obstructive sleep apnea damages the

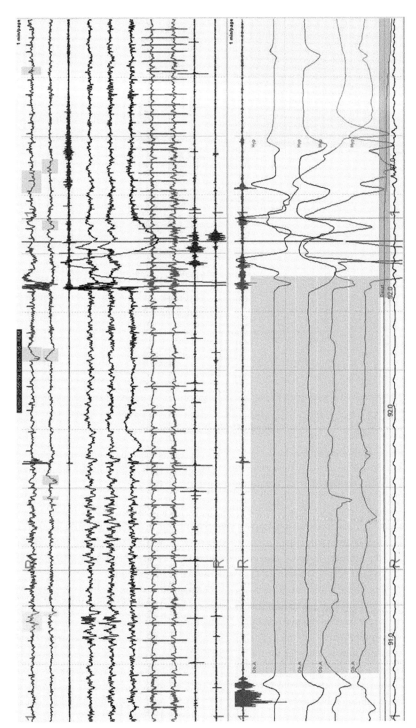

Figure 44.2 Polysomnogram of a patient in rapid eye movement sleep. It shows an obstructive apnea that is followed by an arousal and atrial fibrillation with a rapid ventricular rate. Abbreviations used in figure: EEG, electroencephalogram; EKG, electrocardiogram; EMG, electromyogram; EOG, electrooculogram; NP$_\sim$, nasal pressure transducer. Original content courtesy of Meredith Peters MD. See plate section for color version.

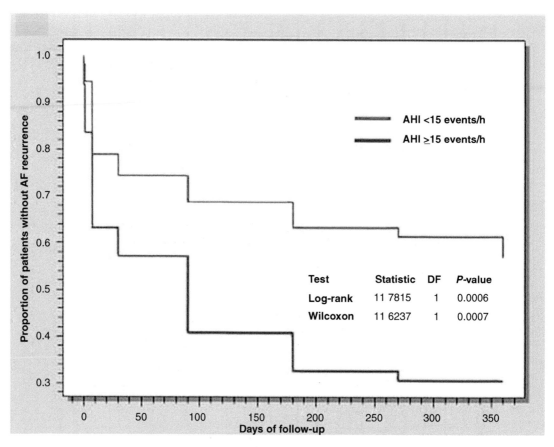

Figure 44.3 Kaplan–Meier curves showing survival free of atrial fibrillation recurrence according to dichotomized apnea/ hypopnea index (< 15 / ≥ 15 events per hour). Abbreviations used in figure: AF, atrial fibrillation; AHI, apnea/hypopnea index. Data from Mazza A, Bendini MG, Cristofori M, et al.[4] See plate section for color version.

cardiovascular system through the cycle of obstruction, hypoxia, and activation of the sympathetic nervous system to open the upper airway, trigger hyperpnea, and restore oxygen levels (Figure 44.4). During the obstructive event, there is increased negative intrathoracic pressure, which increases transmural pressure. This may increase pressure in the pulmonary vasculature leading to pulmonary edema. The increased transmural pressure makes it harder for the ventricle to pump during systole, reducing the ejection fraction. Hence there is increased workload and myocardial oxygen consumption during obstructive events,

increasing the risk for myocardial ischemia. Acutely this may cause infarction. Over time, these mechanisms lead to ventricular hypertrophy, heart failure, and pulmonary hypertension.

Through direct and indirect mechanisms, hypoxia impairs systolic and diastolic function contributing to congestive heart failure and causes the release of arrhythmogenic and inflammatory chemicals that promote remodeling and atherosclerosis. Activation of the sympathetic nervous system occurs during obstructive respiratory events and is triggered by the effects of hypercapnia and hypoxemia on

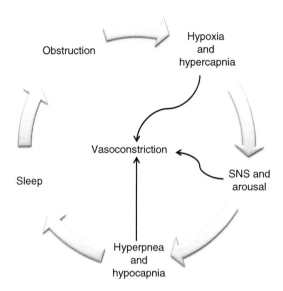

Figure 44.4 Vicious cycle of obstructive sleep apnea. Obstruction leads to hypoxia and hypercapnia, followed by activation of the sympathetic nervous system (SNS) and arousal. The SNS surge triggers hyperpnea and hypocapnia ensues. The direct and indirect consequences of the initial obstruction work to produce systemic and pulmonary vasoconstriction, which is likely to contribute to the long-term cardiovascular sequelae of OSA.

chemoreceptors in the brain and carotid bodies respectively.[7] These lead to vasoconstriction of the arterial vasculature, resulting in increased blood pressure and heart rate. Hypoxia and hypercapnia also cause pulmonary vasoconstriction and increased pulmonary arterial pressures, which gradually lead to pulmonary hypertension and/or cor pulmonale. Hypoxemia followed by hyperpnea causes reoxygenation leading to free radical damage of the tissues. Hyperpnea after obstruction leads to hypocapnia, which causes additional vasoconstriction by shifting the oxygen dissociation curve to the left, further impairing oxygen delivery.[7] Overall, the complex pathogenesis of OSA impairs cardiac function acutely and chronically, leading to cardiovascular disease though neural, physical, and biochemical mechanisms.

Understanding the cardiac dysfunction that occurs as a result of OSA, practitioners should carefully evaluate patients for cardiovascular symptoms and disease. Physical exam may elucidate signs of heart failure, such as rales on the lung exam, elevated jugular venous distention, arrhythmias, heart murmurs, and lower extremity edema. Review of previous electrocardiograms and echocardiograms may be helpful to clarify any abnormalities that may be explained by OSA, such as arrhythmias, heart failure, and pulmonary hypertension. If symptoms, history, or significant physical exam findings raise or confirm suspicions of cardiovascular disease, unattended cardiopulmonary monitoring during sleep (home studies) are not appropriate for evaluation, due to their lowered sensitivity for OSA.

Discussion and main points

As in the daytime, nocturnal cardiac physiology is governed by competing parasympathetic and sympathetic influences. In non-rapid eye movement (NREM) sleep, the parasympathetic tone is high, which lowers the heart rate and blood pressure. Sympathetic nerve activity falls during the transition from wakefulness to NREM and continues to do so as the stages progress up until rapid eye movement (REM) sleep. At the transition to REM sleep, asystole and bradycardia may occur due to increased parasympathetic tone via the vagal nerve, and in disease states a patient can be at risk for arrhythmias such as torsades de pointes.[7] In patients with Long QT and Brugada syndrome, lethal arrhythmias usually occur while sleeping.[7] Vagally mediated AF is a type of neurohormonal AF that occurs during rest or sleep and is caused by the increased activity of the parasympathetic nervous system. In REM sleep there are increased bursts of sympathetic activity with elevations of heart rate and blood pressure that mirror those of wakefulness. Sympathetic drive in REM sleep may cause ventricular arrhythmias, which are exacerbated by hypoxemia and arrhythmogenic chemokines released in response to increased heart rate and blood pressure.[7] Thus, although sleep seems like an unlikely time for a cardiac arrhythmia or sudden death, clinicians must be mindful of the competing influences that occur and their lethal potential. Practitioners must be careful to review the overnight electrocardiogram thoroughly for arrhythmias that may not be present during wakefulness.

As the obesity epidemic continues, OSA will remain highly prevalent as well. Among the increasing numbers of patients with AF, undiagnosed OSA will be common. Due to the increased risk for stroke and heart disease associated with both OSA and AF, effective screening for these conditions should be encouraged. Screening for OSA should be considered in any patient diagnosed with AF. Conversely, sleep specialists should recognize that review of a polysomnogram offers the chance to assess for AF and other arrhythmias that may have gone unnoticed during wakefulness. In patients with AF, attended polysomnography and effective titration should be considered prior to any planned cardioversion, to reduce the risk of AF recurrence, especially in those with severe OSA and nocturnal hypoxemia. Although the exact severity of our patient's OSA is unknown, his untreated OSA is a likely contributor to his recurrent AF. He should undergo an attended polysomnogram and establish adherent use of CPAP prior to his cardioversion to reduce his risk of AF recurrence.

REFERENCES

1. Gami AS, Gregg P, Caples S, et al. Association of atrial fibrillation and obstructive sleep apnea. *Circulation* 2004;**110**:364–7.

2. Gami AS, Hodge DO, Herges RM, et al. Obstructive sleep apnea, obesity, and the risk of incident atrial fibrillation. *J Am Coll Cardiol* 2007;**49**:565–71.

3. Mehra R, Benjamin E, Shahar E, et al. Association of nocturnal arrhythmias with sleep-disordered breathing. *Am J Respir Crit Care Med* 2006;**107**:910–16.

4. Mazza A, Bendini MG, Cristofori M, et al. Baseline apnoea/hypopnea index and high-sensitivity C-reactive protein for the risk of recurrence of atrial fibrillation after successful electrical cardioversion: a predictive model based upon the multiple effects of significant variables. *Europace* 2009;**11**:902–9.

5. Kanagala R, Murali NS, Friedman PA, et al. Obstructive sleep apnea and the recurrence of atrial fibrillation. *Circulation* 2003;**107**:2589–94.

6. Naruse Y, Tada H, Satoh M, et al. Concomitant obstructive sleep apnea increases the recurrence of atrial fibrillation following radiofrequency catheter ablation of atrial fibrillation: clinical impact of continuous positive airway pressure therapy. *Heart Rhythm* 2013;**10**:331–7.

7. Kryger M, Roth T, Dement W, eds. *Principles and Practice of Sleep Medicine*, Fifth Edition. St Louis, MO: Elsevier; 2010, pp. 1353–415.

45

Sleep apnea in the acute stroke setting

Devin Brown

Case

A 77-year-old woman with a history of hypertension, diabetes, and hyperlipidemia awoke one morning with dysarthria and left-sided weakness. Specifically, she recalls difficulty when she tried to use her left arm and when she walked. She lives with her daughter who was not at home when the patient awakened. When the daughter returned in the evening, she noted her mother's left-sided hemiparesis as well as dysarthria. The patient described improvement in her symptoms throughout the day; her left arm strength completely normalized.

On presentation, her exam showed that her blood pressure was 202/98 mmHg. Her heart rate was 87 beats per minute and regular. Her body mass index was 22 kg/m^2 (normal). She was awake, alert, and fully oriented. She had no word finding difficulty, and was able to name objects. She had a noticeable dysarthria. On cranial nerve examination, she had subtle left lower facial droop, without other abnormalities. On motor examination, she had normal bulk and tone throughout the upper and lower extremities. Her upper extremity strength appeared symmetric bilaterally and no drift in the left upper extremity was found. In the lower extremities, she had full strength in the right leg. In the left leg, there was some subtle weakness of left hip flexion, with 5/5 strength distally. Reflexes were 2 in the brachioradialis, 2 in the biceps, 3 in the patellas, and absent at the Achilles tendon and symmetric bilaterally. The plantar responses were flexor. Sensory examination demonstrated a gradient loss to vibratory and temperature sensation in the lower extremities from the knees to the toes, such that vibration sensation was virtually undetectable in the toes. Coordination testing with fine finger movements and finger–nose–finger did not demonstrate any ataxia. The Romberg sign was positive. On gait examination, casual gait demonstrated circumduction of her left leg with frequent falling toward the left. She was able to stand on her heels and on her toes. Tandem gait was not attempted.

Head computed tomography (CT) performed in the Emergency Department did not reveal any acute abnormalities. An electrocardiogram was unremarkable. She was admitted to a stroke unit and underwent magnetic resonance imaging (MRI) of the brain that revealed a small left lateral medullary infarction on diffusion-weighted images (Figure 45.1). No significant stenoses were detected on non-invasive blood vessel images of the head and neck. A transthoracic echocardiogram showed normal left ventricular systolic dysfunction with grade I diastolic dysfunction. No inter-atrial shunt was identified with administration of agitated saline.

The patient enrolled in a sleep apnea treatment clinical trial. On the day after her stroke symptom onset, she had questionnaires administered and overnight diagnostic polysomnography performed at her bedside in the hospital. Her Epworth Sleepiness Scale score was 1 on a scale that ranges from 0 to 24; her

Common Pitfalls in Sleep Medicine, ed. Ronald D. Chervin. Published by Cambridge University Press. © Cambridge University Press 2014.

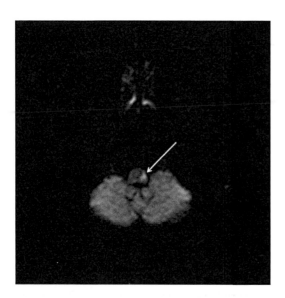

Figure 45.1 Diffusion-weighted axial magnetic resonance imaging (MRI) brain shows acute infarction in left lateral medulla (arrow).

score suggested no subjective excessive daytime sleepiness. Her Sleep Disorders Questionnaire – Sleep Apnea subscale was 21 (normal). Her Barthel index was 50, indicative of moderate dependence for activities of daily living. Her sleep study showed obstructive sleep apnea, with an apnea/hypopnea index of 9 events per hour of sleep, and a minimum oxygen saturation of 82%. The study showed no central apneas. She was randomized to 3 months of treatment with continuous positive airway pressure (CPAP) and she was titrated on CPAP 3 days after her stroke onset.

She was transferred to an inpatient rehabilitation facility 2 days after her stroke onset. She stayed for approximately 3 weeks, with good progress. Her diet advanced from a dysphagia level I diet to a regular diet with swallowing precautions. She was discharged home under her daughter's supervision and with continued outpatient therapies.

She used CPAP for 1 month but then completely stopped its use. At 3 months post stroke, her Barthel index by telephone was 95, indicative of little dependency on others for activities of daily living.

Discussion

Almost uniformly, studies performed in the acute or subacute setting have identified sleep apnea in over half of ischemic stroke patients, with obstructive sleep apnea much more common than central sleep apnea.[1] Despite this high prevalence, sleep apnea is not routinely investigated pre or post stroke, and not surprisingly, patients often underestimate their own risk.[2] Although the example described above was of mild sleep apnea, previously undetected sleep apnea in stroke patients is often more severe. For example, one study of consecutive ischemic stroke patients admitted within a week of stroke found an AHI ≥ 10 in 58%, ≥ 20 in 31%, and ≥ 30 in 17%.[3] Although the above case presented an example of sleep apnea after a brainstem infarction, no specific infarction location has been associated with sleep apnea.[4] Similarly, no ischemic stroke subtype has been exclusively associated with sleep apnea risk, though large artery atherosclerotic disease in comparison to other stroke subtypes may have a stronger association with sleep apnea.[3]

In the community setting, obstructive sleep apnea is associated with male gender, obesity, sleepiness, and snoring. However, in the stroke population, these associations are much weaker or not present.[5] This case identified sleep apnea in a normal weight woman without excessive daytime sleepiness, and with a normal score on a validated sleep apnea questionnaire. To date, no reliable non-physiologic instrument has been identified to screen for or diagnose obstructive sleep apnea in post-stroke patients. While full polysomnography remains the gold standard, for logistical reasons that include better tolerance in the acute stroke population and limited inpatient resources, stroke research studies often use portable devices to detect sleep apnea.[1] Few studies have validated a portable device against polysomnography in stroke patients, but one that did demonstrated a high correlation.[3]

Obstructive sleep apnea is an important risk factor for poor stroke outcomes, including both poor functional outcome and increased mortality.[6] Furthermore, observational data have shown that CPAP use is associated with reduced mortality post stroke.[7] Interestingly, while obstructive sleep apnea is associated with higher mortality, central sleep apnea may not be.[8] If obstructive sleep apnea does worsen stroke outcomes, the mechanism could involve intermittent hypoxemia, stimulation of the sympathetic nervous system, or another factor, but remains unknown. Although it is intuitive that treatment of sleep apnea may improve stroke outcomes, this is not yet supported by definitive randomized, controlled trial data, and clinical equipoise that would allow such trials still exists.[9]

Sleep apnea and stroke do share some risk factors in common, such as obesity. Furthermore, sleep apnea may cause stroke through its association with hypertension. Nonetheless, sleep apnea has been determined to represent an independent risk factor for stroke; even when potential confounders are accounted for, sleep apnea remains a risk factor for the development of incident ischemic stroke.[10] This association has been found in numerous studies that include sleep laboratory-based and epidemiologic studies, though the association is better established in men than women.[11] While the relationship between sleep apnea and incident stroke has been studied, the relationship between sleep apnea and recurrent stroke is largely unknown.

Although the causal pathway between sleep apnea and incident stroke remains unclear, many possibilities exist: sleep apnea is known to exacerbate inflammation, trigger coagulation, and is associated with deleterious cerebral hemodynamics.[12] Currently only observational studies have been performed to demonstrate the association between CPAP use and reduced development of combined cardiovascular and cerebrovascular events.[13] Randomized controlled trial data are not yet available to address whether CPAP prevents incident or recurrent stroke.

Given that sleep apnea is an independent risk factor for stroke, and that no particular infarction location has been linked to sleep apnea, sleep apnea likely often predates stroke. Stroke may however also exacerbate sleep apnea, as several studies have shown that sleep apnea severity typically improves after the first several months post stroke.[3] Nonetheless, the prevalence of sleep apnea in chronic stroke patients remains quite high.

In the general sleep apnea population, CPAP is not uniformly tolerated, and in the stroke population, acceptance and tolerance appear to be further reduced.[3] Even with intensive troubleshooting, usage remains poor.[14] Special practical treatment considerations include selection of masks, interfaces, and headgear that can be used by patients with a dysfunctional arm.[15] Consideration of these factors may help an individual patient and caregiver, but are not likely to improve usage substantially in most post-stroke patients.[16]

As the use of CPAP in stroke patients may be limited, alternatives to CPAP need to be investigated further for the stroke population with sleep apnea. Preliminary work has suggested that positional therapy designed to avoid the supine position may have a modest effect on sleep apnea severity.[17] However, further research into CPAP alternatives in the stroke population is needed.

Main points

This case is illustrative of many characteristics of sleep apnea after stroke: (i) sleep apnea is very common after stroke; (ii) obstructive sleep apnea is much more common than central sleep apnea after stroke; (iii) sleep apnea in stroke patients may not be reliably detected with questionnaires, and therefore a physiologic test is needed; and (iv) stroke patients often do not tolerate CPAP well.

FURTHER READING

Sleep apnea and stroke outcomes

Turkington PM, Allgar V, Bamford J, Wanklyn P, Elliott MW. Effect of upper airway obstruction in acute stroke on functional outcome at 6 months. *Thorax* 2004;**59**:367–71.

Sleep apnea as a stroke risk factor

Yaggi HK, Concato J, Kernan WN, et al. Obstructive sleep apnea as a risk factor for stroke and death. *N Engl J Med* 2005;**353**:2034–41.

Characteristics of sleep apnea post stroke and treatment with CPAP

Bassetti CL, Milanova M, Gugger M. Sleep-disordered breathing and acute ischemic stroke: diagnosis, risk factors, treatment, evolution, and long-term clinical outcome. *Stroke* 2006;**37**:967–72.

REFERENCES

1. Broadley SA, Jorgensen L, Cheek A, et al. Early investigation and treatment of obstructive sleep apnoea after acute stroke. *J Clin Neurosci* 2007;**14**:328–33.

2. Skolarus LE, Lisabeth LD, Morgenstern LB, Burgin W, Brown DL. Sleep apnea risk among Mexican American and non-Hispanic White stroke survivors. *Stroke* 2012;**43**: 1143–5.

3. Bassetti CL, Milanova M, Gugger M. Sleep-disordered breathing and acute ischemic stroke: diagnosis, risk factors, treatment, evolution, and long-term clinical outcome. *Stroke* 2006;**37**:967–72.

4. Bassetti C, Aldrich M, Quint D. Sleep-disordered breathing in patients with acute supra- and infratentorial strokes: a prospective study of 39 patients. *Stroke* 1997;**28**: 1765–72.

5. Arzt M, Young T, Peppard PE, et al. Dissociation of obstructive sleep apnea from hypersomnolence and obesity in patients with stroke. *Stroke* 2010;**41**:e129–34.

6. Turkington PM, Allgar V, Bamford J, Wanklyn P, Elliott MW. Effect of upper airway obstruction in acute stroke on functional outcome at 6 months. *Thorax* 2004;**59**:367–71.

7. Martinez-Garcia MA, Soler-Cataluna JJ, Ejarque-Martinez L, et al. Continuous positive airway pressure treatment reduces mortality in patients with ischemic stroke and obstructive sleep apnea: a 5-year follow-up study. *Am J Respir Crit Care Med* 2009;**180**:36–41.

8. Sahlin C, Sandberg O, Gustafson Y, et al. Obstructive sleep apnea is a risk factor for death in patients with stroke: a 10-year follow-up. *Arch Intern Med* 2008;**168**:297–301.

9. Brown DL, Anderson CS, Chervin RD, et al. Ethical issues in the conduct of clinical trials in obstructive sleep apnea. *J Clin Sleep Med* 2012;**7**:103–8.

10. Yaggi HK, Concato J, Kernan WN, et al. Obstructive sleep apnea as a risk factor for stroke and death. *N Engl J Med* 2005;**353**:2034–41.

11. Redline S, Yenokyan G, Gottlieb DJ, et al. Obstructive sleep apnea hypopnea and incident stroke: The Sleep Heart Health Study. *Am J Respir Crit Care Med* 2010;**182**:269–77.

12. Brown DL. Sleep disorders and stroke. *Semin Neurol* 2006;**26**:117–22.

13. Marin JM, Carrizo SJ, Vicente E, Agusti AG. Long-term cardiovascular outcomes in men with obstructive sleep apnoea-hypopnoea with or without treatment with continuous positive airway pressure: an observational study. *Lancet* 2005;**365**:1046–53.

14. Hsu CY, Vennelle M, Li HY, et al. Sleep disordered breathing after stroke. A randomized controlled trial of continuous positive airway pressure. *J Neurol Neurosurg Psychiatry* 2006;**77**:1143–9.

15. Brown DL, Concannon M, Kaye AB, Zupancic M, Lisabeth LD. Comparison of two headgear systems for sleep apnea treatment of stroke patients. *Cerebrovasc Dis* 2009;**27**: 183–6.

16. Brown DL, Chervin RD, Kalbfleisch JD, et al. Sleep apnea treatment after stroke (SATS) trial: is it feasible? *J Stroke Cerebrovasc Dis* 2011 [Epub ahead of print].

17. Svatikova A, Chervin RD, Wing JJ, et al. Positional therapy in ischemic stroke patients with obstructive sleep apnea. *Sleep Med* 2011;**12**:262–6.

46

A missed diagnosis of obstructive sleep apnea can have a critical adverse impact in the postoperative setting

Satya Krishna Ramachandran

Case

A 32-year-old patient developed a surgical site infection following a laminectomy and open decompression of a lumbar nerve root. Following unsuccessful outpatient antibiotic therapy, the patient was scheduled for surgical drainage of the infection. The past medical history was significant for morbid obesity (body mass index of 44.8 kg/m^2), hypertension, and type 2 diabetes mellitus. General anesthesia with tracheal intubation was planned given the expected prone position for surgery. Premedications included sodium bicitrate 30 cc by mouth, ranitidine 50 mg intravenously (IV), metoclopramide 10 mg IV, and midazolam 2 mg IV. Anesthesia medications included lidocaine mg 40 mg IV, propofol 250 mg IV, fentanyl 300 μg IV, succinylcholine 160 mg IV, vecuronium 10 mg IV, dexamethasone 10 mg IV, ondansetron 4 mg IV, clindamycin 900 mg IV, neostigmine 4 mg IV, and glycopyrrolate 0.8 mg IV. Following uneventful anesthesia and surgery, a morphine patient-controlled analgesia (PCA) pump was commenced to control postoperative pain. The original PCA order called for morphine at 1 mg/ml, demand dose of 1 mg, lockout interval of 8 minutes, a planned increase in dose by 0.5 mg if pain is not controlled, with a 4-hour limit of 30 mg. At about 9:30 PM, the patient was transferred from the post-anesthesia care unit to the floor bed. Shortly thereafter, the acute pain nurse noted the patient's complaint of inadequate analgesia, and increased the PCA settings to demand dose morphine 1.5 mg, lockout interval of 6 minutes, planned increase of PCA dose to 2 mg if pain not controlled, with a 4-hour limit of 45 mg. Postoperative vitals were taken at 10:00 PM and 11:00 PM with no remarkable findings. A nursing evaluation noted that on arrival to floor, the patient was comfortable, wide awake and freely mobile in bed. At approximately 1:30 AM, the nurse walked into the room to start an antibiotic dose and found the patient unresponsive and pulseless. Despite full cardiopulmonary resuscitation, there was no return of spontaneous circulation and the patient was declared dead 45 minutes later. Autopsy examination was largely unremarkable and cardiac arrhythmia was cited as probable cause of death. On further questioning, the family members reported that the patient had been tested for obstructive sleep apnea (OSA) but was not using the positive airway pressure (PAP) device. Additionally, previous anesthesia records were accessed and revealed that the patient received lower doses of morphine for pain relief after the lumbar laminectomy. Expert review also identified serum bicarbonate level to be 34 mEq/l.

This case highlights several challenges to the perioperative management of known or suspected sleep apnea and obesity hypoventilation syndrome: preoperative screening, preoperative testing and fitting for PAP, postoperative monitoring standards, thresholds for initiating PAP postoperatively, and postoperative analgesic strategies. Various specialty organizations have proposed practice guidelines for management of patients with known or suspected OSA.

Preoperative screening for OSA

It is estimated that over 80% of patients with OSA are undiagnosed.[1] Several clinical screening tools have been described in literature, as recently evaluated in a systematic fashion by Ramachandran et al.[2] The summary findings of this study indicate that it is possible to predict severe OSA with a high degree of accuracy by clinical methods. In that study, the Berlin questionnaire was the most accurate questionnaire, whereas morphometry was the most accurate clinical model. Significantly, test accuracy has poor reproducibility in repeated validation studies of the same screening tool. Based on false negative rates, it is possible that all of the studied questionnaires and most of the clinical models will fail to identify a significant proportion of patients with OSA. The large heterogeneity in accuracy of any single test limits the value of screening tools for treatment decisions. Several protocols have been described to manage patients at high risk of OSA, with many using screening tools such as the STOP–Bang questionnaire,[3] the Sleep Apnea Clinical Score (SACS)[4], and the American Society of Anesthesiologists (ASA) screening tool.[5]

One of the better validated screening tools is the STOP–Bang model (Table 46.1), which functions more dependably than the abbreviated STOP questionnaire.[3] On repeated testing, the STOP–Bang tool was shown to have excellent sensitivity for severe OSA with acceptable positive predictive value. Although the authors suggest a threshold of 3 or greater points, an important practical consideration is the number of patients that will screen as high risk. A STOP–Bang threshold of 5 or greater occurs in roughly 30% of the surgical population, and is associated with significantly increased odds of OSA. The odds ratios (95% confidence intervals) were 3.98 (2.38–6.66) for mild OSA, 4.75 (2.81–8.03) for moderate OSA, and 10.39 (4.45–24.26) for severe OSA.[6]

A threshold of 5 or more points is suggested to identify patients who need additional investigation and optimization of coexisting medical conditions before surgery.[7]

An additional consideration in screening algorithms for OSA is the time constraint imposed by the

Table 46.1 STOP–Bang questionnaire

1. **S**noring: Do you snore loudly (loud enough to be heard through closed doors)?	Yes/No
2. **T**ired: Do you often feel tired, fatigued, or sleepy during daytime?	Yes/No
3. **O**bserved: Has anyone observed you stop breathing during your sleep?	Yes/No
4. Blood **P**ressure: Do you have or are you being treated for high blood pressure?	Yes/No
5. **B**ody mass index (BMI): BMI > 35 kg/m^2?	Yes/No
6. **A**ge: Age over 50 years old?	Yes/No
7. **N**eck circumference: Neck circumference >40 cm?	Yes/No
8. **G**ender: Male?	Yes/No
STOP–Bang total points (add all 'yes' responses)	

impending surgical procedure and the likelihood of achieving satisfactory patient participation in a process that involves two visits at minimum: one for diagnostic polysomnography combined with PAP titration (a so-called "split-night" study), and another visit for clinical evaluation, patient education, and receipt of PAP equipment. Several models have been proposed and our dedicated preoperative fast-track sleep laboratory process currently aims to achieve this within 7–14 days of an initial appointment at the preoperative clinic. More efficient usage of home testing and automatically adjusting PAP (auto-PAP) devices, in appropriate candidates, may further help reduce delays related to scheduling.

Preoperative PAP therapy

There is no prospective trial-based evidence of benefit with preoperative PAP therapy, or on the duration of therapy needed to modify surgical risk. However, several potential mechanisms for risk modification with preoperative PAP therapy include reduced sympathetic tone resulting in significant reduction of episodic hypertension, improved heart rate variability, reduced hypoxemia, reduced arrhythmias, and reduced risk of post-cardioversion atrial fibrillation.[8-11] More crucially, cessation of PAP therapy is associated with an instantaneous increase in sympathetic activity,[12] pointing to the significance of reinforcing the need for adherence with PAP therapy in patients undergoing surgery. Preoperative PAP therapy may have complex and seemingly opposing effects on peripheral and central chemosensitivity.[13–15] A reduced peripheral oxygen chemosensitivity may be a side effect of continuous positive airway pressure (CPAP) therapy. The normocapnic hypoxic ventilatory response was reduced after a month of treatment with nasal CPAP (nCPAP) in one study, suggesting potential increased risk of opioid induced respiratory depression.[14] On the other hand, reduction in diurnal hypercapnia seen with non-invasive ventilation in patients with severe obesity hypoventilation syndrome has been shown to improve central apneas.[16] Similarly, PAP therapy for 2 weeks caused a significant increase in hypercapnic ventilatory responses in OSA patients.[15] Thus, initiation of CPAP therapy may influence risk of postoperative respiratory depression by either increasing or decreasing the ventilatory responses to hypercapnia and hypoxia.

A recent study reported a 40% adherence with treatment and median CPAP usage of just 2.5 hours among users.[17] Thus, treatment adherence remains the single biggest challenge to risk modification for preoperative PAP therapy. It is important to note that continuation of PAP therapy is crucial to maintain perioperative benefit. Compared with continuing CPAP, 2 weeks of CPAP withdrawal was associated with a significant increase in morning blood pressures and heart rate, and an increase in urinary catecholamines.[18] The fact that the index case described above was not compliant with use of a PAP device in the preoperative period may increase the likelihood of hypoxemia-related arrhythmias. The timing of sudden death in the postoperative period largely mirrors the nocturnal predominance of sudden cardiac death in patients with OSA.[19,20] Additionally, lower vigilance levels and a limitation of arousal mechanisms during sleep could contribute to this increased risk of nocturnal sudden death in postoperative patients with OSA. Despite this concern, the actual incidence of this dreaded complication may be low even among patients with OSA. Protective

physiologic mechanisms may intervene to enhance arousal including pain and audible monitor alarms.

Postoperative PAP therapy

There is robust evidence to support early treatment of postoperative hypoxemia using CPAP therapy. In a randomized controlled trial of PAP therapy versus face mask oxygen therapy for treatment of hypoxemia after major elective abdominal surgery, PAP treatment was associated with a 10-fold reduction in intubation rates and a 5-fold reduction in pneumonia rates.[21] Direct evidence of benefit of postoperative PAP therapy in patients with OSA is unclear, but postoperative PAP is often considered to be a standard of care for patients with OSA. We use an electronic health record-based paging alert system to activate perioperative OSA protocols and respiratory therapy teams, with associated improvement in outcomes.[22] Development of thresholds for PAP therapy is challenging, as some hospitals require intensive care unit admission for PAP therapy in a previously undiagnosed OSA patient. One potential approach is to link screening tools for OSA with early postoperative desaturation to identify patients needing PAP therapy.[4] However, whether this approach is associated with improved outcomes remains largely unknown. Additional considerations need to include duration of PAP therapy, post-discharge polysomnographic testing, billing requirements, and follow-up pathways. In the case above, use of PAP therapy may have reduced risk for postoperative decline through improved risk for postoperative hypoxemia and arrhythmias.

Postoperative monitoring

Several recent publications from expert societies address the need for monitoring strategies to detect significant drug-induced respiratory depression in the postoperative period. However, as the majority of surgical procedures are performed on an outpatient ambulatory care-basis, postoperative monitoring is typically limited to hospitalized patients and current monitoring protocols often do not extend past

24 hours into the highest risk period for postoperative hypoxemia. The first postoperative day represents the highest risk period for analgesia-related unanticipated respiratory events.[20] However, sleep-related breathing disorders typically peak on the third postoperative night, and the concept of rapid cye movement (REM) rebound has been proposed to explain the mechanisms of related increases in hypoxemia. Extending monitoring to cover this period is typically not feasible because the majority of admitted patients are discharged by then, and evidence does not exist that extended monitoring periods are associated with improved outcomes. Continuous pulse oximetry is superior to intermittent spot-check monitoring, but the clinical significance of postoperative episodic hypoxemia is still unclear, especially during opioid analgesic therapy. Previous studies have failed to demonstrate significant outcome improvement in postoperative patients with continuous pulse oximetry monitoring alone. However, when such monitoring was linked to patient surveillance systems that work by notifying desaturation and pulse rate abnormalities using threshold-based alert pages to nurses, improvements in rescue events and intensive care unit transfers were observed.[23] Inadequate consideration for thresholds for such alarms contribute to technologic intensification and the risk of alarm fatigue related to alarm overload, loss of communication of alarm data to paging interfaces, nuisance alarms, and lack of clarity on thresholds for escalation of care. In summary, the risks of technologic intensification need to be balanced against the benefits of postoperative monitoring methods. In the index case reported above, the use of continuous monitoring may have alerted nurses to a sudden decline in respiration. Our institution currently has a surveillance system that pages nurses when monitor alarms are breached for > 30 seconds.

Postoperative analgesic strategies

Patients with OSA may be at elevated risk of opioid-induced respiratory depression. Opioids are associated with dose-dependent increases in central apneas,

ataxic breathing and postoperative breathing disturbances.[24] Expert bodies call for use of non-opioid or opioid-reduction strategies in patients with OSA. However, reducing opioid dosage alone has not shown benefit in prospective studies. In children, prospective opioid dose reduction was not associated with reduced postoperative hypoxemia.[25] Similarly, in adults, opioid reduction strategies were not associated with change in respiratory disturbances after surgery.[26] These studies highlight the limitation of using opioid-sparing techniques as the sole method of risk modification in patients with OSA. The index case likely had obesity hypoventilation syndrome related to the high bicarbonate levels, severe OSA, and morbid obesity. This potentially increased the propensity to opioid-induced respiratory depression and subsequent death.

Main points

Sleep disorders and OSA in particular are important to consider before and after operative procedures that involve anesthesia. Risk of postoperative respiratory failure may be reduced if OSA can be identified and then treated, both before and after these procedures. The highest risk for exacerbation of OSA may occur after most patients, including those who have inpatient surgery, are discharged. Central sleep apnea is also a concern in the setting of opioid analgesia. Hospital protocols to reduce perioperative risk from sleep apnea are employed increasingly, though more research is clearly needed to define which approaches will have optimal and cost-effective outcomes.

REFERENCES

1. Young T, Palta M, Dempsey J, et al. The occurrence of sleep-disordered breathing among middle-aged adults. *N Engl J Med* 1993;**328**:1230–5.
2. Ramachandran SK, Josephs LA. A meta-analysis of clinical screening tests for obstructive sleep apnea. *Anesthesiology* 2009;**110**:928–39.

3. Chung F, Yegneswaran B, Liao P, et al. STOP questionnaire: a tool to screen patients for obstructive sleep apnea. *Anesthesiology* 2008;**108**:812–21.

4. Gali B, Whalen FX, Jr., Gay PC, et al. Management plan to reduce risks in perioperative care of patients with presumed obstructive sleep apnea syndrome. *J Clin Sleep Med* 2007;**3**:582–8.

5. Munish M, Sharma V, Yarussi KM, et al. The use of practice guidelines by the American Society of Anesthesiologists for the identification of surgical patients at high risk of sleep apnea. *Chron Respir Dis* 2012;**9**:221–30.

6. Chung F, Subramanyam R, Liao P, et al. High STOP–Bang score indicates a high probability of obstructive sleep apnoea. *Br J Anaesth* 2012;**108**:768–75.

7. Joshi GP, Ankichetty SP, Gan TJ, Chung F. Society for Ambulatory Anesthesia consensus statement on preoperative selection of adult patients with obstructive sleep apnea scheduled for ambulatory surgery. *Anesth Analg* 2012;**115**:1060–8.

8. Abe H, Takahashi M, Yaegashi H, et al. Efficacy of continuous positive airway pressure on arrhythmias in obstructive sleep apnea patients. *Heart Vessels* 2010;**25**:63–9.

9. Belozeroff V, Berry RB, Sassoon CS, Khoo MC. Effects of CPAP therapy on cardiovascular variability in obstructive sleep apnea: a closed-loop analysis. *Am J Physiol Heart Circ Physiol* 2002;**282**:H110–21.

10. Kanagala R, Murali NS, Friedman PA, et al. Obstructive sleep apnea and the recurrence of atrial fibrillation. *Circulation* 2003;**107**:2589–94.

11. Ryan CM, Usui K, Floras JS, Bradley TD. Effect of continuous positive airway pressure on ventricular ectopy in heart failure patients with obstructive sleep apnoea. *Thorax* 2005;**60**:781–5.

12. Somers VK, Dyken ME, Clary MP, Abboud FM. Sympathetic neural mechanisms in obstructive sleep apnea. *J Clin Invest* 1995;**96**:1897–904.

13. Redolfi S, Corda L, La Piana G, et al. Long-term non-invasive ventilation increases chemosensitivity and leptin in obesity-hypoventilation syndrome. *Respir Med* 2007;**101**:1191–5.

14. Spicuzza L, Bernardi L, Balsamo R, et al. Effect of treatment with nasal continuous positive airway pressure on ventilatory response to hypoxia and hypercapnia in patients with sleep apnea syndrome. *Chest* 2006;**130**:774–9.

15. Tun Y, Hida W, Okabe S, et al. Effects of nasal continuous positive airway pressure on awake ventilatory responses to hypoxia and hypercapnia in patients with obstructive sleep apnea. *Tohoku J Exp Med* 2000;**190**:157–68.

16. Aurora RN, Chowdhuri S, Ramar K, et al. The treatment of central sleep apnea syndromes in adults: practice parameters with an evidence-based literature review and meta-analyses. *Sleep* 2012;**35**:17–40.

17. Guralnick AS, Pant M, Minhaj M, Sweitzer BJ, Mokhlesi B. CPAP adherence in patients with newly diagnosed obstructive sleep apnea prior to elective surgery. *J Clin Sleep Med* 2012;**8**:501–6.

18. Kohler M, Stoewhas AC, Ayers L, et al. Effects of continuous positive airway pressure therapy withdrawal in patients with obstructive sleep apnea: a randomized controlled trial. *Am J Respir Crit Care Med* 2011;**184**:1192–9.

19. Gami AS, Howard DE, Olson EJ, Somers VK. Day–night pattern of sudden death in obstructive sleep apnea. *N Engl J Med* 2005;**352**:1206–14.

20. Ramachandran SK, Haider N, Saran KA, et al. Life-threatening critical respiratory events: a retrospective study of postoperative patients found unresponsive during analgesic therapy. *J Clin Anesth* 2011;**23**:207–13.

21. Squadrone V, Coha M, Cerutti E, et al. Continuous positive airway pressure for treatment of postoperative hypoxemia: a randomized controlled trial. *JAMA* 2005;**293**:589–95.

22. Ramachandran SK, Kheterpal S, Haas CF, Saran KA, Tremper KK. Automated notification of suspected obstructive sleep apnea patients to the perioperative respiratory therapist: a pilot study. *Respir Care* 2010;**55**:414–18.

23. Taenzer AH, Pyke JB, McGrath SP, Blike GT. Impact of pulse oximetry surveillance on rescue events and intensive care unit transfers: a before-and-after concurrence study. *Anesthesiology* 2010;**112**:282–7.

24. Walker JM, Farney RJ, Rhondeau SM, et al. Chronic opioid use is a risk factor for the development of central sleep apnea and ataxic breathing. *J Clin Sleep Med* 2007;**3**:455–61.

25. Brown KA, Laferriere A, Lakheeram I, Moss IR. Recurrent hypoxemia in children is associated with increased analgesic sensitivity to opiates. *Anesthesiology* 2006;**105**:665–9.

26. Blake DW, Yew CY, Donnan GB, Williams DL. Postoperative analgesia and respiratory events in patients with symptoms of obstructive sleep apnoea. *Anaesth Intensive Care* 2009;**37**:720–5.

Sleep in children

Insight into children's sleep and sleep disorders has provided some of the most exciting developments in sleep medicine within recent years. Although many of the same sleep disorders found in adults also affect children, children are now understood to have, almost invariably, markedly distinct presentations, comorbidities, assessment requirements, and optimal approaches to treatment. In many cases the underlying pathophysiology is quite different from that found among adults.

As for adults, pediatricians and subspecialists from the widest conceivable range of backgrounds, in addition to the many general sleep specialists who see patients of all ages, have made distinct contributions toward the effort to better understand and address childhood sleep disorders. The chapters in this section have been contributed by a pediatric neurologist, general pediatrician, child psychologist,

behavioral/developmental pediatrician, pediatric pulmonologist, and neonatal neurologist.

The specific patient cases covered in this section each highlight at least one commonly misunderstood, or seldom recognized yet important issue about sleep problems in children. Obstructive sleep apnea is emphasized because, as in adults, it represents the most common and one of the most threatening sleep disorders in childhood. However, insomnia that results largely from interactions between parents and their children gives rise to sleep complaints even more commonly. Furthermore, children of specific ages or with particular types of neurologic, psychiatric, other medical, or environmental challenges can present with sleep disorders that must be recognized and addressed. Missing such opportunities at these young ages can have substantial consequences not only during childhood but for a subsequent lifetime.

47

Sleepiness in childhood obstructive sleep apnea may be subtle but significant

Timothy F. Hoban

Case

A 7-year-old boy was brought to the pediatric sleep medicine clinic to investigate whether an underlying sleep disorder might be contributing to his problems with inattention at school. Although he was doing reasonably well in his third grade classes, teachers reported varying degrees of concern regarding inattention and remaining on task. He generally performed well on tests and quizzes, but had difficulty completing and turning in homework and other assignments. The boy's mother also reported frequent episodes of staring or "zoning out" from which he could be alerted by voice or touch.

Assessment of sleep-related symptoms revealed that the boy frequently exhibited loud snoring and mouth breathing during sleep, particularly when nasal congestion was present. No restlessness, diaphoresis, or enuresis were apparent during sleep. The boy's parents and teachers reported no obvious sleepiness apart from transient grogginess upon morning waking. Daytime napping was observed only during particularly lengthy automobile rides.

The patient's medical history was otherwise notable only for allergic rhinitis, which had responded partially to treatment with fexofenadine and fluticasone nasal spray. Family medical history was significant for allergic rhinitis affecting both parents and dyslexia affecting a brother, with no known family history of obstructive sleep apnea (OSA) or attention-deficit/hyperactivity disorder (ADHD).

Physical examination revealed an alert, healthy-appearing third grader whose weight of 52 pounds (23.6 kg) ranked at the 45th percentile for age and whose body mass index of 14.4 kg/m^2 ranked at the 17th percentile. General physical exam revealed a drooping facial appearance consistent with adenoid facies, Dennie–Morgan creases, and allergic shiners. Intranasal exam demonstrated boggy turbinates without rhinorrhea. Intraoral exam was notable for a crowded posterior oropharynx with 3+ cryptic tonsils but no palatal or occlusal abnormalities. Brief neurologic examination was unremarkable.

The clinical impression was that the constellation of symptoms and exam findings were suggestive of OSA, and a baseline nocturnal polysomnogram was ordered for further assessment. This study demonstrated OSA that became severe during rapid eye movement (REM) sleep. The apnea/hypopnea index (AHI, events per hour of sleep) was 26 for the study as a whole, rising to 75 during REM sleep. Respiratory disturbances were characterized primarily by hypopneas associated with arousals and sleep fragmentation (an arousal index of 28 per hour of sleep), but only mild desaturation of SpO$_2$ levels from baseline (nadir 87%) (Figure 47.1).

What treatment would you recommend?

Adenotonsillectomy and nasal continuous positive airway pressure (CPAP) both represent first-line

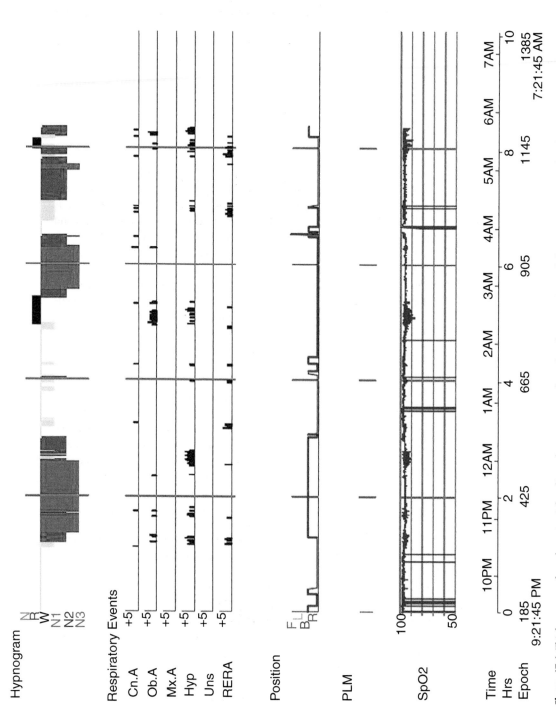

Figure 47.1 This hypnogram from the patient's baseline polysomnogram reflects sleep fragmentation and obstructive respiratory disturbances during rapid eye movement (REM) sleep in a child with obstructive sleep apnea (OSA). Abbreviations used in figure: N, unspecified non-REM; R, REM; W, wake; N1, N2, N3, non-REM stages N1, N2, N3; Cn.A, central apneas; Ob.A, obstructive apneas; Mx.A, mixed apneas; Hyp, hypopneas; Uns, unscored events; RERA, respiratory effort-related arousals; F, front; L, left lateral; B, back; R, right lateral; PLM, periodic leg movements; SpO2, oxygen saturation by finger oximetry; Hrs, hours. See plate section for color version.

treatments for OSA in children. Adenotonsillectomy is chosen more frequently than CPAP, in part because the procedure is relatively straightforward and offers the potential for surgical cure in cases where airway obstruction is primarily related to adenotonsillar hypertrophy. This procedure is not uniformly successful, however, and recent research suggests that respiratory parameters during sleep fully normalize in only 25–50% of children treated in this fashion.[1,2] In addition to the possibility of residual OSA, other potential risks and side effects related to surgery and anesthesia must also be considered.

Nasal CPAP is also considered a first-line treatment for childhood OSA. Continuous positive airway pressure is non-surgical, relatively safe, and effective in alleviating airway obstruction related to factors beyond adenotonsillar hypertrophy. Most side effects such as skin irritation or pressure intolerance are mild and self-limited, although acquired maxillary retrusion has been rarely reported as a complication of long-term use in younger children.[3] Acclimation to routine nightly use can be challenging, however, particularly for younger children or those with developmental disabilities.

For the patient described above, the major treatment options and their relative tradeoffs were discussed in detail with both parents during a subsequent clinic appointment. They expressed concern regarding the potential risks of adenotonsillectomy and were more comfortable proceeding with a trial of nasal CPAP. We discussed pragmatic aspects of CPAP with the child and parents, who all agreed to extend their best effort to use CPAP nightly for 2 months following the sleep laboratory CPAP titration, with the understanding that we would meet and reassess progress of treatment at that point.

The CPAP titration assessed pressure settings of 4–8 cm of water, and demonstrated that a setting of 6 cm of water provided good control of respiratory disturbances during sleep. Fragmentation of sleep architecture was considerably improved, sleep was increased, and periods of wakefulness were diminished in comparison to the baseline study (Figure 47.2). The CPAP induced near-normalization of the arousal index (score of 10) and percentage of stage R sleep (15%).

The family returned to clinic several months following the CPAP trial and reported that the patient had taken only 4 days to become comfortable with use of CPAP at bedtime and that he had used it nightly since then. Snoring and restlessness during sleep had largely resolved following initiation of treatment. No problems with comfort or side effects were reported, apart from noise secondary to water condensation in the plastic tubing. On rare occasions, the noise would wake the child during the night.

The mother reported being "very impressed" by several unexpected but dramatic areas of improvement. Whereas the boy had previously been groggy and difficult to awaken on school days, he was now waking independently and fully refreshed – sufficiently early that he now routinely had time to play on his computer before going to school. Daytime alertness and level of energy were visibly better, staring spells had resolved, and the family received an unprompted telephone call from his teacher reporting that attention in class had also improved.

Discussion

This case vividly illustrates how daytime sleepiness in children with OSA may be expressed in subtle or intermittent fashions. Whereas most adults with OSA present with sleepiness as an obvious and easily referable daytime symptom, affected children are more likely to exhibit inattention, hyperactivity, or behavioral dysregulation during the daytime. Such behaviors are often attributed to alternative causes such as ADHD, and are often not recognized as symptoms of an underlying sleep disorder. This results in many children receiving stimulants or other treatments for ADHD and behavioral disorders rather than receiving appropriate testing and treatment for their underlying sleep-disordered breathing.

Careful examination of the daytime symptoms described in this case yields important insights regarding how daytime sleepiness is expressed in children with OSA. Grogginess upon morning waking is uncommon in preadolescent children who receive habitually sufficient sleep, but frequent among

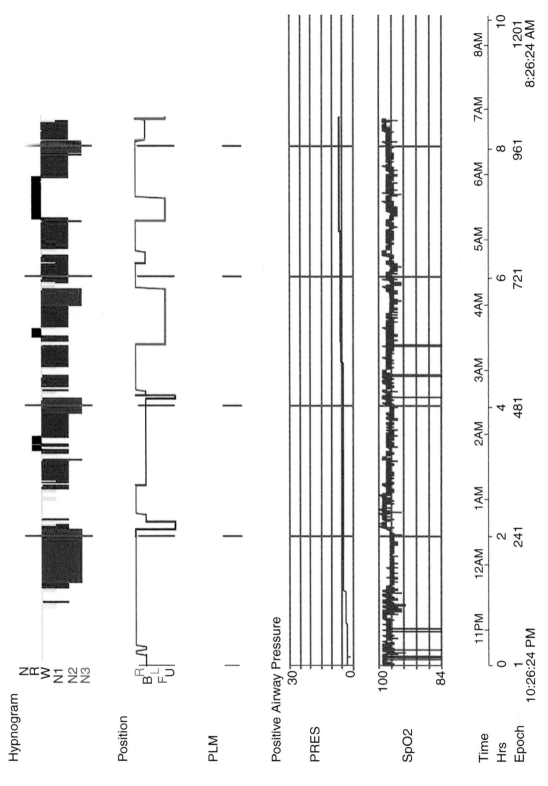

Figure 47.2 The patient's hypnogram, from the initial titration on continuous positive airway pressure (CPAP), reflects increased sleep and improved sleep when obstructive sleep apnea is treated. Abbreviations used in figure: N, unspecified non-REM; R, REM; W, wake; N1, N2, N3, non-REM stages N1, N2, N3; R, right lateral; B, back; L, left lateral; F, front; U, undetermined position; PLM, periodic leg movements; PRES, CPAP pressure setting in centimeter of water; SpO2, oxygen saturation by finger oximetry; Hrs, hours. See plate section for color version.

younger children with moderate or severe OSA, even when sleep duration is lengthened. Daytime inattention, staring, or "zoning out" in school represent common symptoms of sleepiness in school-aged children, symptoms that are often overlooked or misattributed to other causes unless the child appears obviously somnolent. Impaired daytime alertness and performance in children with OSA are often subtle and pervasive to the point that the full extent and severity of symptoms become apparent only in retrospect after treatment is initiated. This was the case for the child described above, whose parents had not appreciated significant sleepiness prior to the diagnosis of OSA, but who subsequently reported dramatic improvements in alertness, level of energy, and school performance following initiation of treatment.

This case also demonstrates that CPAP can be effectively used as first-line treatment for OSA in young children as an alternative to the more commonly selected adenotonsillectomy. Several factors helped augment CPAP compliance and effectiveness for the child described in this case. Both parents were motivated to successfully implement use of CPAP due to their concerns regarding potential side effects of adenotonsillectomy and possible risks of general anesthesia. They worked consistently and effectively to incorporate CPAP use into the nightly bedtime routine and portray CPAP use in a positive fashion for their son. The fact that the child and parents quickly recognized the positive clinical benefits of CPAP treatment further reinforced their belief in the importance of continued treatment and their commitment to regular use.

Successful use of CPAP in children is most likely when the child and parents are motivated and willing to devote effort to its use. Although acclimation to use of CPAP can be more challenging for developmentally disabled or very young children, use of behavioral desensitization techniques sometimes permits gradual introduction to treatment and eventual entrainment to long-term use.[4]

Main points

- Symptoms of daytime sleepiness in children with OSA are more often characterized by inattention,

hyperactivity, and staring spells than by frank somnolence.
- Daytime neurobehavioral symptoms of childhood OSA are often misattributed to ADHD or other conditions.
- Nasal CPAP represents a feasible first-line treatment for many children with OSA in addition to adenotonsillectomy.

FURTHER READING

Sleepiness, ADHD, and neurobehavioral manifestations of childhood OSA

Chervin RD. Attention deficit, hyperactivity, and sleep disorders. In Sheldon SH, Ferber R, Kryger MH, eds. *Principles and Practice of Pediatric Sleep Medicine*. Philadelphia, PA: Elsevier Saunders;2005, pp. 161–9.

CPAP treatment of childhood OSA

Marcus CL, Rosen G, Ward SL, et al. Adherence to and effectiveness of positive airway pressure therapy in children with obstructive sleep apnea. *Pediatrics* 2006;**117**: e442–51.

References

1. Tauman R, Gulliver TE, Krishna J, et al. Persistence of obstructive sleep apnea syndrome in children after adenotonsillectomy. *J Pediatrics* 2006;**149**:803–8.
2. Guilleminault C, Huang YS, Glamann C, et al. Adenotonsillectomy and obstructive sleep apnea in children: a prospective survey. *Otolaryngol Head Neck Surg* 2007;**136**:169–75.
3. Li KK, Riley RW, Guilleminault C. An unreported risk in the use of home nasal continuous positive airway pressure and home nasal ventilation in children: mid-face hypoplasia. *Chest* 2000;**11**:916–18.
4. Rains JC. Treatment of obstructive sleep apnea in pediatric patients. Behavioral intervention for compliance with nasal continuous positive airway pressure. *Clin Pediatr (Phila)* 1995;**34**:535–41.

48

Clinically significant upper airway obstruction may be present in children even when the polysomnogram is normal by adult standards

Timothy F. Hoban

Case

An 8-year-old girl with Russell–Silver syndrome was referred to a Pediatric Sleep Medicine clinic for evaluation of restless, unrefreshing sleep, and pervasive daytime tiredness. On a typical night, the child would retire at 9:30 PM in a bedroom shared with an older sister. Following sleep onset near 10:15 PM, she reported frequent but brief periods of spontaneous waking during the night, although she would typically remain in bed until morning waking at 8:30–9:00 AM. Both she and her mother noted that nighttime sleep was seldom refreshing, even when sleep duration was lengthened. In addition, they both reported pervasive daytime tiredness that peaked during the afternoon hours. Daytime napping had stopped at about age 6 or 7, and was not currently observed even during long automobile rides.

The family had not observed habitual snoring and reported only minimal soft snoring when the child was ill. She was described as a restless and sweaty sleeper, even when room temperature was optimal. There were no complaints of growing pains or of leg restlessness or dysesthesias near bedtime.

Past medical history was notable for Russell–Silver syndrome associated with intrauterine growth retardation, failure-to-thrive, renal tubular acidosis, and gastroesophageal reflux disease requiring gastrostomy and nighttime tube feedings. There had been numerous medical hospitalizations for dehydration during intercurrent illness, but no history of significant adenotonsillar or pulmonary disease. Family history was notable for leg restlessness, affecting the child's mother, which resolved when underlying iron deficiency was identified and treated. On review of systems, the family reported that the child was doing reasonably well in her third grade home-schooling program apart from fatigue or an afternoon headache that occasionally interrupted scheduled activities. No significant external stressors or disturbances of mood were reported.

Physical examination revealed an alert, articulate girl of small stature who exhibited typical physical features of Russell–Silver syndrome, including a thin mouth, small and narrow chin, and clinodactyly of the fifth fingers. Her weight of 41 pounds (18.7 kg) and body mass index of 12.0 kg/m^2 both ranked below the 2nd percentile for age, while her height of 4 feet, 1 inch (124 cm) ranked at the 25th percentile. Intraoral exam was notable for micrognathia and a mildly high-arched palate without tonsillar hypertrophy. Cardiac, pulmonary, and limited neurologic exams were normal.

The initial clinical impression was that daytime symptoms were potentially consistent with either fatigue or sleepiness and that no precise cause was immediately evident. The presence of excessive night waking and the fact that sleep was seldom refreshing were felt to be potentially consistent with an underlying sleep disturbance such as periodic limb movement disorder, with sleep-disordered breathing considered less likely. Insufficient sleep duration and sleep disruption secondary to nocturnal tube feedings were felt to represent possible contributing factors, although the family considered this unlikely.

Initial diagnostic testing

As daytime fatigue can represent a symptom of anemia or thyroid disorders, and periodic limb movement disorder is sometimes associated with underlying iron deficiency states, laboratory screening for these conditions was performed immediately following the initial appointment. Although complete blood count and thyroid function tests were normal, the percent transferrin saturation was mildly low at 13.1% (normal 20–50%) and the ferritin level of 12.0 was in the range thought to be associated with increased risk for restless legs syndrome (RLS) and periodic limb movement disorder (PLMD).

A nocturnal polysomnogram was performed to screen for sleep disorders that might disturb the quality or continuity of sleep. The study did not identify any significant respiratory disturbances. The pediatric apnea/hypopnea index (AHI, events per hour of sleep) of 0.4 was within normal limits as determined by both pediatric and adult standards (AHI < 1 and AHI < 5, respectively) and no snoring or significant desaturations of SpO_2 were observed. Periodic limb movements were minimally elevated at a rate of 5.1 per hour during sleep. None of these movements were associated with arousal. Analysis of sleep architecture was notable for low sleep efficiency of 60% and short total sleep time of 284 minutes due to prolonged sleep onset latency and increased wakefulness after sleep onset, for increased stage 1 sleep (13%), and for decreased stage rapid eye movement (REM) sleep (12%).

A Multiple Sleep Latency Test was performed on the day following the polysomnogram to objectively measure daytime sleepiness. This study recorded sleep during two of five 20-minute nap opportunities. No sleep-onset REM periods were observed. The calculated mean sleep latency of 18.6 minutes was normal as determined by both pediatric and adult standards.[1]

What treatment or additional testing would you recommend?

Establishing optimal treatment for a child who presents with poor sleep quality and daytime fatigue can be challenging when initial assessments fail to identify a clear-cut cause that is proportionate to symptoms. In this case, it was unclear whether modestly low transferrin saturation and ferritin levels in the absence of anemia were sufficient to fully explain the child's symptoms. Although mild iron deficiency states may be associated with increased risk for RLS or PLMD, this child reported no symptoms suggestive of RLS, and her symptoms and her polysomnogram findings only marginally attained the criteria necessary (five or more periodic leg movements per hour of sleep) for a diagnosis of pediatric PLMD.[2]

As no other immediately evident sleep disorders were apparent apart from possible PLMD, a trial of iron supplementation (3 mg/kg per day of elemental iron) was recommended. Although the frequency and severity of daytime headaches improved considerably during treatment with ferrous sulfate, and transferrin saturation levels normalized, there was no improvement in nocturnal restlessness or sleep quality, which continued to be described by the family as "horrible." A subsequent trial of pramipexole at doses of up to 0.125 mg before bedtime was stopped due to lack of efficacy and the dose-limiting side effect of nausea.

A repeat polysomnogram was then performed using esophageal pressure (Pes) monitoring to screen for subtle forms of airway obstruction that are not always demonstrable with standard polysomnography. This study demonstrated findings consistent with increased upper airway resistance. Esophageal pressure fluctuations with respiration were tonically abnormal at −12 to −15 cm of water (normal 0 to −10 cm of water) (Figure 48.1). Cortical arousals from sleep also were common, despite a normal AHI of 0.8 and normal SpO_2 levels. Furthermore, gradual increases in Pes readings, suggestive of increased work of breathing, were not commonly leading to arousals, defined as respiratory effort-related arousals and now commonly added to the respiratory disturbance index. Evidence of more broadly disrupted sleep architecture did

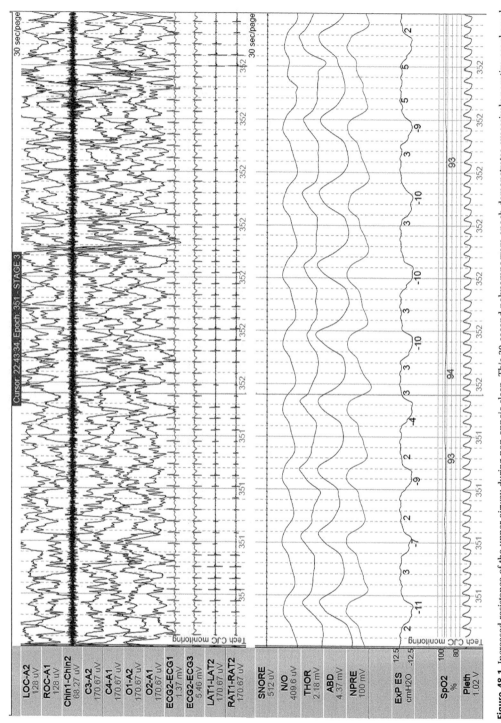

Figure 48.1 Increased resistance of the upper airway during non-apneic sleep. This 30-second polysomnogram epoch demonstrates excessively negative esophageal pressure fluctuations with inspiration (measured peak-to-trough on the ExPes channel), indicative of increased work of breathing. Mildly low baseline SpO2 levels are also evident. Abbreviations used in figure: LOC-A2, ROC-A1, left and right electrooculograms; Chin1-Chin2, chin surface electromyogram; C3-A2, C4-A1, O1-A2, O2-A1, central and occipital electroencephalograms; ECG2-ECG1, ECG2-ECG3, electrocardiograms; LAT1-LAT2, RAT1-RAT2, left and right anterior tibialis surface electromyograms; SNORE, snoring microphone; N/O, nasal–oral airflow by thermocouple; THOR, ABD, thoracic and abdominal excursion as indicated by piezoelectric belts; NPRE, nasal pressure; ExPES, esophageal pressure; SpO2, oxygen saturation by finger oximetry; Pleth, plethysmography signal from oximeter.

remain evident however, with reduced sleep efficiency of 76.2%, increased stage 1 sleep (16.0%), and markedly reduced stage REM sleep (3.3%). No periodic limb movements of sleep were recorded.

A CPAP trial performed using Pes monitoring tested pressure settings of 4, 5, 6, 7, and 8 cm of water. A CPAP setting of 5 cm of water provided optimal control of respiratory disturbances during sleep and was associated with normalization of respiration-associated esophageal pressure fluctuations (Figure 48.2). Use of home CPAP was initially complicated by skin irritation and breakdown which resolved after replacing the nasal mask interface with nasal pillows. After 8 months of regular CPAP use (and ongoing iron supplementation), the family reported that night waking, nighttime sleep quality, and daytime alertness had all improved.

Discussion

This case demonstrates that clinically significant airway obstruction during sleep may be present in children even when respiratory findings on standard polysomnography are normal by both adult and pediatric standards. Increased upper airway resistance, in the form of chronic rather than intermittent airway obstruction, disturbs sleep quality but may give rise to few scorable respiratory events on standard polysomnography. Esophageal pressure monitoring in such cases provides valuable quantitative data on upper airway resistance and work of breathing.

Upper airway resistance syndrome (UARS) was a term formerly used to describe a condition in which gradually increasing negative Pes swings – largely in the absence of more obvious apneas or hypopneas – do lead to arousals. Upper airway resistance syndrome in children is associated with symptoms similar to those observed in classic childhood OSA[3] and treatment strategies are comparable as well. This terminology (UARS) was largely supplanted when the second edition of the International Classification of Sleep Disorders (ICSD-2) was published in 2005 and the American Academy of Sleep Medicine Scoring Manual

appeared in 2007; these references expanded the nosology of airway obstruction and OSA to include respiratory effort-related arousals, identified by nasal pressure flow monitoring or esophageal manometry, when deriving the respiratory disturbance index. The respiratory disturbance index, with a sensitive threshold as low as one event per hour of sleep, can now be used to assist in the identification of symptomatic children with pediatric OSA.

Although this child's clinical presentation initially seemed consistent with periodic limb movement disorder, the lack of response to treatment trials of ferrous sulfate and pramipexole led to appropriate consideration of alternative conditions that could also cause nocturnal restlessness and poor sleep quality. The presence of fragmented sleep architecture on the initial polysomnogram represented an important clue that extrinsic disruption of sleep was present in spite of seemingly normal respiratory parameters on standard monitoring using thermocouple and nasal pressure flow sensors.

It is important to note that obstructive sleep-disordered breathing was ultimately identified in this patient in the absence of obvious snoring or typical risk factors such as adenotonsillar hypertrophy or obesity. The symptoms of sleep-disordered breathing in children may be subtle or non-specific and sometimes evolve insidiously over time. Although adenotonsillar hypertrophy is frequently present in children with symptomatic airway obstruction, its presence is neither necessary nor sufficient for diagnosis. Predisposition to upper airway obstruction during sleep may also be associated with other factors such as craniofacial anatomy or underlying genetic or medical disorders.

This case also illustrates the utility of Pes monitoring to augment the sensitivity of standard polysomnography for the detection of subtle partial airway obstruction during sleep. It is thought that children are more likely than adults to experience chronic airway obstruction during sleep as opposed to the intermittent hypopneas or obstructive apneas seen in classic obstructive sleep apnea. The use of Pes in this case facilitated detection of upper airway obstruction that was not demonstrable on standard

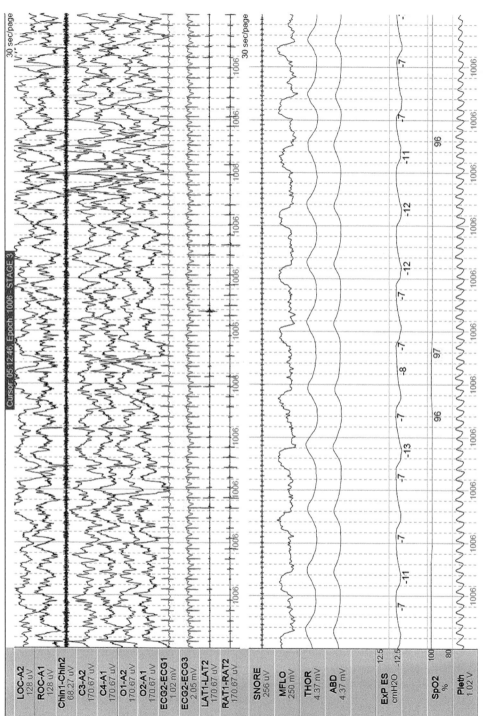

Figure 48.2 Normalization of increased upper airway resistance with continuous positive airway pressure (CPAP). This 30-second polysomnogram epoch demonstrates improved, normal esophageal pressure fluctuations with inspiration (measured peak-to-trough on the Exp ES channel during treatment with CPAP). Baseline SpO2 levels have also normalized. Abbreviations used in figure: LOC-A2, ROC-A1, left and right electrooculograms; Chin1-Chin2, chin surface electromyogram; C3-A2, C4-A1, O1-A2, O2-A1, central and occipital electroencephalograms; ECG2-ECG1, ECG2-ECG3, electrocardiograms; LAT1-LAT2, RAT1-RAT2, left and right anterior tibialis surface electromyograms; SNORE, snoring microphone; THOR, ABD, thoracic and abdominal excursion as indicated by piezoelectric belts; ExPES, esophageal pressure; SpO2, oxygen saturation by finger oximetry; Pleth, plethysmography signal from oximeter.

polysomnogram and confirmed that treatment with CPAP was effective in eliminating that obstruction.

Technically, Pes monitoring is performed using a thin, flexible, water or air-filled tube attached to a pressure transducer. The technique assesses respiratory effort via measurement of negative intrathoracic pressure fluctuations during inspiration, with excessively negative fluctuations being indicative of increased upper airway resistance and work of breathing. Although the minimally invasive nature of Pes has limited widespread adoption, the technique has negligible impact on sleep quality and substantially improves the sensitivity of polysomnogram for the detection of chronic partial airway obstruction.[4]

Alternative methods used in the assessment of chronic partial upper airway obstruction in children include end-tidal or transcutaneous carbon dioxide monitoring. These methods assess for hypoventilation, and provide quantitative data. However, neither technique is as accurate as blood gas monitoring, which is rarely feasible during an outpatient sleep study. Furthermore, published data on head-to-head comparison of carbon dioxide monitoring to Pes monitoring has suggested that the latter technique is more sensitive to upper airway resistance.

Main points

- Clinically significant airway obstruction is sometimes present in children whose standard polysomnogram is normal by adult or even pediatric standards.

- Esophageal pressure monitoring augments the sensitivity of polysomnography for detection of otherwise subtle airway obstruction during sleep.
- Upper airway resistance syndrome can affect children in the absence of snoring or traditional risk factors such as tonsillar hypertrophy or obesity.

FURTHER READING

Upper airway resistance syndrome

Guilleminault C, Khramtsov A. Upper airway resistance syndrome in children: a clinical review. *Semin Pediatr Neurol* 2001;**8**:207–15.

References

1. Hoban TF, Chervin RD. Assessment of sleepiness in children. *Semin Pediatr Neurol* 2001;**8**:216–28.
2. American Academy of Sleep Medicine. Periodic limb movement disorders. In *International Classification of Sleep Disorders. Diagnostic and Coding Manual*, Second Edition. Westchester, IL: American Academy of Sleep Medicine 2005, pp. 182–6.
3. Guilleminault C, Pelayo R, Leger D, et al. Recognition of sleep-disordered breathing in children. *Pediatrics* 1996;**98**:871–82.
4. Chervin RD, Aldrich MS. Effects of esophageal pressure monitoring on sleep architecture [see comment]. *Am J Respr Crit Care Med* 1997;**156**:881–5.

49

Low socioeconomic conditions can create substantial challenges to adequate sleep for young children

Katherine Wilson

Case

A 3-year-old girl presented to the pediatric sleep clinic with persistent difficulty initiating sleep and maintaining sleep for the past year, and particularly over the past 6 months. She had previously been diagnosed with moderate obstructive sleep apnea on overnight polysomnography and underwent an adenotonsillectomy for treatment. On follow-up polysomnography after surgery, her obstructive sleep apnea had resolved. However, since treatment of her obstructive sleep apnea, her mom has not noted any improvements in her ability to fall asleep or maintain sleep. Her mother reports no symptoms of residual obstructive sleep apnea.

The child's bedtime routine usually starts around 7:30 PM and consists of a light snack followed by brushing her teeth. Bedtime is at 8:00 PM with the child taking up to 4 hours to fall asleep at night. She typically falls asleep on the couch while watching television and will sleep there the rest of the night. She has her own bedroom but rarely sleeps in it. Her mother is typically present and sitting on the couch when the child falls asleep. The child has nightly nocturnal arousals, which require a brief intervention from mom about 6–8 times each night in order for her to fall back asleep. The child awakens about 7:00 AM, after an estimated 8 hours of sleep each night. Her mother estimates that the child takes a 2-hour nap at daycare a few days per week.

What additional questions about the sleeping environment might be helpful?

When further asked about the child's sleeping environment, mom reports that the bedroom is located in the basement and during the winter months it is too cold for her to sleep there. Therefore, during the winter she sleeps on the couch in the living room. Mom also reports that they live near the railroad tracks and that the train may also affect the child's sleep at night. The child's bedroom is dark; however, when she sleeps on the couch there is light from the television. Mom reports that they plan to move to a new apartment in the next few months so that the child will have a warm bedroom. Mom hopes that the move will also eliminate the environmental noise from the train.

At a 6-month follow-up visit, the family has moved to their new apartment and the child has a new bedroom that is kept at a comfortable temperature. The bedroom is also dark and quiet. Her mother has prioritized having her child sleep in her new bedroom and reports significant improvements in the child's sleep. Mom feels that bedtime is less stressful and that the child falls asleep much more easily. She takes about 30 minutes to fall asleep currently compared to several hours previously. She is falling asleep in her own room on most nights of the week; occasionally she will still fall asleep on the couch. However, she is no longer watching television when she falls asleep and she is able to fall asleep without her mom present.

Mom also notes that she is able to sleep through the night on most nights of the week. Occasionally, she will have 1–2 nocturnal awakenings but is able to fall back asleep more easily with less intervention required from mom. Her mother now estimates 9.5–10 hours of sleep each night. The child continues to take a nap a few days per week at daycare. Mom continues to report no residual symptoms of obstructive sleep apnea.

Discussion

Poor sleep has been associated with daytime consequences such as behavior problems and poor school performance in children, which tend to improve with restoration of sleep.[1,2] Children living in low-income households are particularly vulnerable to a variety of sleep problems, including increased bedtime resistance, insufficient sleep duration,[3] and obstructive sleep apnea[4] as illustrated by this case. Low-income children are also more likely to have poor sleep hygiene practices such as not having a regular bedtime routine[5] or watching television while falling asleep.[6] These poor sleep hygiene practices can prevent adequate sleep.[7] For example, children without a regular bedtime routine tend to sleep less each night. Similarly, evening television use by children is associated with more sleep problems. This is especially true for low-income children who are more likely to have a television in the bedroom, which is associated with shorter sleep duration[8] and more sleep disturbances.[6] Little information is available about possible associations between sleep environments and sleep problems or sleep duration. However, anecdotally, there are concerns that sleep environment, including room temperature, noise level, and bright lights, can impair children's ability to obtain adequate sleep. This may be especially relevant for some low-income families.

As presented in this case, the child had a number of environmental factors that were affecting her sleep, including sleeping on the couch due to a cold bedroom, use of television, and environmental noise from a nearby train. As a result this child was not getting adequate sleep. Mom initially estimated that she obtained about 8 hours of sleep per night

Table 49.1 National Sleep Foundation recommendations for sleep in children[9]

Age	Hours sleep
Toddlers	12–14
Preschoolers	11–13
School-aged	10–11
Teenagers	8.5–9.25

plus a 2-hour daytime nap several days per week. For preschool-age children the National Sleep Foundation recommends 11–13 hours of sleep (Table 49.1).[9] However, like this child, many children do not get the targeted amount of sleep each night. The growing sleep debt can start early in childhood and is estimated to be even worse for older children, with high school students obtaining on average 2 hours less than the recommended amount of sleep. Fortunately, at follow-up, this child's sleep duration had improved to 9.5–10 hours of sleep per night, which illustrates the importance of addressing environmental factors with families.

This case history also illustrates behavioral insomnia of childhood, which is common in the preschool age group and affects an estimated 10–30% of young children.[7] There are two types of behavioral insomnia of childhood: sleep-onset association type and limit-setting type. Sleep-onset type is defined as the need for certain conditions to be present in order for the child to fall asleep initially and, in particular later on, following nocturnal awakenings. Examples of conditions include parental presence, rocking or other movements, or use of television. Limit-setting type is defined as poor limit-setting by parents with regard to bedtime and typically manifests as the child delaying or refusing to go to bed. This child had sleep-onset association type because she required her mom's presence to fall asleep initially and then later in the night to fall back asleep after an arousal. Treatment for behavioral insomnia of childhood generally starts with a recommendation of good sleep hygiene habits, along with a regular bedtime and bedtime routine. Different approaches, including extinction and graduated extinction, are discussed with families to transition the child to be able to fall asleep independently. Specifically for this case, we discussed good sleep hygiene, such as elimination of television at bedtime, nightly practice of the child falling sleep in her own bedroom, and use of a regular bedtime and bedtime routine. In addition, mom was encouraged to use graduated extinction to slowly limit her presence at bedtime so that the child became accustomed to falling asleep on her own. These recommendations became easier once they moved to their new apartment and the child had a bedroom that promoted better sleep. For many children, the practice of falling asleep independently at sleep onset reduces the need for parental presence with nocturnal awakenings. This child's nocturnal awakenings – or at least those that her mom was aware of – also improved with her improved ability to fall asleep independently. For this family, moving to a new apartment was a crucial factor in improving the child's sleep.

This case also illustrates the overlap of two or more sleep disorders in many children, as this child also had a diagnosis of obstructive sleep apnea. As seen in this case, the first-line treatment for obstructive sleep apnea in children is usually adenotonsillectomy. In contrast, continuous positive airway pressure (CPAP) is the first-line treatment for most adults. While this child's obstructive sleep apnea resolved with surgery, for many children this may not be the case. Adenotonsillectomy was previously thought to be curative in the majority of children, with reported cure rates of about 80%. However, more recently, adenotonsillectomy is reported to be curative in about 50% of children. The decrease in efficacy may reflect increased numbers of obese children, who in comparison to their peers may be less likely to achieve complete resolution of obstructive sleep apnea after adenotonsillectomy. In addition, refined monitoring and scoring of pediatric apneic events, and increased sensitivity of the modern definition for pediatric obstructive sleep apnea may have had impact on reported surgical cure rates.

Despite these changes, adenotonsillectomy can still offer benefit by a reduction in the severity of sleep apnea for many children. Adenotonsillectomy is therefore still recommended, for appropriate candidates, as a first-line treatment in children. The American Academy of Sleep Medicine (AASM) guidelines[10] recommend a polysomnogram for diagnosis of obstructive sleep apnea prior to surgical treatment in children suspected of sleep-disordered breathing. For children with mild obstructive sleep apnea, the AASM recommends a postoperative clinical evaluation for residual symptoms of obstructive sleep apnea, and a follow-up polysomnogram when symptoms persist. For children with moderate to severe obstructive sleep apnea preoperatively, obese children, or children with predisposing medical conditions (e.g. cranio-facial anomalies, Down syndrome, or Prader–Willi syndrome) the AASM recommends repeating the polysomnogram postoperatively. These recommendations highlight the concern for residual obstructive sleep apnea following surgery in some pediatric patients. For children with residual obstructive sleep apnea on a polysomnogram following adenotonsillectomy, CPAP is generally recommended for treatment. However, some patients may benefit from additional surgical evaluation.

Diagnoses

1. Inadequate sleep hygiene, including: (a) falling asleep with the television on; (b) environmental factors such as a cold bedroom necessitating use of the couch to sleep in the winter; and (c) increased noise level of the nearby train, which may have contributed to the child's inability to fall asleep and maintain sleep. The poor sleep hygiene practices and environmental factors largely improved with moving to a new apartment.

2. Insufficient sleep duration of 8 hours each night plus 2-hour naps several days per week, as compared to 11–13 hours recommended for this age group. The child's short sleep duration was likely secondary to inadequate sleep hygiene and environmental factors that affected her ability to get adequate sleep. Her sleep duration had increased at the follow-up visit to 9.5–10.0 hours at night, due in part to improvements in her sleep hygiene and sleep environment.

3. Behavioral insomnia of childhood (sleep-onset association type), with mom's presence required to fall asleep at bedtime and then again during

nocturnal arousals. The insomnia improved with behavioral intervention and good sleep hygiene practices.

4. History of obstructive sleep apnea that has been treated with adenotonsillectomy.

Main points

- Sleep hygiene and environmental challenges that may be particularly common among low-income families can affect a child's ability to obtain sufficient or adequate quality sleep. Clinicians should ask about the household dynamics and sleeping environments as they can be significant but addressable contributors to sleep problems in many children.

- Insufficient sleep duration is common among children of all ages and clinicians should be aware of age-based sleep recommendations.

- Behavioral insomnia of childhood is seen in about 10–30% of young children and can be addressed with a number of behavioral techniques. Initial treatment usually focuses on good sleep hygiene, a regular bedtime, and a regular bedtime routine as an initial starting point. If the child has residual difficulty with behavioral insomnia of childhood, referral to a sleep specialist may be helpful to address more specific needs.

- Clinicians should evaluate children for residual obstructive sleep apnea following treatment with adenotonsillectomy.

REFERENCES

1. Sadeh A, Gruber R, Raviv A. Sleep, neurobehavioral functioning, and behavior problems in school-age children. *Child Dev* 2002;**73**:405–17.

2. Chervin R, Ruzicka DL, Giordani BJ, et al. Sleep-disordered breathing, behavior, and cognition in children before and after adenotonsillectomy. *Pediatrics* 2006;**117**:e769–78.

3. Crabtree VM. Cultural influences on the bedtime behaviors of young children. *Sleep Med* 2005;**6**:319–24.

4. Spilsbury J. Neighborhood disadvantage as a risk factor for pediatric obstructive sleep apnea. *J Pediatr* 2006;**149**:342–7.

5. Hale L, Berger LM, LeBourgeois MK, Brooks-Gunn J. Social and demographic predictors of preschooler's beditme routines. *J Dev Behav Pediatr* 2009;**30**:394–402.

6. Owens J, Maxim R, McGuinn M, et al. Television-viewing habits and sleep disturbance in school children. *Pediatrics* 1999;**104**:e27.

7. Mindell J, Owens, JA. *A Clinical Guide to Pediatric Sleep: Diagnosis and Management of Sleep Problems*. Philadelphia, PA: Lippincott Williams and Wilkins;2003.

8. Mindell J. Developmental aspects of sleep hygiene: findings from the 2004 National Sleep Foundation Sleep in America poll. *Sleep Med* 2009;**10**:771–9.

9. National Sleep Foundation. *Children and Sleep* http://www.sleepfoundation.org/article/sleep-topics/children-and-sleep. Accessed May 5, 2012.

10. Aurora RN, Zak RS, Karippot A, et al. Practice parameters for the respiratory indications for polysomnograph in children. *Sleep* 2011;**34**:379–88.

50

Inadequate sleep hygiene is a common cause of sleepiness in adolescents

Dawn Dore-Stites

A 15-year-old high school freshman describes falling asleep in class over the past 9 months. She initially presented to her pediatrician, who ran thyroid tests and iron studies, which were within normal limits. She denied symptoms of sleep-disordered breathing including snoring, morning headaches, and restlessness. She described difficulties initiating and maintaining sleep.

What is her current sleep schedule?

She typically went to her bedroom at 10:00 PM; however, sleep was often not initiated until approximately 12:30 AM. She described often waking around 3:30 AM and was unable to identify a trigger. She estimated remaining awake for approximately an hour. As she was trying to return to sleep during an awakening, she would play games on her cell phone. She described being "bored" during these periods of wakefulness and wanting to pass time while waiting to fall back asleep. On school days, she needed to wake by 6:00 AM and was very difficult to rouse. This often led to her being late to her first hour of classes.

On weekends, she would typically retire to her bedroom at 11:00 PM and would initiate sleep within 10–15 minutes. If allowed to wake independently, she would often sleep until 10:00 AM. She sustained wakefulness throughout weekend days; however, on school days, she would often nap after school until her parents returned home from work at 6:00 PM (approximately 3 hours).

What was her daytime routine, and was she engaging in sleep inhibiting behaviors?

She noted that her most difficult portion of the day included her morning classes. She would typically consume caffeinated beverages (coffee or soda) throughout the morning to attempt to stay awake. She did not have any caffeinated beverages at lunch, but she would often drink caffeinated sodas at dinner after her nap.

In middle school, she was involved in several sports, but her participation was halted when she sustained an injury to her knee. As a result her physical activity decreased from at least an hour per day to its current level of minimal activity. Many of her friends continued to participate in sports and were not available after school for social activities.

What was her bedtime routine, and what purposes do the routines serve?

Prior to going to her room on school nights, she would generally brush her teeth and wash her face. She would then typically do homework for an hour while lying in bed. After homework was completed, she would text friends or go on social media sites until she felt drowsy. She stated that she preferred to text friends at this time of night since her parents were asleep and she felt as if she could be undisturbed. Late

Common Pitfalls in Sleep Medicine, ed. Ronald D. Chervin. Published by Cambridge University Press. © Cambridge University Press 2014.

evenings were also the only time her friends were available to talk due to their sports schedules. On weekends, her curfew was 11:00 PM and she was with friends right up until she returned home. Upon returning home, she would generally go to her room and initiate sleep quickly.

Discussion

Adolescents are at risk for several sleep problems including insomnia secondary to anxiety and delayed sleep phase. In addition, they are more prone to engage in activities prior to bed that may delay sleep, all while having more limited parental monitoring. These variables can lead to cases that appear similar on the surface, but require further clinical assessment in order to generate an appropriate differential diagnosis.

Delayed sleep phase, or a tendency to be a "night owl" is common in adolescence due to biologic changes at this time of development.[1] Often, teenagers will engage in compensatory behaviors to manage their difficulties with sleep initiation. Many of these behaviors are consistent with poor sleep hygiene. However, managing the sleep hygiene concerns alone rarely alleviates the delayed sleep phase. This patient's ability to fall asleep quickly on weekends despite a relatively similar bedtime on weekdays provides evidence against delayed sleep phase.

It is also not uncommon for adolescents to struggle with various forms of insomnia. While improved sleep hygiene is a part of most empirically supported insomnia treatments, little evidence exists to support its use as a singular treatment.[2] In this case, the patient's description of boredom during nocturnal arousals does not support a diagnosis of psychophysiological insomnia.

For this patient, the most appropriate diagnosis is one of inadequate sleep hygiene, as evidenced by the description of erratic sleep patterns and several sleep inhibiting behaviors prior to bedtime. Research demonstrates that individuals without underlying medically based sleep disorders can struggle with sleepiness as a result of adopting unhealthy sleep behaviors.[2]

Inadequate sleep hygiene is one of the most common sleep problems of childhood and adolescence.[3] Sleep hygiene refers to a collection of behaviors all of which promote good sleep patterns. Several rules of sleep hygiene are widely circulated, but comparatively few empirical data exist to indicate which rules are most critical, and the lists vary from text to text.[2,4] Debate continues on which behaviors to include, but in general, most lists incorporate the following recommendations: routine sleep–wake times, avoidance of caffeine and nicotine, calming bedtime routines, avoidance of electronics at bedtime and during the targeted sleep period, regulation of light exposure, and exercise during the day (Table 50.1).

Management of sleep hygiene problems

Careful clinical assessment is critical to management of sleep hygiene-related problems for a variety of reasons. First, there is some individual variability with sleep hygiene practices and it is important to understand what purpose the behavior has for the patient rather than exclusively focus upon the superficial description of the behavior. For one person, having a television on in a room may be sleep promoting as it blocks out ambient noise. For others, a television is too stimulating and promotes wakefulness. Careful assessment of how an individual patient responds to the behavior is an important component of sound information gathering.

Secondly, it is essential to fully assess the patient's motivation for making changes to her sleep. Specifically, the changes needed (removal of naps; absence of electronics at bedtime; cessation of caffeine use at dinner) may present as significant and distressing disruptions to the patient and her family. In addition, if the parents are unwilling or unable to establish and maintain consistent limits on the changes, the resulting behavior could be worse than what initially presented.

Eliciting an understanding from the adolescent about the positive changes that may result from improved sleep hygiene may improve adherence to treatment recommendations. As an example, asking the adolescent what they would gain from being able to remain awake after school may reveal factors that can be used to sustain motivation across this and later

Table 50.1 Common sleep hygiene goals for adolescents, and suggested approaches that can help to identify suboptimal sleep habits and reasons for them

Sleep hygiene goal	Useful questions	Further comments
Adopt regular sleep schedule	Does the patient take naps to escape conflict at home or to engage in unmonitored activities at night?	Asking the patient what he or she enjoys about being up at night may provide clues about secondary gain for poor sleep schedules
	Does the parent(s) go to bed before the adolescent?	Asking the patient about their day-to-day schedule (rather than just weekdays and weekends) may reveal significant variability
	Do sports or homework schedules preclude routine bedtimes?	
Avoid caffeine and nicotine	Does the patient know what beverages include caffeine?	Ask about specific beverages he or she consumes after dinner
	Does the patient smoke cigarettes or chew tobacco?	After asking the parent to leave the room, asking the adolescent about the last time he or she smoked a cigarette may lead to discussion of nicotine use
Avoid electronics prior to bedtime	What electronic devices does the patient have in his or her room (television, laptop, etc.)?	Asking parents about established limits on Internet access (e.g. turning off router for wireless) may spark discussion about methods to limit use
	Does the patient have access to the Internet?	
	Does the patient receive texts throughout the night?	Determining why the patient feels he or she needs to receive texts throughout the night may identify possible barriers to removal of the phone from the room
	Does the patient require electronic devices to complete homework?	
Limit bright light exposure	Does the adolescent have a night-light due to fears of the dark?	Determine whether the night-light is a habit or related to fears at night
	Does the patient do homework or read in his or her room prior to bed?	Discuss possible strategies to limit bright light exposure such as smaller lamps or lower wattage bulbs

changes. In addition, focus upon one change at a time may prevent the patient from feeling overwhelmed with the need to change several factors all at once.

For the above patient, the primary target behaviors include reduction of napping after school, reduction or change in timing of caffeine use, decreased use of electronics at bedtime, and increased physical activity at appropriate times of the day. With the varied array of target behaviors, identifying an initial step for the patient often presents the first challenge in treatment. Selection of a behavior can be influenced by what the patient and the family identify as a manageable initial goal, as well as what the clinician views as the most efficacious. For this patient, regulating the sleep–wake cycle by removal of naps may yield carryover effects in other areas – namely reduced nocturnal arousals due to increased sleep

consolidation and shorter latency to sleep onset. Therefore, if possible within the family system, limiting naps would be an appropriate first-line treatment target.

Using the principles above, querying the patient about what behaviors she could engage in after school that would elicit wakefulness and what benefits she could derive from the activities would be a reasonable first step. In addition, asking the parents to monitor and establish limits on napping in order to help the patient maintain a more appropriate schedule is crucial to success.

After regulation of the sleep schedule, the likely next treatment targets would include eliminating electronics at bedtime. For this patient, use of electronics appears to be stimulatory, yielding increased latency to sleep onset and extending the duration of nocturnal arousals. Again, the parents' ability to establish clear limits and maintain consistency in regulation of rules around electronics would be imperative to the success of the intervention, as an adolescent is unlikely to self-regulate.

Targeting daytime behaviors that perpetuate poor sleep hygiene would be the final step in treatment. For some patients, further education on how caffeine use and exercise affect sleep patterns would be necessary so that the patients can understand why these would be incorporated into treatment. Healthy sleep habits do not just include nighttime behaviors, and adoption of healthy practices throughout the day can be helpful to a lifetime of good sleep.

Main points

Inadequate sleep hygiene is a common contributor to daytime sleepiness in children and adolescents.

Careful assessment is critical to the differential diagnosis and allows identification of variables amenable to intervention.

REFERENCES

1. Crowley S, Acebo C, Carskadon MA. Sleep, circadian rhythms and delayed sleep phase in adolescence. *Sleep Med* 2007;**8**:602–12.
2. Stepanski E, Wyatt J. Use of sleep hygiene in the treatment of insomnia. *Sleep Med Rev* 2003;**7**:215–25.
3. Moore M. Behavioral sleep problems in children and adolescents. *J Clin Psychol Med Settings* 2012;**19**:77–83.
4. Posner D, Gehrman, P. Sleep hygiene. In Perlis M, Aloia M, Kuhn B, eds. *Behavioral Treatments for Sleep Disorders: A Comprehensive Primer of Behavioral Sleep Medicine Interventions*. New York, NY: Academic Press;2011, pp. 119–26.

51

Sleep and attention-deficit/hyperactivity disorder in children

Barbara T. Felt and Lauren O'Connell

Case

A 6-year-old boy, Joey, presented for an attention-deficit/hyperactivity disorder (ADHD) evaluation. The parents reported that concerns about Joey's overactivity started in preschool and persisted through kindergarten. The first grade teacher expressed more concern, and stated Joey was off-task, failed to complete assignments, interrupted others, and was often out of his seat. A classroom observation by school staff demonstrated that Joey was off-task 40% of the time compared to his peers at 10%. The parents described having similar concerns at home over the last 2–3 years. Behavioral rating scales from parents and the teacher demonstrated significant levels of concern in domains consistent with ADHD combined-type. Recently, the teacher expressed concern that Joey's behaviors could affect his learning and his parents have noticed problems for Joey getting along with his peers.

What further information is needed?

In the evaluation of ADHD, it is essential to obtain a thorough review of other behavioral and medical symptoms, as well as past medical, social, and family history. A sleep history should document sleep duration and continuity, and any symptoms related to breathing, movements, and daytime functioning of the patient.

The parents denied any changes in Joey's health, mood, or home circumstances. Family history revealed

ADHD and obstructive sleep apnea (OSA) for the father and restless legs syndrome (RLS) for the mother. Parents reported Joey's bedtime was 8:00 PM but sleep onset was often an hour later. He reported uncomfortable sensations in his legs at bedtime that made it hard to get to sleep. Joey didn't describe any waking after sleep onset but parents noted he had loud snoring and was restless and sweaty most nights. Joey always seemed tired when they woke him at 7:30 AM and he was often irritable in the later afternoon. Sometimes he napped on the way to soccer practice after school.

A polysomnogram demonstrated OSA, with an apnea/hypopnea index of 5.4 apneic events per hour of sleep, sleep efficiency 75%, no significant hypoxia, and 8 periodic limb movements of sleep (PLMS) per hour. He was referred to otolaryngology and adenotonsillectomy (AT) was recommended. Several months after surgery, the parent reported that Joey's snoring and sleep quality were improved. However, he still had problems getting to sleep and being tired during the day. His teacher noted behavioral improvements but his attention in class remained poor.

Laboratory studies of iron status were obtained and showed: serum ferritin 10 µg/l (ref. range 18–320 µg/l); percent transferrin saturation 12.0 (ref. range 20–50%); serum iron 90 µg/dl (ref. range 33–150 µg/dl), and hemoglobin 12.8 g/dl (ref. range 11.5–16.0 g/dl). These results were judged consistent with iron deficiency. No anemia was found. An iron supplement was recommended. After 3 months, all iron measures were within the normal range, and in particular, serum ferritin was

52 µg/l. Joey's leg discomfort at bedtime, daytime functioning, and attention had now improved. Behavioral ratings by parents and Joey's teacher no longer supported a diagnosis of ADHD.

Discussion

Attention-deficit/hyperactivity disorder is a common neuropsychiatric disorder that usually presents in childhood. Inattentiveness, impaired executive functioning, motoric hyperactivity, and impulsive actions result in patterns of functionally significant symptoms that are currently classified within three ADHD subtypes. Children with predominantly inattentive ADHD have difficulty staying on task, forgetfulness, and poor organization. Meanwhile, impulsivity, fidgeting, and overactivity are typical of the predominantly hyperactive-impulsive subtype of ADHD. Children with combined-type ADHD have symptoms from both subtypes. These symptoms significantly interfere with a child's ability to learn, to participate in home and school activities, and to maintain developmentally appropriate, positive relationships. Attention-deficit/ hyperactivity disorder affects 5–10% of school-aged children and adolescents.[1]

Sleep problems also occur commonly in childhood, affecting 11–40% of school-age children. In children with ADHD, the prevalence is even higher, at 25–50%. A relationship between ADHD and sleep problems has been acknowledged for decades, and evidence strongly supports associations between disorders of sleep and ADHD. However, it remains challenging to tease apart this multifaceted interface.[2,3] On the one hand, insufficient or poor-quality sleep can lead to daytime sleepiness, poor behavioral regulation, and decreased executive function, and these symptoms could mimic or exacerbate ADHD. At the same time, ADHD symptoms can manifest as poor sleep hygiene and bedtime resistance, leading to shortened sleep duration and insufficient, inefficient sleep. In addition, sleep problems may simply co-occur with ADHD in the same patient, without a causal relationship. Last, it is also possible that ADHD and certain sleep disorders share a common antecedent. Common anatomic pathways,

neurotransmitter secretion patterns, and environmental factors are all potential contributors to a neurobiologic overlap between sleep disorders and ADHD.

The case illustrates two specific medical conditions that can affect sleep quality or duration and have overlap with ADHD: sleep-disordered breathing (SDB) and RLS. Sleep-disordered breathing describes a range of conditions from primary snoring (without gas exchange abnormalities) to OSA (marked by recurrent episodes of reduced to no air flow). Restless legs syndrome symptoms include the urge to move one's legs, associated with uncomfortable sensations when sitting or lying, that usually occur in the evening and are relieved by movement. To meet the full criteria, children should describe the feeling of discomfort or urge to move, or have two of three other factors: sleep disturbance, a positive family history, or periodic limb movement disorder.[4]

Sleep-disordered breathing and attention-deficit/hyperactivity disorder

A relationship between SDB and ADHD symptoms is strongly supported by the literature. For example, parents of children with ADHD, in comparison to parents of children without ADHD, are more likely to report that their children have habitual snoring. In addition, children with parental reports of high SDB symptom scores also have more inattention and hyperactivity symptoms.[5] A similar association between SDB and ADHD symptoms is demonstrated in general pediatric clinic settings.[6] In addition, about a third of children scheduled to have AT for SDB symptoms are found to meet the diagnostic criteria for ADHD.[7]

Nonetheless, several aspects of the relationship between SDB and ADHD require further investigation.[8] First, no clear "dose–response" relationship exists between the two disorders. Obstructive sleep apnea may be more common in children with mild ADHD symptoms than in those with more severe ADHD symptoms. Conversely, children with ADHD may be most likely to have subtle SDB, rather than severe OSA.[9] In addition, the effects of SDB on ADHD symptoms are not necessarily concurrent; children who are habitual snorers are more likely than their peers to develop symptoms of ADHD 4 years later.[10] The effects of SDB also appear to extend beyond ADHD symptoms. Bullying and mood problems are reported frequently among children with SDB.[11] Sleep-disordered breathing also appears to affect cognitive domains, including reaction time, task vigilance, visual spatial functioning, and other aspects of neurobehavioral functioning.[12,13]

The pathways that mediate relationships between SDB and ADHD are not well-established but several hypotheses have emerged. Fragmented sleep related to SDB contributes to sleep disruption that in turn may affect daytime attention. Fragmented sleep may also manifest as excessive sleepiness in children with SDB. An independent effect of shorter sleep duration is also hypothesized. Another proposed link is that chronic hypoxemia affects the development of brain structures related to attention and executive functioning, and promotes expression of proinflammatory markers. Genetic predisposition and the environment could also play roles. In addition, the duration and timing of SDB relative to a child's development may affect ADHD symptoms.[12,14]

Taken together, the overall consensus is that parents who report more SDB symptoms for their children also report that their children have more ADHD symptoms. Fortunately, it appears that AT surgery improves both the SDB and ADHD symptoms for many patients. Among children who meet ADHD criteria prior to AT, studies demonstrate that half or more do not meet ADHD criteria 6–12 months after surgery.[7,15] Further, studies suggest that AT for children with mild OSA may improve ADHD symptoms more than psychostimulant treatment.[16] However, as not all children will see resolution of ADHD symptoms, and risk remains for residual SDB, clinicians should remain vigilant for both SDB and ADHD symptoms after surgery and over time.

Restless legs syndrome and attention-deficit/hyperactivity disorder

Childhood RLS is associated with ADHD symptoms. About 12–35% of school age children with ADHD meet criteria for RLS.[4,17] Among children with RLS symptoms, in comparison to children without RLS symptoms, a greater percentage have hyperactive behavior (18% vs. 11%).[6] Other studies demonstrate symptoms of inattention in one-fourth of children with RLS,[18] and higher conduct problems associated with symptoms of RLS and PLMS.[19] Among children with five or more PLMS per hour of sleep, 44% have co-occurring ADHD.[9]

A number of hypotheses are proposed to explain the association between RLS and ADHD. Children with RLS may appear to be more hyperactive because they can't sit still due to leg discomfort. The overactivity or discomfort may in turn lead to inattention during the day. Others hypothesize that sleep disruption or shortened sleep duration as a result of RLS or PLMS creates poorer daytime functioning, poorer emotion regulation, inattention, and overactivity. Some have proposed that sleepy children paradoxically appear hyperactive in an attempt to maintain alertness. Abnormalities in central dopaminergic systems are also proposed as a common link between these conditions and ADHD, and iron deficiency may be a common underlying factor. Iron is a cofactor in the synthesis of catecholamines, which include dopamine, a neurotransmitter thought to play an important role in both RLS and ADHD. In addition, a common genetic link among these conditions has been proposed.[4,20]

A limited period of iron supplementation, with follow-up for an appropriate response, is commonly recommended for RLS that is associated with iron deficiency. Similar to findings in adults, children with RLS in comparison to their peers more often have serum ferritin $< 50 \ \mu g/l$.[18] Iron supplementation alleviates symptoms in some children.[17] In addition, one double-blinded study suggests improvement of ADHD symptoms with iron supplementation.[21]

Tips

Screen for SDB, RLS, or any other primary sleep disorders in all children with ADHD symptoms. Treatment of SDB is likely to improve comorbid ADHD. Pre- and postsurgical ADHD evaluation across multiple settings is recommended. Restless legs syndrome that is associated with an underlying iron deficiency may improve with iron supplementation.

REFERENCES

1. Subcommittee on Attention-Deficit/Hyperactivity Disorder, Steering Committee on Quality Improvement and Management. ADHD: clinical practice guideline for the diagnosis, evaluation, and treatment of attention-deficit/hyperactivity disorder in children and adolescents. *Pediatrics* 2011;**128**:1007–22.

2. Owens JA. The ADHD and sleep conundrum: a review. *J Dev Behav Pediatr* 2005;**16**:312–22.

3. Cortese S, Faraone SV, Konofal E, Lecendreux M. Sleep in children with attention-deficit/hyperactivity disorder: meta-analysis of subjective and objective studies. *J Am Acad Child Adolesc Psychiatry* 2009;**48**:894–908.

4. Picchietti MA, Picchietti DL. Advances in pediatric restless legs syndrome: iron, genetics, diagnosis and treatment. *Sleep Med* 2010;**11**:643–51.

5. Chervin RD, Dillon JE, Bassetti C, Ganoczy DA, Pituch KJ. Symptoms of sleep disorders, inattention and hyperactivity in children. *Sleep* 1997;**20**:1185–92.

6. Chervin RD, Archbold KH, Dillon JE, et al. Inattention, hyperactivity, and symptoms of sleep-disordered breathing. *Pediatrics* 2002;**109**:449–56.

7. Dillon JE, Blunden S, Ruzicka DL, et al. DSM-IV diagnoses and obstructive sleep apnea in children before and 1 year after adenotonsillectomy. *J Am Acad Child Adolesc Psychiatry* 2007;**46**:1425–36.

8. Youssef NA, Ege MM, Angly SS, Strauss JL, Marx CE. Is obstructive sleep apnea associated with ADHD? *Ann Clin Psych* 2011;**23**:213–24.

9. O'Brien LM, Holbrook CR, Mervis CB, et al. Sleep and neurobehavioral characteristics of 5- to 7-year-old children with parentally reported symptoms of attention-deficit/hyperactivity disorder. *Pediatrics* 2003;**111**:554–63.

10. Chervin RD, Ruzicka DL, Archbold KH, Dillon JE. Snoring predicts hyperactivity four years later. *Sleep* 2005;**28**: 885–90.

11. O'Brien LM, Lucas NH, Felt BT, et al. Aggressive behavior, bullying, snoring, and sleepiness in schoolchildren. *Sleep Med* 2011;**12**:652–8.

12. Owens JA. Neurocognitive and behavioral impact of sleep disordered breathing in children. *Pediatr Pulmonol* 2009;**44**:417–22.

13. Gozal D. Obstructive sleep apnea in children: implications for the developing central nervous system. *Semin Pediatr Neurol* 2008;**15**:100–6.

14. Beebe DW. Neurobehavioral effects of obstructive sleep apnea: an overview and heuristic model. *Curr Opin Pulm Med* 2005;**11**:494–500.

15. Li HY, Huang YS, Chen NH, Fang TJ, Lee LA. Impact of adenotonsillectomy on behavior in children with sleep-disordered breathing. *Laryngoscope* 2006;**116**:1142–7.

16. Huang YS, Guilleminault C, Li HY, et al. Attention-deficit/hyperactivity disorder with obstructive sleep apnea: a treatment outcome study. *Sleep Med* 2007;**8**:18–30.

17. Picchietti MA, Picchietti DL. Restless legs syndrome and periodic limb movement disorder in children and adolescents. *Sem Pediatr Neurol* 2008;**15**:91–9.

18. Kotagal S, Silber MH. Childhood-onset restless legs syndrome. *Ann Neurol* 2004;**56**:803–7.

19. Chervin RD, Dillon JE, Archbold KH, Ruzicka EL. Conduct problems and symptoms of sleep disorders in children. *Am Acad Child Adolesc Psychiatry* 2003;**42**:201–8.

20. Reif A. Is NOS1 a genetic link between RLS and ADHD? *J Psychiatric Res* 2009;**44**:60–1.

21. Konofal E, Cortese S, Marchand M, et al. Impact of restless legs syndrome and iron deficiency on attention-deficit/hyperactivity disorder in children. *Sleep Med* 2007;**8**:711–15.

52

Obstructive sleep apnea can occur without prominent snoring among children with Trisomy 21

Fauziya Hassan

Obstructive sleep apnea syndrome (OSAS) is a common condition in children with a prevalence of 1–6%.[1-3] It is described as a disorder of breathing during sleep, characterized by intermittent partial or complete upper airway obstruction or by prolonged partial obstruction. Either pattern interferes with normal ventilation during sleep and often affects sleep as well.[4] Typical symptoms noted with OSAS are snoring, possible snort arousals, gasping arousals, and restless or disrupted sleep. Some children sleep with their neck arched, and occasionally among children with underlying syndromes, sleeping in a tripod position is noted. Signs associated with OSAS can include midface hypoplasia, retrognathia, micrognathia, enlarged tongue, adenoid facies, or pectus excavatum. The daytime consequences of OSAS can include impact on cognitive functioning, behavioral problems,[5] cardiac dysrrthymias, hypertension, failure to thrive, and systemic inflammation.[2,6,7] Among the more serious sequelae of OSAS are pulmonary hypertension and right-sided heart failure.

The OSAS is diagnosed by overnight polysomnography, a monitored study conducted in a sleep lab. The typical parameters that are monitored include several electroencephalographic (EEG) leads, two electrooculographic (EOG) leads that detect eye movements, and chin surface electromyographic (EMG) leads. These three types of data – EEG, EOG, and EMG – permit subsequent sleep and wake staging, in 30-second epochs, by sleep technologists. Several other types of equipment or leads are also used, including nasal pressure cannulae and oro-nasal thermistors to record for airflow, thoracic, and abdominal belts that monitor excursion with breathing, two electrocardiographic (ECG) leads, surface EMG of the legs, and pulse oximetry with a 3-second or less averaging time for the signal. The apnea/hypopnea index (AHI, events per hour of sleep) is assessed during the sleep study; this is the number of apneas (generally obstructive, central, or mixed) and hypopneas per hour of recorded sleep. An AHI>1 can support a diagnosis of OSAS[8] though some specialists use slightly higher thresholds (e.g. 1.5 or 2.0). Hypopneas are scored as such when there is a 30% drop in airflow, for at least 2 respiratory cycles (for children), culminating in arousal, awakening, or ≥3% drop in oxygen saturation from the baseline. Obstructive apneas are scored when there is a >90% drop in airflow, for at least 2 respiratory cycles in children, despite continued effort as reflected by excursion in the thoracic and abdominal belts. Snoring is also monitored during the sleep study. In certain patient populations, there may be no evidence of snoring. Snoring is caused typically by vibration of the soft palate. In the presence of hypotonia vibration of the soft palate may be absent.

Trisomy 21 (Down syndrome) is a one of the most common genetic conditions. The syndrome is characterized by features such as an enlarged tongue, midface hypoplasia, hypotonia, and in some children, hypothyroidism. There is a high likelihood of obstructive sleep apnea among children with Trisomy 21; the prevalence is thought to lie between 50 and 80%. One

Common Pitfalls in Sleep Medicine, ed. Ronald D. Chervin. Published by Cambridge University Press. © Cambridge University Press 2014.

study reviewed snoring children with Trisomy 21, aged 4.9 years on average, and found almost all of them (97%) had obstructive sleep apnea with a mean AHI of 12.9.[9] Another study in a tertiary care center found that among 56 children with Trisomy 21 who completed overnight polysomnograms (PSG) between the ages of 2 and 4 years, 57% had underlying obstructive sleep apnea.[10] It is currently recommended that all children with Down syndrome undergo a PSG.

Case

A 6-month-old boy with Trisomy 21 presented to the pediatric pulmonology clinic in a tertiary care center with a chief complaint of chronic cough and wheezing. He had been diagnosed previously with bronchiolitis and the symptoms were responsive to oral steroids and bronchodilators. Snoring was not initially reported but upon detailed history taking, as the patient did have Trisomy 21, the symptom was endorsed. His mother reported snoring to be present occasionally, not habitually. When present, the snoring was characterized as soft and typically occurred only during upper respiratory tract infections (URIs). No snorting or gasping arousals and no witnessed apneas were reported. His mother also did not report restless sleep, sleeping with the neck arched, or sleeping in a tripod position. Frequent awakenings were not present. Typically cough and wheezing were noted with upper respiratory tract infections. Mother reported his sleep to be restful and quiet and said that the child would wake up in the morning feeling refreshed. There were no symptoms of gastroesophageal reflux disease. Birth history was notable for full-term delivery with no complications. Family history was positive for asthma in various immediate family members. On physical examination typical Trisomy 21 features were noted. These included macroglossia, midface hypoplasia, and a short neck. No tonsillar hypertrophy was present. On chest examination pectus excavatum was noted and the air entry was clear. No wheezing or crackles were noted. There was no murmur noted and abdominal exam was benign. Neurologic exam revealed mild hypotonia.

The differential diagnosis considered for cough and wheezing included asthma, airway malacia, post-viral hyperreactivity, and airway inflammation from secondary aspiration. Given a history of positive response to bronchodilators and oral steroids in the past, the child was started on bronchodilators and inhaled corticosteroids. At a follow-up visit 2 months later, interim history revealed that the child had two URIs that necessitated oral antibiotic treatment and bronchodilator therapy, with no significant symptomatic improvement. On further detailed history taking, snoring persisted during URIs, but again was noted to be occasional and not habitual. The physical exam during this visit was not significantly different from that of the previous visit with the exception of mild prominence of pectus excavatum.

With the suboptimal response to bronchodilators, and no difference in symptoms of cough and wheezing after use inhaled corticosteroids, flexible bronchoscopy to evaluate for airway malacia was discussed. The parents did not want to proceed with an invasive procedure. With the history of some snoring (though occasional) and the pectus excavatum along with enlarged tongue and the accompanying midface hypoplasia associated with Down syndrome, the decision was made to move forward with a baseline PSG. The PSG in fact showed severe OSAS with an AHI of 23 and frequent, moderate snoring. Oxygen desaturations to a nadir of 86% were noted and OSAS was noted to be worse during REM sleep. After subsequent treatment for OSAS with supplemental oxygen, a flexible laryngoscopy by a pediatric otolaryngologist was scheduled. This did not reveal adenotonsillar hypertrophy. The boy subsequently underwent a flexible bronchoscopy and rigid bronchoscopy under sedation for assessment of the upper and lower airway. Moderate tracheomalacia and mild to moderate bronchomalacia were noted during the procedure.

Discussion

This case highlights several important points. Snoring is not as good a predictor of OSAS severity as is often assumed.[11] In children with OSAS, snoring can be soft as typically there is prolonged partial obstruction. Other factors that can affect parental or family report of snoring can be parental presence at bedtime or during sleep, the distance of the parents' bedroom from the child's, and whether intervening doors are kept open or closed. Therefore, and again in particular among patients with hypotonia, snoring cannot be taken as a strong predictor for the diagnosis of OSAS. Other symptoms and signs should be taken into consideration. These can include restless sleep, frequent nighttime arousals, and diaphoresis. Pectus excavatum can be noted among children with OSAS.

The main treatment option for obstructive sleep apnea among children is adenotonsillectomy. Among children with craniofacial syndromes practitioners should be aware that though adenotonsillectomy is the first treatment option, residual obstructive sleep apnea often persists as the obstruction may occur at multiple sites. In addition, more severe OSAS raises the chance of residual OSAS after adenotonsillectomy.[12] Children with syndromes or severe OSAS should be monitored closely after adenotonsillectomy. This often includes overnight observation in the hospital. The American Academy of Pediatrics recommends a baseline sleep study or objective testing for OSAS among all children prior to adenotonsillectomy.[13] All children with OSAS should be reevaluated clinically after surgery and those with high-risk conditions or residual signs and symptoms of OSAS should have repeat objective testing including a repeat baseline PSG if available.[13] In addition, surgery for such individuals should be performed in centers that are equipped to handle high-risk pediatric cases during and after surgery.

If residual OSAS persists after adenotonsillectomy, then positive airway pressure (PAP) either in the form of continuous positive airway pressure (CPAP) or bi-level positive airway pressure (Bi-PAP) is the preferred treatment option. Among children, especially with underlying syndromes, there is a better chance of tolerance of masks used for positive airway pressure if mask desensitization is performed prior to the PAP titration study. Acclimatization to mask and PAP therapy may take months and a formal desensitization program is often required to achieve success. Among

infants and toddlers with Trisomy 21, in whom adeno-tonsillar hypertrophy is not noted, otolaryngology evaluation is required to determine the site of airway obstruction. Airway malacia has higher prevalence among children with Trisomy 21. Oxygen supplementation may also be a consideration to treat OSAS in these children, as risk for development of midface hypoplasia has been reported with chronic use of a facial mask.

Major points

Clinicians should maintain a high index of suspicion for OSAS among children with Trisomy 21. Polysomnography should be performed to assess for objective evidence of OSAS. Follow-up PSG should be done after surgical intervention such as adenotonsillectomy, as OSAS may persist.

REFERENCES

1. Bixler EO, Vgontzas AN, Hung-Mo L, et al. Sleep disordered breathing in children in a general population sample: prevalence and risk factors. *Sleep* 2009;**32**:731–6.
2. O'Brien LM, Holbrook CR, Mervis CB, et al. Sleep and neurobehavioral characteristics of 5- to 7-year-old children with parentally reported symptoms of attention-deficit/hyperactivity disorder. *Pediatrics* 2003;**111**:554–63.
3. Vianello A, Bevilacqua M, Salvador V, Cardaioli C, Vincenti E. Long-term nasal intermittent positive pressure ventilation in advanced Duchenne's muscular dystrophy. *Chest* 1994;**105**:445–8.
4. American Thoracic Society. Standards and indications for cardiopulmonary sleep studies in children. *Am J Respir Crit Care Med* 1996;**153**:866–78.
5. Rosen CL, Storfer-Isser A, Taylor HG, et al. Increased behavioral morbidity in school-aged children with sleep-disordered breathing. *Pediatrics* 2004;**114**:1640–8.
6. Capdevila OS, Kheirandish-Gozal L, Dayyat E, Gozal D. Pediatric obstructive sleep apnea: complications, management, and long-term outcomes. *Proc Am Thorac Soc* 2008;**5**:274–82.
7. Rothstein R, Paris Y, Quizon A. Pulmonary hypertension. *Pediatr Review* 2009;**30**:39–46.

8. Erler T, Paditz E. Obstructive sleep apnea syndrome in children: a state-of-the-art review. *Treat Respir Med* 2004;**3**:107–22.

9. Fitzgerald DA, Paul A, Richmond C. Severity of obstructive apnoea in children with Down syndrome who snore. *Arch Dis Child* 2007;**92**:423–5.

10. Shott SR, Amin R, Chini B, et al. Obstructive sleep apnea: Should all children with Down syndrome be tested? *Arch Otolaryngol Head Neck Surg* 2006;**132**:432–6.

11. Blunden S, Lushington K, Lorenzen B, et al. Symptoms of sleep breathing disorders in children are underreported by parents at general practice visits. *Sleep Breath* 2003;**7**:167–76.

12. Gottschall J. Evaluation of adenotonsillectomy for obstructive sleep apnea using pre- and post-op polysomnograms. *AAP Grand Rounds* 2008;**19**:8–9.

13. Marcus CL, Brooks LJ, Draper KA, et al. Diagnosis and management of childhood obstructive sleep apnea syndrome. *Pediatrics* 2012;**130**:576–84.

53

Familiarity with infant sleep and normal variants can prevent extensive but unnecessary testing and intervention

Renée A. Shellhaas

Overview

Newborn infants have a relatively limited repertoire of external signs of neurologic health or illness. A healthy neonate spends about two-thirds of each day asleep, with increasingly consolidated sleep bouts evolving over the first year of life. Therefore, understanding the normal patterns of movements during sleep, as well as normal and abnormal mental status, is essential for the clinical assessment of very young infants. Unusual paroxysmal movements often raise concern for seizures and underlying significant brain dysfunction. However, the differential diagnosis of newborns' unusual movements is quite broad and not uniformly ominous. Knowledge of benign and worrisome diagnoses, and their associated features, especially in the context of expected behaviors during wakefulness and sleep, can lead to a parsimonious evaluation and save the patient from unnecessary treatment.

Case: unusual neonatal movements: worrisome or not?

A 15-day-old full-term infant boy presents to the pediatrician due to concerning jerking movements. The infant has sudden, brief, jerking movements of the arms more than the legs, which occur in 1–5-minute episodes. Sometimes the right arm is most affected, but at other times the left seems more involved. Between events, he appears well. He alerts with minimal stimulation and maintains an awake state for up to 1 hour at a time, following which he sleeps for 1 or 2 hours. He feeds well every 3 hours and appears well hydrated.

Review of the infant's history reveals that he was born at 39 weeks gestation via spontaneous vaginal delivery to a primigravida mother. The pregnancy was uncomplicated. His birth weight was 7.61 pounds (3450 g). He was discharged home at 48 hours of life, after routine perinatal care. He breast-feeds well and takes no medications. He regained his birthweight within a week.

At the pediatrician's office, the infant appears well, weighs 8.16 pounds (3700 g), and has normal vital signs (including normal temperature). The infant is sleeping quietly in his mother's arms when he suddenly has a series of arrhythmic twitching movements of the right arm, followed by the left arm and leg. The pediatrician moves him to the examining table and undresses him. He cries and the movements cease.

What are the diagnostic possibilities?

Among newborn infants, focal seizures can be the first sign of serious systemic or neurologic illness. Therefore, they should prompt an emergent evaluation with immediate treatment of the underlying cause. However, many paroxysmal neonatal movements are not, in fact, seizures (Table 53.1). Since the diagnostic evaluation of neonatal seizures is often invasive, and anticonvulsant medications can have significant side

Table 53.1 Differential diagnosis of paroxysmal movements among newborn infants*

Diagnosis	Clinical signs	Diagnostic tests	Treatment
Central nervous system infection	Altered mental status Focal seizures Bulging fontanel	CSF analysis Blood culture	Antibiotics Anticonvulsant medication
Electrolyte abnormalities	Depressed mental status Poor feeding/dehydration Focal seizures	Measurement of serum electrolytes and glucose	Normalize sodium, calcium, glucose No anticonvulsants typically required
Stroke	Focal seizures Hemiparesis (may be subtle) Variable altered mental status	Brain MRI	Supportive treatment Anticonvulsant medication for acute symptomatic seizures
Gastroesophageal reflux	Poor feeding, failure to thrive Irritability, especially during/after feeds Arching	None, or pH probe	Ranitidine or other antireflux medication Thickened feeds
Hyperekplexia	Exaggerated startle response to minimal external stimulation (while awake)	Clinical diagnosis, with or without genetic confirmation	None, or clonazepam if infant is highly symptomatic
Neonatal abstinence syndrome	Irritability Jittery or myoclonic movements while awake and/or asleep Gastrointestinal dysfunction	History of prenatal drug exposure (illicit or prescribed)	Non-pharmacologic measures (swaddling, quiet environment) Methadone taper
Benign neonatal sleep myoclonus	Myoclonic movements which resolve upon awakening Otherwise healthy infant	None	Reassurance
Normal infant body movements	Erratic, arrhythmic but symmetric movements, with obvious normal reflexes (e.g. Moro reflex) in an otherwise healthy infant	None	Reassurance
Normal infant eye movements	Prominent Bell's phenomenon, with upward eye deviation under semi-closed lids, as a normal infant falls into active asleep	None	Reassurance

* This list is not meant to be exhaustive. Rather, it is designed to demonstrate the range of diagnostic considerations for neonates with unusual paroxysmal movements.
CSF, cerebrospinal fluid; MRI, magnetic resonance imaging.

effects, awareness of common non-seizure etiologies of paroxysmal movements is critical for the primary care physician.

Which tests are required? Which are not?

In our case, the history of myoclonic jerks that only occur during sleep, in the context of a completely healthy infant, is sufficient for the diagnosis of benign neonatal sleep myoclonus. The key element of history is that the events occur **only during sleep**. Neonatal sleep states are classified into quiet and active sleep (Table 53.2), or when necessary, indeterminate sleep. Classically, neonatal sleep myoclonus is described during quiet (non-rapid eye movement), but not active, sleep. However, some newer data suggest that benign myoclonus can also occur during active sleep

Table 53.2 Neonatal sleep–wake states

State	Body movements	Eye movements	Breathing pattern
Active sleep (rapid eye movement [REM] sleep precursor)	Some brief twitching movements	REMs	Irregular
Quiet sleep	Nearly still, with only rare twitches	None	Regular
Wakefulness	*Active alert*: Symmetric, irregular but smooth movements, with occasional startles	*Active alert*: Eyes open ± fix and follow	*Active alert*: Irregular
	Quiet alert: Few movements	*Quiet alert*: Eyes open and focused	*Quiet alert*: Regular

and during transitions from sleep to wakefulness. The myoclonus can be symmetric and synchronous, or have a focal semiology. Classically, the arms are the most involved, but myoclonus of the legs, face, and trunk can also occur. There is no associated apnea, cyanosis, or eye deviation. Sometimes, there are provoking factors, such as repetitive sounds, tactile stimuli, or rocking during sleep.

The classic teaching is that movements caused by seizures cannot be suppressed by gentle restraint of the limb, while non-seizure movements can be easily extinguished. For example an infant who is simply jittery, such as a newborn with neonatal abstinence syndrome, will have excessive low-amplitude and high frequency limb movements and an exaggerated Moro reflex. The jittery movements increase in response to internal and external stimuli, but are calmed by gentle restraint. Contrary to this classic teaching, the movements of benign neonatal sleep myoclonus often continue despite restraint of the limb. Waking the infant, and observing the cessation of myoclonic movements, is the key feature of both the history and examination.

If the diagnosis is in question then a full evaluation is warranted. Reasons to question the diagnosis of benign neonatal sleep myoclonus include an ill-appearing infant, abnormal vital signs, abnormal mental status or focal neurologic abnormalities on physical examination, risk factors for infection (such as maternal group B streptococcal infection), etc. Seizures can occur during both wakefulness and sleep, another key diagnostic distinction.

For any infant in whom a diagnosis of neonatal seizures is being considered, a full sepsis evaluation is strongly recommended (to include cultures of blood, urine, and cerebrospinal fluid) and antibiotics should be administered until the cultures are proven to be negative. Electrolyte and glucose levels should also be measured, and corrected if abnormal. However, anticonvulsant medications are not always immediately mandatory. If the episodes in question are not clinically felt to be definite seizures, then antiseizure treatment can sometimes be deferred until a definite diagnosis is made (sepsis evaluation should not be postponed, however).

The optimal diagnostic test to confirm or refute the diagnosis of neonatal seizures is electroencephalography (EEG). Once the event of concern is recorded, it can be determined if it is a seizure (if yes, then initiation of antiseizure treatment should be expedited). If the event is not a seizure, but the infant is encephalopathic or the EEG is not completely normal, then continued EEG monitoring might reveal subtle or subclinical seizures. Indeed, > 50% of neonatal seizures are entirely subclinical and so cannot, by definition, be diagnosed by bedside clinical observation alone. That these seizures are subclinical should not be surprising since a non-verbal infant cannot describe a visual hallucination or a rising epigastric sensation, hallmarks of focal occipital or temporal lobe seizures.

If the infant in our case discussion had experienced events that were described slightly differently, then additional testing would have been required. For example, had the events been described as focal clonic jerking, rather than arrhythmic myoclonus, then evaluation for seizures would have been necessary. In our infant's case, the EEG would have been normal, as would the entire diagnostic evaluation. By causing sedation, administration of anticonvulsant medication could have exacerbated the sleep myoclonus.

Discussion

Benign neonatal sleep myoclonus is most commonly reported among healthy infants in the third through fifth weeks of life, although signs often begin in the first few days of life. Myoclonus typically resolves by 6 months of age. In rare cases the myoclonus persists into the second year of life. The incidence is difficult to estimate, because very often a formal diagnosis is not sought, but it has been estimated to be 0.8–3.0 cases per 1000 births, nearly identical to that of true neonatal seizures. Although the literature contains reports of mild speech or language disabilities and of mild hypotonia among a few patients with benign neonatal sleep myoclonus, the incidence of these findings may not be any higher than that of the general population. As a rule, benign neonatal sleep myoclonus is just that – a benign condition.

As emphasized in our case, the classic history, in the context of a normal, healthy infant, is sufficient for the diagnosis of benign neonatal sleep myoclonus. Despite the classic history, many infants with benign neonatal sleep myoclonus are evaluated by primary care physicians, and subspecialists, who do not entertain the diagnosis. This is a recurring theme among the many published case series of benign neonatal sleep myoclonus patients. Parents often do not volunteer that the events occur exclusively during sleep and clinicians forget to ask. Misdiagnosis can lead to costly and unnecessary testing, as well as inappropriate and ineffective treatment with anticonvulsant medications.

Benign neonatal sleep myoclonus can be diagnosed relatively easily, in most cases. As children grow older, however, unusual paroxysmal movements in sleep can become more difficult diagnostic dilemmas. For example, frontal lobe epilepsy typically presents with erratic but stereotyped hypermotor seizures that arise out of non-rapid eye movement sleep. Children with myoclonic epilepsy syndromes may have a combination of normal sleep myoclonus and epileptic myoclonus as they fall asleep, because epileptiform discharges are often activated during drowsiness. In these instances, diagnostic testing with EEG can be necessary in order to determine which events are seizures, and which antiseizure medications are likely to be most effective.

Main points

Although newborn infants can display a range of unusual movements during sleep and wakefulness, most are not seizures. Recognizing patterns of neonatal movements, key elements of the history, and the relation of the events to sleep and wakefulness can lead to an accurate diagnosis of benign neonatal sleep myoclonus, without costly testing or unnecessary treatment.

FURTHER READING

Coulter DL, Allen RJ. Benign neonatal sleep myoclonus. *Arch Neurol* 1982;**39**:191–2.

Kaddurah AK, Holmes GL. Benign neonatal sleep myoclonus: history and semiology. *Pediatr Neurol* 2009;**40**:343–6.

Maurer VO, Rizzi M, Bianchetti MG, Ramelli GP. Benign neonatal sleep myoclonus: a review of the literature. *Pediatrics* 2010;**125**:e919–24.

54

Obstructive sleep apnea in patients with neuromuscular disorders

Fauziya Hassan

Obstructive sleep apnea is particularly common among certain high-risk groups of patients, including those with neuromuscular disorders. However, the symptoms of sleep-disordered breathing can be subtle. There may be an increase in the number of awakenings at night, daytime sleepiness, or morning headaches. Cardiac involvement is commonly seen among children with Duchenne muscular dystrophy, and cardiac disease is the second most common cause of mortality in this patient population. Almost 10–20% of these patients die from cardiac failure. Dilated cardiomyopathy and left-sided heart failure as well as pulmonary hypotension and right-sided heart failure are noted. Cardiac arrhythmias can also be diagnosed. Cardiovascular comorbidities are also found in association with obstructive sleep apnea;[1] prominent examples include right-sided heart failure, arrhythmias, and systemic hypertension. Therefore, obstructive sleep apnea can be a particular concern in patients whose neuromuscular disorder already raises concern for cardiac problems.

Case

An 8-year-old boy with Duchenne muscular dystrophy was seen in the pediatric pulmonology clinic for the first time. He did not have any previous hospitalizations. Over the past year his muscle strength had declined and he had become non-ambulatory and wheelchair bound. He had not had any respiratory complications. Upper respiratory tract infections would last about a week and he had no prolonged cough. His cough was somewhat weak. He had no wheezing during respiratory infections. He had no history of previous pneumonias or frequent respiratory infections. The family used a vest for airway clearance on a daily basis but used the cough-assist device only as needed. He did not have any trouble swallowing foods. He had no choking with oral food intake.

With regard to sleep symptoms, he had some difficulty with sleep initiation, with mildly increased latency to sleep of about 45 minutes. No snoring was noted by his mother. In addition, no witnessed apneas, diaphoresis, or frequent nocturnal awakenings were reported. The patient had no complaints of morning headaches. He did have mild restlessness during sleep. He complained of some daytime tiredness but not sleepiness. He had received good grades in school. His mother reported that a sleep study done at an outside institution showed normal findings.

On physical exam, the patient was wheelchair bound with significant hypotonia. He had mild contractures of his knees bilaterally. There was no scoliosis. The rest of the physical exam did not reveal any other pertinent positives such as a crowded oropharynx or significant adenotonsillar hypertrophy. End-tidal carbon dioxide ($ETCO_2$) during the clinic visit was 34 mmHg and oxygen saturation on room air was 96%. Maximal inspiratory pressure (MIP) was –28 cm of water and maximal expiratory pressure (MEP) was 37 cm of water. His spirometry was normal

Common Pitfalls in Sleep Medicine, ed. Ronald D. Chervin. Published by Cambridge University Press. © Cambridge University Press 2014.

but the efforts were variable and did not meet American Thoracic Society (ATS) criteria for reproducibility. Arm span was not used as a proxy for height for the spirometry; rather, parent-reported measurement was used for height. In many instances where the patient is wheelchair bound and height cannot be measured, reported height is used, which can lead to error in estimation of lung function. In this case the spirometry was interpreted as normal but with variable efforts. No further testing or change in treatment regimen was recommended during the clinic visit.

The patient had a follow-up clinic visit 6 months later. He had done well in the interim. He had one upper respiratory tract infection, over the winter season, lasting < 5 days. He was using the cough assist and vest with bronchodilator therapy for airway clearance twice a day. He did not have a significant decline in his muscle strength. He did not have any reported snoring or frequent arousals. His mother did not report gasping or snorting arousals, or any witnessed apneas. He still had difficulty in sleep initiation and his mother reported sounds at night that sounded like whimpering. The MIP value during this visit was –18 cm of water and MEP was 12 cm of water. The $ETCO_2$ during this clinic visit was 30 mmHg. There was a question about suboptimal efforts during the MIP and MEP maneuvers. Spirometry could not be done during the clinic visit. The decision was made to proceed with a baseline polysomnogram with $ETCO_2$ monitoring given the decline in MIP and MEP values since the prior clinic visit.

Baseline polysomnography performed 3 months later showed severe obstructive sleep apnea with an apnea/hypopnea index (AHI, events per hour of sleep) of 39, an arousal index of 53, and oxygen desaturations to a nadir of 75%. Frequent moderate to loud snoring was noted during the study. Sleep fragmentation was noted. The study did not show sleep-related hypoventilation. The $ETCO_2$ values during the sleep study were 39–41 mmHg during wakefulness and 40–46 mmHg during sleep. He subsequently underwent a titration study that demonstrated high carbon dioxide values on continuous positive airway pressure (CPAP) therapy. He was transitioned to bi-level positive airway pressure (Bi-PAP) but was unable to trigger a transition from lower expiratory PAP (EPAP) to higher inspiratory PAP (IPAP) during events that resembled hypopneas. He was started on Bi-PAP with spontaneous timed (ST) mode and a setting of IPAP 16 cm of water, EPAP 4 cm of water, and a backup rate of 16 breaths per minute. This resolved his obstructive sleep apnea and on this therapy $ETCO_2$ values were in the low 40s.

The patient was evaluated 2 months later in clinic. He was using Bi-PAP with a full face mask every night. He reported higher energy levels during the day and his sleep quality had improved, with significant reduction in restlessness. There were no interval illnesses. The $ETCO_2$ values during the clinic visit were 36–37 mmHg. Spirometry showed severe restriction but with variable effort noted during the maneuvers. The study was done using arm span as a proxy measurement for height.

Discussion

This case highlights the fact that a report of snoring in a child is dependent on parental knowledge that may not be accurate. Under-reporting of this symptom is common.[2] The presence of hypotonia may also cause diminished inspiratory effort and soft palate vibration, and the minimal snoring that results may not be proportionate to the severity of the underlying obstructive sleep apnea. In this case there was no parental report of snoring but frequent moderate snoring was recorded on the sleep study. The treatment of obstructive sleep apnea in such patients is complicated by the fact that residual obstructive sleep apnea is common, due to hypotonia, after adenotonsillectomy. Pharyngeal walls can collapse due to hypotonia.[3]

Obstructive sleep apnea and hypoventilation become more frequent with reduction in muscle strength that is sufficiently prominent to cause a patient with neuromuscular disorder to become wheelchair bound. The ATS guidelines indicate that patients should be screened for hypoventilation and obstructive sleep apnea when spirometry shows severe restriction, with a forced vital capacity (*FVC*) < 45% of predicted. There are neurocognitive implications of

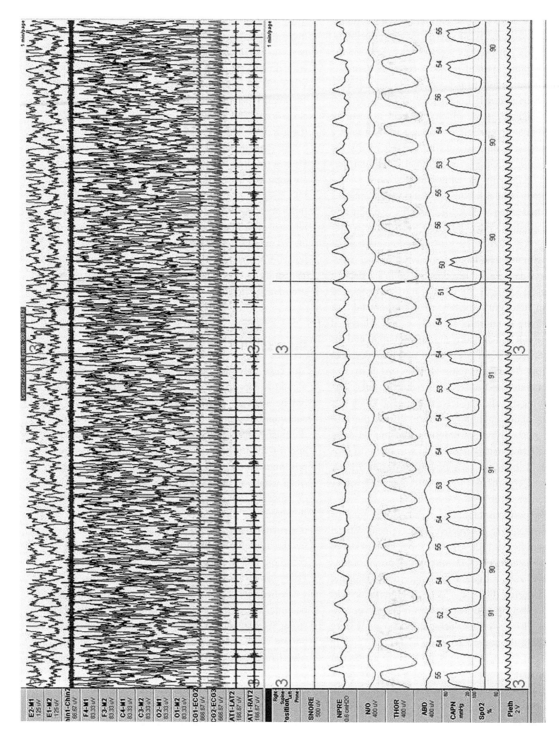

Figure 54.1 Hypoventilation noted during a diagnostic polysomnogram with end-tidal carbon dioxide monitoring. See plate section for color version. Abbreviations: E1 and E2, left and right eye leads; M1 and M2, mastoid leads; O, occipital EEG leads; C, central EEG leads; ECG, electrocardiogram leads; LAT and RAT, left and right anterior tibialis leads; NPRE, nasal pressure; N/O, oro-nasal thermistor; THOR, thoracic belt; ABD, abdominal belt; CAPN, capnogram; SpO2, oxygen saturation; Pleth, plethysmography.

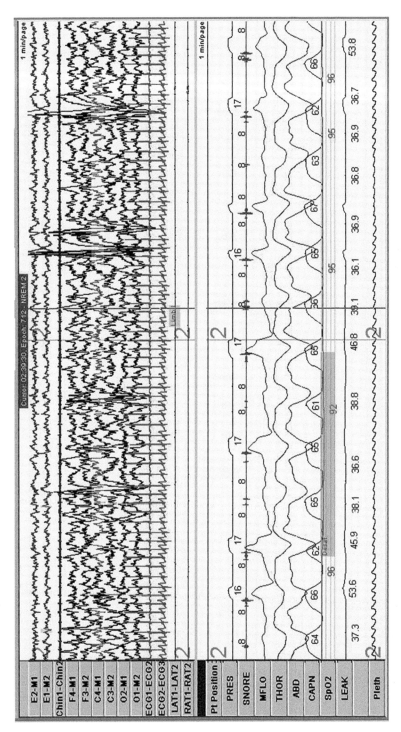

Figure 54.2 Bi-level positive airway pressure (Bi-PAP) with irregular, intermittent inability to trigger jump from expiratory positive airway pressure to a higher inspiratory positive airway pressure (IPAP). This is best reflected in the tracings marked PRES (mask pressure) and MFLO (mask flow). See plate section for color version. Abbreviations: E1 and E2, left and right eye leads; M1 and M2, are mastoid leads; F, frontal electroencephalography (EEG) leads; C, central EEG leads; O, occipital EEG leads; ECG, electrocardiogram leads; LAT and RAT, left and right anterior tibialis leads; NPRE, nasal pressure; N/O, oro–nasal thermistor; THOR, thoracic belt; ABD, abdominal belt; CAPN, capnogram; SpO2, oxygen saturation; Pleth, plethysmography; PRES, bi-level positive airway pressure; MFLO is mask flow.

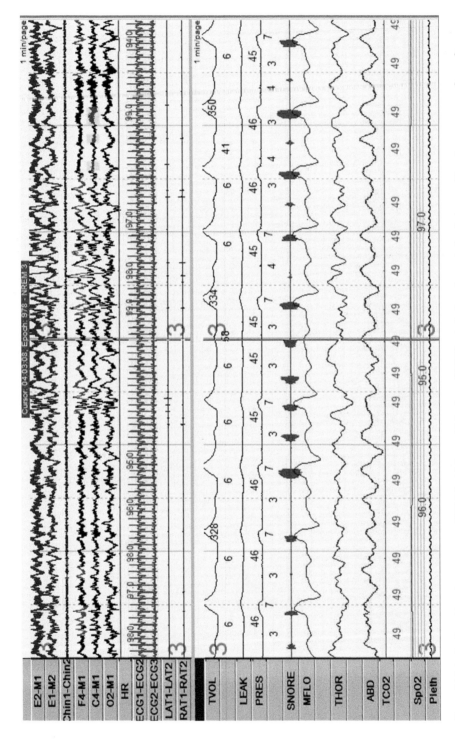

Figure 54.3 Bi-level positive airway pressure (Bi-PAP) with lower tidal volume (TVOL) noted when change to inspiratory positive airway pressure, from a lower expiratory positive pressure, does not occur. See plate section for color version. Abbreviations: E1 and E2, left and right eye leads; M1 and M2, mastoid leads; F, frontal electroencephalography (EEG) leads; C, central EEG leads; O, occipital EEG leads; ECG, electrocardiogram leads; LAT and RAT, left and right anterior tibialis leads; NPRE, nasal pressure; N/O, oro-nasal thermistor; THOR, thoracic belt; ABD, abdominal belt; CAPN, capnogram; SpO2, oxygen saturation; Pleth, plethysmography; TVOL, tidal volume; TCO2, transcutaneous carbon dioxide monitoring.

muscular dystrophy; maneuvers to perform spirometry may not always be possible, and therefore MIP and MEP should be considered. A high risk of hypoventilation exists when the patient becomes wheelchair bound, and when indicated sleep studies in this patient population should include end-tidal or transcutaneous carbon dioxide monitoring.[3] Annual evaluation for sleep-disordered breathing among wheelchair users is recommended. In one study sleep hypoventilation was predicted by awake partial pressure of arterial carbon dioxide ($PaCO_2$) $\geq$ 45 mmHg.[4] Forced expiratory volume in 1 second (FEV_1) values < 20% of predicted are associated with daytime hypoventilation. Stabilization of pulmonary function along with improvement in survival can be seen after the initiation of non-invasive positive pressure ventilation (NIPPV).[5,6]

As noted with this case, CPAP (and supplemental oxygen) may have limited roles in treatment of sleep-disordered breathing among patients with neuromuscular disorders, as the problem is not just obstruction of the upper airway, but also a component of underlying hypoventilation (Figure 54.1). Bi-level PAP, unlike CPAP, is able to generate higher tidal volumes by virtue of pressure support (PS, equal to the difference between IPAP and EPAP) (Figures 54.2 and 54.3). In some patients with kyphoscoliosis and stiffness of the chest wall, uncontrolled administration of CPAP may be harmful because it can increase functional residual capacity (*FRC*). In patients with severe restrictive lung disease, PS as high as 20 cm of water may be needed to treat hypoventilation. This can lead to a high mask leak as well as difficulty tolerating NIPPV.

Main points

When children with muscular dystrophy become wheelchair bound, they have a higher likelihood of obstructive sleep apnea and hypoventilation. Close monitoring and annual evaluation is needed to assess for sleep-disordered breathing. Non-invasive positive pressure ventilation is frequently needed for treatment, and Bi-PAP with ST mode is frequently required.

REFERENCES

1. Capdevila OS, Kheirandish-Gozal L, Dayyat E, Gozal D. Pediatric obstructive sleep apnea: complications, management, and long-term outcomes. *Proc Am Thorac Soc* 2008;**5**:274–82.

2. Blunden S, Lushington K, Lorenzen B, et al. Symptoms of sleep breathing disorders in children are underreported by parents at general practice visits. *Sleep Breath* 2003;**7**:167–76.

3. American Thoracic Society. Respiratory care of the patient with Duchenne muscular dystrophy. *Am J Respir Crit Care Med* 2004;**170**:456–65.

4. Hukins CA, Hillman DR. Daytime predictors of sleep hypoventilation in Duchenne muscular dystrophy. *Am J Respir Crit Care Med* 2000;**161**:166–70.

5. Phillips MF, Smith PEM, Carroll N, Edwards RHT, Calverley PMA. Nocturnal oxygenation and prognosis in Duchenne muscular dystrophy. *Am J Respir Crit Care Med* 1999;**160**:198–202.

6. Vianello A, Salvador V, Cardaioli C, Vincenti E. Long-term nasal intermittent positive pressure ventilation in advanced Duchenne's muscular dystrophy. *Chest* 1994;**105**:445–8.

Sleep in older persons

Complaints about sleep are common at all ages, but become particularly prevalent among older persons. As this age demographic rapidly accounts for an increasing proportion of the population, physicians of all types are likely to be confronted with increasing numbers of patients who would like nothing more than a good night's sleep, for themselves and often for their caregivers as well. At stake is not only health and well-being, but also substantial and growing costs of care during a newly expanded lifespan. Although older persons are subject to virtually all the sleep disorders that can affect patients at younger ages, presentations can become different and sometimes unique to the context of chronic comorbidities and vulnerabilities of the aged.

The chapters in this section are written by a cognitive disorders specialist, two geriatricians,

and a neurologist with specific expertise in sleep problems of older persons. The specific cases highlight interactions between aging, cognition, dementia, delirium, risk for falls and hip fractures, and sleep disorders. They emphasize special considerations when it comes to medications used for sleep as well as other chronic medical conditions in older patients. The authors of these chapters portray the complexities of a growing sleep medicine subfield that will assume increasing importance in coming years. Only a handful of sleep specialists currently specialize in aging. More such individuals will clearly be needed, not only to see patients, but to investigate key remaining questions that have scarcely been explored, and to educate the rest of us on their findings.

55

Cognitive effects of untreated sleep apnea

Judith L. Heidebrink

Case

A 55-year-old woman has noted problems with her memory over the past few years. She misplaces her car keys and misses turns when driving, even though she recognizes her surroundings. She forgets to check on the laundry or on food she is preparing. She loses her train of thought in the middle of a sentence and seems slower to process what others say to her. Her general examination is unremarkable. She recalls accurately what she weighed at her annual exam a week ago. She is fully oriented to time and place. Her language and copying abilities are intact. She repeats three words and remembers two of them after a brief delay, the third with a prompt. She makes an error when subtracting from 20 by 3s. Brain imaging does not reveal significant atrophy or hippocampal abnormalities. She wonders if she should take a medication to help her memory.

What additional historical information would you obtain?

Although the patient is concerned about her memory, her symptoms and her cognitive performance suggest that her primary difficulty is with attention rather than memory per se. The history should explore potential causes of inattention. This includes inquiring about lifelong difficulties with attention, current symptoms of depression or other mood disturbances, use of medications that could impair attention, and indications of insufficient or ineffective sleep.

The patient reports that she can sleep for 9 hours at night but still feels tired in the morning. She falls asleep readily in sedentary situations. She has tried to use a timer to remind herself about tasks, but she falls asleep before setting the timer. She snores regularly and loudly.

What testing do you recommend?

The patient has non-refreshing sleep, excessive daytime sleepiness, and loud snoring. These symptoms are typical of untreated sleep apnea. You recommend a polysomnogram, which reveals severe obstructive sleep apnea (OSA) with 71 apnea/hypopnea events per hour of sleep and frequent oxygen desaturations.

Discussion

Cognitive complaints are common among adults with untreated OSA. Such individuals experience forgetfulness, slowed cognitive processing and response times, and an inability to concentrate that impacts their daily functioning. These cognitive difficulties can be sufficiently disruptive that a medical evaluation is sought. Despite the increased prevalence of OSA with age, older adults complaining of "memory loss" are not routinely asked about symptoms of OSA, such as daytime sleepiness or snoring. Unless a sleep history is

Common Pitfalls in Sleep Medicine, ed. Ronald D. Chervin. Published by Cambridge University Press. © Cambridge University Press 2014.

obtained, cognitive symptoms due to OSA may be misdiagnosed as Alzheimer's disease or another neurodegenerative disorder. Patients may undergo unnecessary brain imaging or other diagnostic tests and be started inappropriately on dementia medications.

The prevalence of cognitive impairment among individuals with OSA is not known precisely. Cognitive impairment is related to OSA severity, but the relationship is not linear. Limited or no cognitive impairment may be detected if OSA is mild and not accompanied by sleepiness. However, substantial cognitive impairment has been noted in over 25% of older adults with newly diagnosed OSA.[1] This number should be viewed with caution, though, since studies using sleep center populations may not reflect the general community of persons with OSA. Individuals with greater impairments are more likely to seek clinical evaluation. In addition, persons with OSA may have comorbid health conditions that contribute to their cognitive impairment. Nonetheless, even when controlling for these factors, several specific cognitive impairments have been described in adults with untreated OSA. Table 55.1 summarizes the most commonly reported findings from tests of cognitive performance.[2]

Untreated OSA is associated with impaired attention, particularly sustained attention (vigilance). As in the case history, patients report being easily distracted or losing their focus while engaged in tasks carried out over a period of time. However, attentional impairments may not be readily apparent during a routine medical assessment. Bedside tests (e.g. serial subtractions) may be too brief to detect inattention, as errors

tend to increase with task duration. Sustained attention can be formally measured by the Psychomotor Vigilance Task (PVT) or similar tests. In the PVT, subjects are asked to press a button whenever a stimulus appears on a screen, such as the red dot shown in Figure 55.1.

The red dot appears randomly for a few seconds at a time, and responses are assessed over 10 minutes. Both speed of response and frequency of failing to respond are measured. As a group, patients with untreated OSA have slower response times and more failures to respond than normal controls. To provide some clinical perspective, the PVT was used to compare subjects with OSA (average age 47) to healthy, non-sleepy adults (average age 27) who had consumed increasing amounts alcohol. On average, a subject with OSA had comparable or worse performance than a younger individual who was "legally drunk."[3]

Neuropsychological testing has also demonstrated impairments in executive function in adults with untreated OSA. Executive function refers to the ability to perform and regulate goal-directed behavior. It includes planning, sequencing, forming concepts, monitoring, and making adjustments as needed. Tests of executive function include Trails B, in which subjects are timed as they connect alternating numbers and letters in sequential order (1–A–2–B, etc.), and the Wisconsin Card Sorting Test, in which subjects use

Table 55.1 Cognitive performance in adults with untreated obstructive sleep apnea

Cognitive domain	Impairment
Attention/vigilance	+
Executive function	+
Memory	±
General intelligence	−
Language	−
Visual perception	−

Figure 55.1 Test of sustained attention. Subjects are asked to press a button whenever the red dot appears on the screen. See plate section for color version.

feedback to determine card matching rules. Individuals with untreated OSA routinely underperform on these types of tasks compared to healthy controls. They also perform more poorly on certain tests of psychomotor function, particularly those involving fine motor coordination.

Memory tests in persons with untreated OSA have yielded mixed results. Impaired recall of word lists or pictures is inconsistently found across studies. It is not known whether elderly individuals are more susceptible to memory disturbances from OSA. However, age does not appear to modify the general profile of cognitive impairment observed with OSA. That is, when cognitive impairments are detected, they characteristically fall within the domains of attention, executive function, and memory. Obstructive sleep apnea is not typically associated with impairments in language, visual perception, or general intelligence. Thus, individuals with OSA who have evidence of declining general intellect need further evaluation to determine the cause of their cognitive impairment.

The biologic processes underlying cognitive impairment in OSA remain under investigation. Experimental models focus on the effects of hypoxemia and sleep fragmentation. A leading theory is that hypoxemia contributes to a cerebral microvasculopathy through multiple potential mechanisms. Selective vulnerability of the prefrontal cortex and subcortical white matter has been proposed, which would account for the pattern of cognitive deficits observed in OSA. The concept of "frontal dysfunction" is also supported by functional imaging studies in OSA. Clinical–pathological correlations are being explored, such as whether memory impairment is more likely when OSA is accompanied by significant hypoxemia.

Continuous positive airway pressure (CPAP) corrects both the sleep fragmentation and the hypoxemia of OSA and in most circumstances is the treatment of choice. The goals of CPAP therapy are to improve patient quality of life and to reduce the morbidity associated with OSA. This includes amelioration of cognitive impairment. Anecdotally, patients have described substantial improvements in cognition following treatment of OSA, declaring, "My mind is

back." An earlier, qualitative analysis of OSA treatment reported encouraging improvements in attention/vigilance, executive function, and memory across the majority of studies reviewed.[4] A recent meta-analysis, however, concluded that objective improvements may be more limited.[5] Thirteen randomized controlled studies of CPAP, comprising 554 patients with OSA, were analyzed. Small, but measurable improvements in attention were reported in the majority of studies. No other cognitive domain showed consistent improvements with CPAP treatment. Of note, the duration of treatment was < 1 month in several of the studies, and many also had low CPAP adherence rates. Thus, while this analysis may guide expectations for short-term improvement with suboptimal CPAP adherence, it does not contradict studies reporting normalization of memory among optimal CPAP users at 3 months.

In order to address concerns about small sample sizes, short treatment durations, and inadequate control groups, the Apnea Positive Pressure Long-term Efficacy Study (APPLES) randomized nearly 1100 adults with OSA to 6 months of active versus sham CPAP.[6] Cognitive testing was performed at baseline, 2 months, and 6 months. The active CPAP group improved from baseline on a measure of executive function at both 2 months and 6 months, but was statistically different from the sham group only at the 2-month time point. Attention and memory measures did not differ between the two groups. However, there was little evidence of cognitive impairment at baseline in either group.

Despite similar cognitive profiles between older and younger adults with untreated OSA, less is known about the cognitive response to CPAP in persons over age 65. Small treatment studies have shown positive effects, even when the older subjects had preexisting dementia. Yaffe et al.[7] studied the relationship between untreated OSA and the development of cognitive impairment among 298 elderly women. Over 5 years of follow-up, subjects with OSA were nearly twice as likely to develop mild cognitive impairment or dementia. Thus, the benefits of CPAP therapy may include both amelioration of existing cognitive deficits and prevention of future cognitive decline.

Main points

Unaddressed sleep apnea can mimic neurodegenerative disease and lead to unnecessary evaluation and treatment. A sleep history is an important part of the assessment of cognitive complaints.

FURTHER READING

Aloia MS, Zimmerman ME. Sleep-disordered breathing and cognition in older adults. *Curr Neurol Neurosci Rep* 2012;**12**:537–46.

Matthews EE, Aloia MS. Cognitive recovery following positive airway pressure (PAP) in sleep apnea. In Van Dongen HPA, Kerkhof GA, eds. *Progress in Brain Research*. Amsterdam: Elsevier BV;2011, pp. 71–88.

REFERENCES

1. Antonelli Incalzi R, Marra C, Salvigni BL, et al. Does cognitive dysfunction conform to a distinctive pattern in obstructive sleep apnea syndrome? *J Sleep Res* 2004; **13**:79–86.
2. Beebe DW, Groesz L, Wells C, et al. The neuropsychological effects of obstructive sleep apnea: a meta-analysis of norm-referenced and case-controlled data. *Sleep* 2003;**26**:298–307.
3. Powell NB, Riley RW, Schechtman KB, et al. A comparative model: reaction time performance in sleep-disordered breathing versus alcohol-impaired controls. *Laryngoscope* 1999;**109**:1648–54.
4. Aloia MS, Arnedt JT, Davis JD, et al. Neuropsychological sequelae of obstructive sleep apnea–hypopnea syndrome: a critical review. *J Int Neuropsychol Soc* 2004;**10**:772–85.
5. Kylstra WA, Aaronson JA, Hofman WF, et al. Neuropsychological functioning after CPAP treatment in obstructive sleep apnea: a meta-analysis. *Sleep Med Rev* 2013;**17**:341–7.
6. Kushida CA, Nichols DA, Holmes TH, et al. Effects of continuous positive airway pressure on neurocognitive function in obstructive sleep apnea patients: the Apnea Postive Pressure Long-term Efficacy Study (APPLES). *Sleep* 2012;**35**:1593–602.
7. Yaffe K, Laffan AM, Harrison SL, et al. Sleep-disordered breathing, hypoxia, and risk of mild cognitive impairment and dementia in older women. *JAMA* 2011;**306**:613–19.

56

Obstructive sleep apnea can present with symptoms and findings unique to older age

John J. Harrington

An 81-year-old woman was referred to the sleep medicine clinic by her cardiologist. She has a history of hypertension, paroxysmal atrial fibrillation, hypothyroidism, and dyslipidemia. Intermittent atrial fibrillation often presented as distressing palpitations that could lead to a bedridden state two or three times per month. The patient denied previous diagnostic testing for a sleep disorder and was otherwise generally a healthy and active community-dwelling older woman. Due to reported snoring and the severity and frequency of her recurrent dysrhythmia, and its potential association with occult obstructive sleep apnea (OSA), further consultation was sought.

The patient's sleep–wake routine and reported sleep hygiene were unremarkable. Prior to going to bed she sometimes watched television or played the piano. Her bedroom environment was described as comfortable and her only in-bed activity was a short period of reading, which she found relaxing, just prior to turning her lights out. She was married but her husband slept in another bedroom. Her sleep schedule was not advanced and included going to bed at approximately 11:00 PM and sleeping until 7:00 AM. Her sleep latency was usually under 30 minutes in duration, but the remainder of her nighttime sleep was remarkable for recurrent, transient awakenings. On arising in the morning, more often than not, she described her sleep as unrefreshing. She also complained of mild to moderate sleepiness during the day and often dozed during passive activities. She regularly took short naps in the early afternoon.

What other clinical history information was useful?

She described mild to moderate daytime sleepiness, but on completing a subsequent Epworth Sleepiness Scale (ESS) her score was only 6 out of 24, not suggestive of excessive subjective sleepiness. This discrepancy in these subjective measures of sleepiness is not altogether surprising. In fact, a recent study of older adults by Onen and colleagues found that nearly 60% of participants were unable to answer at least one item on the ESS, and even though all reported excessive daytime sleepiness, only 24% had scores consistent with this complaint (i.e. ESS score > 10).

On further questioning regarding her repeated nighttime awakenings, for which she denied any specific precipitant, she mentioned that during most of these events she would need to urinate prior to falling back to sleep. She did report some mild snoring but did not endorse frequent or loud snoring, gasping arousals, or witnessed apneas.

What were important findings on physical examination?

The patient was normotensive and had a low but regular resting heart rate, consistent with beta-adrenergic blockade. She showed a normal weight with a body mass index (BMI) of 25 kg/m^2. Her oropharyngeal airway was not notably crowded, and she

Common Pitfalls in Sleep Medicine, ed. Ronald D. Chervin. Published by Cambridge University Press. © Cambridge University Press 2014.

had a modified Mallampati Classification grade of II. This is a modification of a visual scoring system first developed to predict difficult endotracheal intubation, and is similarly used as a screening tool for OSA. The modified Mallampati Classification system is a grading system of I–IV, with Classification I representing clear visibility of anatomic oropharyngeal structures (e.g. tonsils, pillars, and soft palate) and Classification IV representing the absence of visibility of these structures.

What diagnostic testing was conducted?

Due to the severity of her noted tachyarrhythmia (which is listed as a "Guideline" for polysomnographic testing by the American Academy of Sleep Medicine) as well as her symptoms of snoring, recurrent nocturnal awakenings with nocturia, unrefreshing sleep, and daytime sleepiness, a baseline polysomnogram in a sleep laboratory was ordered.

She slept for 283 minutes and her sleep efficiency was 87%. Her sleep architecture revealed an absence of N3 sleep and an arousal index of 23 per hour of sleep. She was noted to have OSA with an apnea/hypopnea index (AHI, events per hour of sleep) of 16. These respiratory events occurred more often in non-rapid eye movement (REM) sleep than in REM sleep, and both apneas and hypopneas were equally common. The minimum oxygen saturation was 80%. There were infrequent periodic limb movements. A subsequent continuous positive airway pressure (CPAP) titration study established that a pressure of 7 cm of water optimally controlled her sleep apnea and resulted in an AHI of 0.5 per hour, with normal oxygen saturation.

Discussion

The population of the United States is rapidly aging. In 2009, the percentage of those individuals aged 65 years and older was approximately 13%. By 2030, this age group is expected to comprise 19% of the US population, or 72 million persons. The consequences of these demographic changes will have an important influence on the burden of chronic diseases, including primary sleep disorders.

Reports of sleep difficulty are exceedingly common among older adults. Problems arise from a variety of reasons, including primary sleep disorders and comorbidities frequently noted in this population. These complaints are not necessarily related to aging. Older adults may report sleep impairment because of illness (cardiovascular disease, chronic pain syndromes, mood disorders, and cognitive impairment), frailty, retirement, and poor sleep hygiene. The latter may include decreases in sunlight exposure, decreased physical activity, and frequent napping.

Obstructive sleep apnea, which was identified in this woman, is frequently present in older adults but not always diagnosed. Multiple longitudinal and cross-sectional studies have consistently demonstrated an increased prevalence of sleep-disordered breathing with increasing age. Regardless of what definition of OSA is used, the prevalence estimates of this disorder are significantly higher among the elderly compared to middle-age populations.

Risk factors for OSA in the elderly can differ from those in younger patients. For instance, the importance of obesity markers as predictors of OSA in middle-aged persons is considerably diminished in older adults. Nearly half of older persons with OSA have normal BMIs. However, among obesity-related variables, BMI remains a significant determinant of OSA severity among elderly persons.

The consequences of OSA in older adults also may differ from those in younger age groups. Increased mortality for instance is noted in younger adults with OSA but this has not been demonstrated in the elderly. Postulated reasons for this include less severe OSA, a survival effect, or possibly ischemic preconditioning. Other potential manifestations of OSA, such as nocturia, cognitive impairment, and cardiac arrhythmias – at least two of which are noted in the above clinical vignette – are reported more frequently in older adults. Subjective and objective measures of daytime sleepiness are significantly decreased in older adults, despite more disturbed nighttime sleep, but are important to assess. Subjective symptoms of poor sleep quality and daytime sleepiness in this population are associated with declining quality of life, and poor sleep quality is associated with increased frailty.

The classic symptoms of OSA, namely loud snoring, witnessed apneas, and daytime sleepiness, may be reported less often by older persons than by middle-aged persons. These symptoms may indeed occur less often, or this finding may arise due to the absence of a bed partner, or a bed partner with intact hearing and cognition necessary to monitor for these symptoms. For these reasons, providers should maintain an increased level of suspicion of OSA when potentially related symptoms, such as nocturia, are reported.

Nocturia is commonly ascribed to bladder problems but it is particularly prevalent and bothersome in patients who, likes ours, has OSA. A proposed mechanism for nocturia in sleep-disordered breathing is thought to be related to right-sided cardiac distention due to increased negative intrathoracic pressures. This leads to subsequent release of arterial natriuretic peptide and inhibition of antidiuretic hormone and aldosterone. This may lead to right-sided cardiac distention and subsequent release of atrial natriuretic peptide. In one small study, a majority of older women with nocturia had evidence of OSA, and diluted nighttime urine appeared to be a sensitive marker for sleep-disordered breathing.

The presence of atrial fibrillation is commonly associated with both advancing age and OSA. In one study, subjects with severe sleep-disordered breathing had significantly increased odds of serious cardiac arrhythmias (c.g. atrial fibrillation and non-sustained ventricular tachycardia) than controls even after controlling for potential confounders. Among these arrhythmias, atrial fibrillation is the most strongly associated with sleep-disordered breathing. Further, the presence of untreated sleep apnea is associated with a higher recurrence of atrial fibrillation after cardioversion.

How increasing age contributes to the pathogenesis of OSA remains unclear. The importance of gender as a risk factor of OSA is lost after about the age of 50 years as women go through menopause. The contribution of obesity as a risk factor for OSA increases until the age of 60 years and then decreases thereafter. Proposed anatomic and physiologic factors that

may increase the prevalence of OSA in older adults include lengthening of the soft palate, increased parapharyngeal fat pad size independent of BMI, lower lung volumes, diminished genioglossus negative pressure reflex, and decreased chemosensitivity to hypoxia and hypercapnia.

Compared to polysomnographic findings among younger patients with OSA, sleep studies of older adults tend to show decreased AHI, reduced AHI during REM sleep, prolongation of respiratory events with increased proportion of frank apneas, reduced snoring, and better preserved oxygen saturation. Diminished chemosensitivity along with increased upper airway collapsibility may be explanations for reduced respiratory event-related arousability and increased apnea percentage, respectively. The reduction in apneic events in stage REM sleep may be related to increased upper airway collapsibility that lessens the relative contribution of atonia in stage REM sleep. Other discordant sleep measures include decreased total sleep time, sleep efficiency, increased wake time during sleep, and increased number of awakenings compared to the younger groups.

Treatment options for OSA typically include positive airway pressure, mandibular advancement devices, and surgery. Mandibular advancement may be problematic in older persons due to poor dentition, and surgery has obvious associated risks. Continuous positive airway pressure is usually the treatment of choice for OSA regardless of age. This therapy provides air pressure to the upper airway and acts as a pneumatic splint. As was noted in this patient, relatively modest CPAP adequately treated her OSA, and reduced her AHI, snoring, and oxygen saturation. Continuous positive airway pressure requirements tend to be lower in older patients than in younger patients and may reflect differences in respiratory anatomy and physiology.

Other beneficial effects of CPAP therapy in older adults are less well known because effectiveness studies generally focus on younger subjects. That said, some studies that included older adults demonstrated improvements in cognition, cardiovascular function, and nocturia following CPAP therapy. Continuous positive airway pressure therapy has been noted to be superior when compared to conservative therapy in improving subjective, but not objective, measures of sleepiness in older adults. Limited evidence supports the role of CPAP in improving complaints of snoring and witnessed apneas in older patients. Although CPAP therapy may reduce nighttime urination, no controlled studies have evaluated this outcome.

Non-adherence to CPAP therapy is problematic for all age groups and age alone does not appear to alter compliance. Factors likely to contribute to CPAP non-adherence in older adults may include cognitive impairment, other medical comorbidities, altered manual dexterity, nocturia, and minimal partner support. Important predictors of CPAP non-adherence in older adults are nocturia, current cigarette smoking, symptom persistence, and advanced age at diagnosis. Improvements in CPAP adherence with behavioral intervention have been demonstrated in this population. In a study conducted by Aloia and colleagues, an intervention was evaluated to improve CPAP adherence in an older population. The experimental group underwent two intervention sessions, the first of which educated participants regarding the severity of their sleep apnea, efficacy of CPAP therapy (based on a titration study), and symptoms (including neurobehavioral performance). A subsequent session provided subjects with information on their personal CPAP adherence, assessed changes noticed on CPAP therapy, and individually addressed obstacles while on CPAP therapy. These participants were compared with a control group (matched for education, age, and disease severity). Although adherence was similar in both groups early in follow-up, at 12 weeks, the intervention group demonstrated a significant increase (3.2 hours/night) in adherence.

The patient described above was prescribed CPAP therapy. She had some initial difficulties tolerating CPAP but with a change in CPAP mask (nasal to full face mask), along with the addition of pressure relief on expiration, her adherence was excellent. After instituting nightly CPAP therapy, she reported much less sleepiness (ESS score decreasing from 6 to 1), decreased nocturia, and a feeling of more refreshing sleep upon awakening. Unfortunately, she continued to report occasional episodes of bothersome paroxysmal atrial fibrillation despite medical therapy, and was referred for an electrophysiology consultation.

Main points

Obstructive sleep apnea is common among older adults. Characteristic symptoms of OSA in this population may vary considerably from those of younger adults, as may results of subjective and objective testing, and treatment. Patients should be assured that effective treatments for sleep apnea are available and well tolerated.

FURTHER READING

Aloia MS, Dio LD, Ilniczky N, et al. Improving compliance with nasal CPAP and vigilance in older adults with OSAHS. *Sleep Breath* 2001;**5**:13–22.

Chung S, Yoon IY, Lee CH, et al. Effects of age on the clinical features of men with obstructive sleep apnea syndrome. *Respiration* 2009;**78**:23–9.

Eikermann M, Jordan AS, Chamberlin NL, et al. The influence of aging on pharyngeal collapsibility during sleep. *Chest* 2007;**131**:1702–9.

Mehra R, Stone KL, Blackwell T, et al. Osteoporotic fractures in men study prevalence and correlates of sleep-disordered breathing in older men: osteoporotic fractures in men sleep study. *J Am Geriatr Soc* 2007;**55**:1356–64.

Onen F, Moreau T, Gooneratne NS, et al. Limits of the Epworth Sleepiness Scale in older adults. *Sleep Breath* 2013;**17**:343–50.

Phillips BA. Obstructive sleep apnea in the elderly. In Kryger M, Roth T, Dement W, eds. *Principles and Practice of Sleep Medicine*, Fifth Edition, online. St Louis, MO: Elsevier;2011, Chap. 134.

Weaver TE, Chasens E. Continuous positive airway pressure treatment for sleep apnea in older adults. *Sleep Med Rev* 2007;**11**:99–111.

57

Delirium and sundowning in older persons: a sleep perspective

Mihai C. Teodorescu

Case

You are caring for Mr. D., an 80-year-old man who lives independently with his wife. He presented at the prompting of his wife with strange behaviors in the evenings and at night. He says that he has reluctantly agreed to come in for an assessment. He himself denies problems with memory, which he considers to be normal for his age.

His wife describes that for the past few weeks there are stretches of several evenings in a row when he appears quite disoriented and restless. His wife describes him suddenly yelling and punching in the air when in bed waiting to fall asleep. He has knocked over the bedside lamp and twice struck his wife, so she decided to sleep in a nearby twin bed. About 3 days prior to his clinic visit, in the evening, he told his wife that he was "trying to catch a thief." As he reached over to "grab the villain," he fell to the ground. He found himself on the floor. His wife reports that when these episodes are occurring she ends up sleeping in another room. For the past couple of days, though, he remained calm and pleasant in the evenings, and appeared to his wife "back to usual self."

The patient reports that since he is "retired" there is no "pressing need to follow a schedule." He goes to bed between 10:00 PM and 12:00 AM, "when he feels tired." He sleeps as late as 8:00–10:00 AM in the morning, depending on "how well he slept that night" since "I don't have to go to work." During the day he often spends most of his time in a chair watching television, mainly sports. However, he dozes off in front of

the television multiple times during the day. These episodes may add to 1–2 hours of sleep during the day.

Past medical history does include loss of short-term memory, word-finding problems, and difficulty following directions. These problems began about 3 years ago and have progressed gradually since then. Over the last couple of years, Mrs. D. also had to step in to balance their checkbook and manage their household finances, tasks that he managed without problems over the previous 45 years of his married life. He now requires assistance when taking his medications and supervision with many of the household chores. He appears anxious whenever left alone and has grown emotionally dependent on his wife.

He has a 10-year history of hypertension treated with metoprolol 100 mg twice daily and felodipine 5 mg daily, coronary artery bypass graft in 1990, and depression, treated with fluoxetine 40 mg daily. He has no history of epilepsy. On review of symptoms, he does occasionally report to his wife visual hallucinations. He has no history of falls, but walking is getting to be slower and somewhat unstable.

Clinical examination reveals an alert and comfortable male. He is mildly obese. Blood pressure is 150/70 mmHg lying and 135/60 mmHg standing. Heart exam reveals a regular rhythm with a pulse rate of 80 per minute. He scores 15 out of 30 on a Mini-Mental State Examination (MMSE) and fails the clock-drawing test. He scores 4 out of 15 on the Geriatric Depression Scale. Neurologic examination demonstrates mild cogwheeling and some slowness in movements. The rest of the physical examination is unremarkable.

Routine biochemistry, including blood glucose and hematology tests all show results that are within normal ranges. An electroencephalogram is normal. Computed tomography scans of his head show minimal white-matter changes and no large-vessel or lacunar infarcts.

What is the etiology of Mr. D.'s behavior disturbances?

This patient has probable dementia with Lewy bodies (DLB) according to consensus criteria.[1] Dementia with Lewy bodies is part of the Lewy body spectrum of disorders, in which the clinical presentation varies according to the site of most impactful neuronal loss related to Lewy body formation. In the case of DLB, the limbic cerebral cortex appears to be the primary site involved. Dementia with Lewy bodies does share with Alzheimer's dementia (AD) the features of beta-amyloidosis, senile plaque formation, and cholinergic deficits; however, deficits involving dopamine pathways are thought to be much greater in DLB, resembling Parkinson's disease more than AD.

In DLB, cognitive and functional impairments include visual hallucinations and delusions, parkinsonian features with bradykinesia and rigidity, fluctuating consciousness, and repeated falls. Dementia with Lewy bodies is associated with abnormal control of consciousness throughout the day with fluctuations in arousal and alertness, thought to be related to the subcortical and cortical cholinergic deficits. Alteration in cholinergic activity may underlie the fluctuating level of consciousness observed in about 80% of these patients.[2] Visual hallucinations may be quite common in DLB patients (up to half of patients) while auditory hallucinations may occur in 20%. Dementia with Lewy bodies patients have higher levels of sleepiness and sleep disturbance compared with AD patients and specifically have more abnormalities in control of movements, as reflected for example by periodic limb movements; more bad dreams; and more confusion on waking.[3]

According to his wife, who is his primary caregiver, this patient's agitated and restless behavior is noted predominantly in the evening in a recurrent pattern. No acute precipitating medical condition or drug could be attributed as the cause for his behaviors. This is most consistent with sundowning. Sundowning – the recurring onset of confusion or agitation in some elderly patients in the evening – can constitute a significant clinical problem.[4] Although variability in the peak time of behavioral disruption has been reported, the maximal behavioral disruption most commonly is temporally localized to the later afternoon or evening. Although sundowning is reported to occur in a quarter to a third of AD patients, the prevalence of sundowning in LBD patients is less clear. In an institutionalized population of 30 patients with dementia, there were 8 sundowners, 5 with a diagnosis of probable AD and 1 with LBD.[5] There was a strong association with restlessness and disrupted sleep.[5] In community-dwelling patients, sundowning is associated with significant caregiver stress,[6] likely contributing to an increased risk of institutionalization. Sundowning ranks second, only to wandering, for disruptive behaviors among institutionalized patients.[7]

Sundowning shares similarities with delirium, e.g. attention deficits and activity disturbances, and occurs on a background of cognitive impairment.[7] However, sundowning episodes in comparison to delirium are spread over a longer period of time, have a predictable tendency to occur at specific times of the day (linked to a 24-hour cycle), and may not include phenomenology as severe as those that occur in delirium. Clinical studies have confirmed the temporal occurrence late in the day of the common behaviors of restlessness and increased levels of confusion that characterize sundowning.[8]

Pathogenesis

The pathogenesis of delirium and that of sundowning are not well understood. States of global cognitive dysfunction such as delirium and sundowning are characterized by variable degrees of attention deficit, disorganized thinking, and variable levels of consciousness as well as disorganized patterns of sleep. Sleep is commonly disturbed in delirious and sundowning patients. Researchers are still trying to understand whether a causal link exists between these syndromes and sleep disturbance, or whether the associations with sleep problems result from shared mechanisms.[9] It is likely that the relationship between these states and sleep is bi-directional. Sleep disturbances may be modifiable risk factors in their pathogenesis, but at the same time sleep is likely influenced by their presence.

Normal sleep is characterized by a circadian rhythm and a structured progression through the sleep stages. Patients with dementia, however, tend to have an increased amount of sleep fragmentation with lower sleep efficiency, increased stage N1 sleep, and decreased stage N3 sleep. Expected awake time is characterized by increased daytime sleepiness and napping.[10] Furthermore, patients with DLB in comparison to those with AD tend to have a higher index of disturbed sleep, more movements while asleep, and more abnormal daytime sleepiness.[11]

Circadian rhythms are disrupted in dementia and may play an important role in the pathogenesis of sundowning.[10] Lewy body dementia patients show marked loss of Nucleus Basalis Meynert (NBM) large cholinergic neurons (75–80%) in conjunction with reduced cholinergic activity in the reticular thalamic nucleus leading to hallucinations and fluctuating consciousness.[10] These individuals have decreased activity of the suprachiasmatic nuclei (SCN) and decreased synthesis of melatonin, with eventual disappearance of the circadian melatonin rhythm. Serotonin also appears to show stepwise depletion during the course of the dementia.[12]

External factors may accentuate neurologic vulnerabilities. For example, *zeitgeber* timing and exposure may become more problematic. Patients with dementia tend to have lower exposure to light during the day.[13] As dementia progresses, it may be associated with lower activity levels and more phase delay.[13] In AD, for example, patients have greater motor activity during the nighttime, a phase delay averaging 2 hours, as well as an attenuation of motor activity circadian rhythm compared with healthy elderly patients.[14]

Increases in patient's fatigue, excessive environmental stimulation, and changes in caregiver environment (fatigue, caregiver change, lower caregiver availability) are also reported to contribute to sundowning.[7] For community-based patients, caregiver stress and burnout may lead to conflicts, frustration, and distress that increase the likelihood of sundowning. In the case of institutionalized patients, an increase in the number of patients a caregiver has to care for can diminish the intensity of structured stimulation for patients, increase boredom, and lead to agitation and restlessness.[7]

Uncontrolled medical and psychiatric symptoms that have a circadian rhythm may also contribute to sundowning. Examples can include pain, hunger, and anxiety symptoms. Medications may have anticholinergic effects or induce restlessness. They also may inappropriately change the level of alertness, augmenting sedation during the daytime or excessive alertness during the night. Certain medications used for behavioral changes associated with dementia, such as benzodiazepines (e.g. lorazepam), may actually induce paradoxical agitation, worsen behavioral disinhibition, or increase confusion in certain patients.

Delirium is usually a multifactorial syndrome, rather than one that is triggered by a single factor. Delirium results from the interaction of vulnerability on the part of the patient – as defined by predisposing conditions, such as cognitive impairment, severe illness, or visual impairment – and hospital-related insults such as medications and procedures. A neurotransmitter imbalance between dopamine and acetylcholine is suspected;[9] levels of acetylcholine may be low while those of dopamine are high. Acute changes in medical condition, sleep habits, use of sedatives and other medications, environmental noise, and artificial light can be listed among the main triggers of delirium. An association has been shown between sleep disturbances and the number of chronic diseases, the presence of pain, use of tricyclic antidepressants, and the length of hospital stay.[15]

Medications may increase the propensity for delirium and sundowning. Some of these effects may be mediated by neural circuits underlying both sleep and delirium mechanisms. Benzodiazepines may further weaken the already vulnerable sleep–wake cycle.[10] Benzodiazepines are strong independent risk factors for the development of delirium. These medications adversely affect sleep architecture by decreasing slow-wave sleep and also rapid eye movement sleep.[16] Medications with anticholinergic properties are associated with worse cognitive performance and an increased risk for delirium.[17]

Assessment tools

The increased restlessness that accompanies sundowning or delirium can be confirmed by objective measures of activity using actigraphy.[18] The device can register movement data in minute epochs via the use of a linear accelerometer, and is usually placed on the patient's non-dominant arm for a number of consecutive days. Some models also record light exposure levels.

Actigraphy helps identify periods of increased behavioral disturbance. When physical agitation is present, verbal agitation is most likely also present.[19] Actigraphy allows differentiation between different patterns of increased agitation, such as "weaker agitation rhythms" (having low-grade agitation throughout the 24 hours) as compared to rhythmic periods of agitation and quietness, which tend to show peak agitation in the afternoon.

Recorded actigraphic data allow comparison of daytime activity levels (for example, from 8:00 AM to 4:00 PM) or evening activity levels (e.g. from 4:00 PM to 12:00 AM) to averaged 24-hour activity. Data also allow calculation of the mean time of peak daily activity, which in sundowning patients is likely to occur in the evenings.[18]

Problems of sundowning, delirium, and related sleep disturbance in dementia are a significant cause of distress to caregivers. Agitation is most disruptive to caregivers in the evening hours when the caregivers themselves are tired. In institutional settings, the staff-to-patient ratio is lower during evening and night hours compared to the regular work day hours, and agitation in the evening may be perceived as more disruptive.[19]

Moderate to severe distress was found in 16 out of 17 caregivers for patients with DLB in one study.

Interventions

Confusional states, particularly when associated with increased motor activity, are a significant source of morbidity and mortality as well as caregiver stress and burnout. Caregiver support, such as providing respite care (tailored to individual caregiver needs), and multicomponent interventions directed toward the caregiver (or combined with the patient), can improve caregiver psychosocial health and may diminish need for institutionalization among dementia patients.[20]

A behavioral approach should be always considered as an initial step in managing a patient's symptoms. An algorithm named Treatment Routes for Exploring Agitation (TREA) has been proposed that may provide a systematic methodology for individualizing non-pharmacologic interventions to the unmet needs of the affected patient.[21] The first step toward developing an individualized treatment plan is to attempt to understand the etiology of the agitated behavior. A decision tree protocol can be used while capitalizing on preserved abilities of the affected patient and accounting for deficits, especially those related to sensory perception, cognition, and mobility. Individual past experiences and preferences such as past work, hobbies, important relationships, and sense of identity, may be used to tailor treatment. Accommodation and flexibility are essential elements of intervention.

The spectrum of interventions may include individualized music, family videotapes and pictures, illustrated reading materials, games, toys, employment of massage, pain treatment, and trips. Activities need to be meaningful to the patient, can be easily administered and match the affected individual's level of functioning. Implementation of TREA in a group of 89 nursing home residents in comparison to controls improved agitation, and increased pleasure and interest.[21]

The Hospital Elder Life Program delirium intervention strategy targeted six risk factors (dehydration, sleep deprivation, immobility, visual impairment,

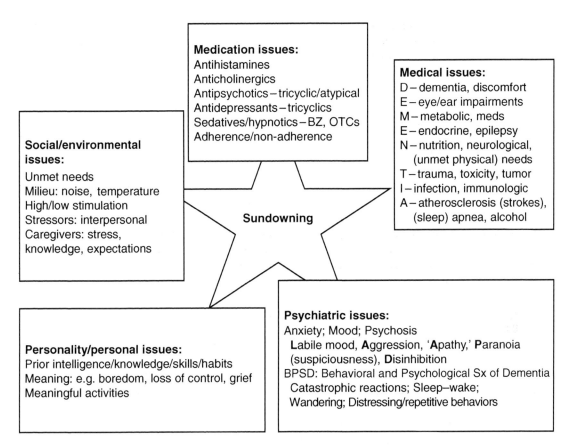

Medication issues:
Antihistamines
Anticholinergics
Antipsychotics – tricyclic/atypical
Antidepressants – tricyclics
Sedatives/hypnotics – BZ, OTCs
Adherence/non-adherence

Medical issues:
D – dementia, discomfort
E – eye/ear impairments
M – metabolic, meds
E – endocrine, epilepsy
N – nutrition, neurological,
　(unmet physical) needs
T – trauma, toxicity, tumor
I – infection, immunologic
A – atherosclerosis (strokes),
　(sleep) apnea, alcohol

Social/environmental issues:
Unmet needs
Milieu: noise, temperature
High/low stimulation
Stressors: interpersonal
Caregivers: stress,
knowledge, expectations

Sundowning

Personality/personal issues:
Prior intelligence/knowledge/skills/habits
Meaning: e.g. boredom, loss of control, grief
Meaningful activities

Psychiatric issues:
Anxiety; Mood; Psychosis
　Labile mood, **A**ggression, '**A**pathy,' **P**aranoia
　(suspiciousness), **D**isinhibition
BPSD: Behavioral and Psychological Sx of Dementia
　Catastrophic reactions; Sleep–wake;
　Wandering; Distressing/repetitive behaviors

Figure 57.1 Sundowning.

cognitive impairment and hearing impairment) at the time of hospital admission.[22] For example, in regard to sleep factors, non-pharmacologic interventions included providing a warm drink (milk or herbal tea) at bedtime, relaxation tapes or music, and back massage. Other strategies included noise-reduction (e.g. silenced pill crushers and beepers, reduced noise in the hallways) and re-scheduled medical care to allow sleep (e.g. timing of medications and procedures).[22] These interventions reduced the number and duration of episodes of delirium, and also the rate of use of sleep medications.

Patients with DLB appear to be particularly sensitive to anticholinergic agents due to their marked cholinergic deficiency.[10] In fact, autopsies of patients who responded well to agents that increased acetylcholine availability showed DLB rather than AD as the etiology for their dementia. Acetyl cholinesterase inhibitors may therefore be quite useful. Improvement in sundowning in a patient with DLB after treatment with donepezil, a cholinesterase inhibitor, has been reported.[18] In another study, a small subgroup treated with rivastigmine was noted to have a reduction in both the Epworth Sleepiness Scale and the Pittsburgh sleep quality index scores, and less troublesome nighttime behaviors such as "bad dreams," periodic limb movements, and confusion on waking.[23]

In regard to medications that should be avoided in DLB patients, besides anticholinergic agents, antipsychotic medications should be very carefully considered, if they are to be used at all. Although they are employed with relative benefits in delirious states

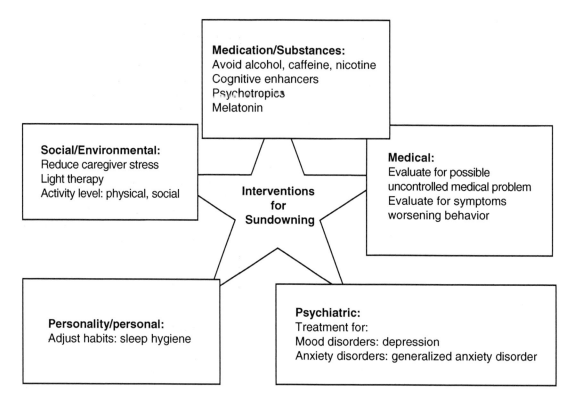

Figure 57.2 Interventions for sundowning.

and symptom management in other dementias, in the case of DLB patients severe neuroleptic sensitivity reactions in up to half of patients can lead to worsening parkinsonism, affect consciousness levels, and induce autonomic disturbances similar to those noted in neuroleptic malignant syndrome, resulting in increased mortality. These effects are thought to be mediated by an acute blockade of D2 receptors.

Other interventions can target the inadequate influence of external *zeitgebers*, such as irregular or reduced light exposure, meals, social interactions, and physical activity. Effects of light therapy on cognition, function, sleep, behavioral disturbances, and psychiatric disturbances associated with dementia were reported to be of unclear benefit in a Cochrane review.[24] The nonsignificant results may have been related to small sample sizes that contribute to insufficient power to detect a difference, if one is present. Differences in

severity of dementia may have also influenced results. The best time of day to offer light therapy remains unknown. Nonetheless, light therapy is generally well tolerated. A multimodel approach is probably best. In a randomized, controlled trial of patients with dementia and their family caregivers, behavioral techniques – specifically sleep hygiene education, daily walking, and increased light exposure – were shown to improve sleep.[25]

Studies of melatonin have shown mixed results. In a randomized, placebo controlled study of nursing home subjects, melatonin administered at 10:00 PM for 10 consecutive nights produced no beneficial effects for sleep, circadian rhythms, or agitation.[26] However, in an open-label study that employed actigraphy, use of melatonin (3 mg) every evening for 3 weeks by community-based patients with day–night rhythm disturbances or sundowning was well tolerated and was associated with complete remission in 4 out of 7 patients.[27] A significant decrease in sundowning was also reported in another study of 11 nursing home patients.[28] A recently published Cochrane meta-analysis of melatonin use in dementia showed significant improvement in psychopathological behavior as reflected by the Alzheimer's Disease Assessment Scale – Non-cognitive (ADAS-NC) and the Neuropsychiatric Inventory (NPI).[29] While the meta-analysis did not support the use of melatonin for treatment of cognitive impairment associated with dementia, the authors did find that melatonin treatment may be effective for other dementia-related disturbances.

Main points

Older, demented patients are at risk for delirium and also sundowning (Figure 57.1), which can create major challenges for caregivers as well. Both conditions can have multiple causes and triggers, which must be dissected within the context of a complete history, examination, review of medications, and additional testing if no cause for dementia has yet been established. Treatment can similarly involve a multipronged approach that includes behavioral intervention, minimization offending environmental and pharmacologic triggers, consideration for use of melatonin, and assistance for caregivers (Figure 57.2).

REFERENCES

1. McKeith IG, Perry EK, Perry RH. Report of the second dementia with Lewy body international workshop: diagnosis and treatment. Consortium on Dementia with Lewy Bodies. *Neurology* 1999;**53**:902–5.
2. Byrne J. Lewy body dementia. *J Royal Soc Med* 1997;**90** (Suppl 32):14–15.
3. Bliwise DL, Mercaldo ND, Avidan AY, et al. Sleep disturbance in dementia with Lewy bodies and Alzheimer's disease: a multicenter analysis. *Dement Geriatr Cogn Disord* 2011;**31**:239–46.
4. Bliwise DL. What is sundowning? *J Am Geriatr Soc* 1994;**42**:1009–11.
5. Lebert F, Pasquier F, Petit H. Sundowning syndrome in demented patients without neuroleptic therapy. *Arch Gerontol Geriatr* 1996;**22**:49–54.
6. Gallagher-Thompson D, Brooks JO, 3rd, Bliwise D, Leader J, Yesavage JA. The relations among caregiver stress, "sundowning" symptoms, and cognitive decline in Alzheimer's disease. *J Am Geriatr Soc* 1992;**40**:807–10.
7. Khachiyants N, Trinkle D, Son SJ, Kim KY. Sundown syndrome in persons with dementia: an update. *Psychiatry Investig* 2011;**8**:275–87.
8. Evans LK. Sundown syndrome in institutionalized elderly. *J Am Geriatr Soc* 1987;**35**:101–8.
9. Watson PL, Ceriana P, Fanfulla F. Delirium: is sleep important? *Best Pract Res Clin Anaesthesiol* 2012;**26**:355–66.
10. Klaffke S, Staedt J. Sundowning and circadian rhythm disorders in dementia. *Acta Neurol Belg* 2006;**106**:168–75.
11. Grace JB, Walker MP, McKeith IG. A comparison of sleep profiles in patients with dementia with lewy bodies and Alzheimer's disease. *Int J Geriatr Psychiatry* 2000;**15**:1028–33.
12. Wu YH, Feenstra MG, Zhou JN, et al. Molecular changes underlying reduced pineal melatonin levels in Alzheimer disease: alterations in preclinical and clinical stages. *J Clin Endocrinol Metab* 2003;**88**:5898–906.
13. Ancoli-Israel S, Klauber MR, Jones DW, et al. Variations in circadian rhythms of activity, sleep, and light exposure related to dementia in nursing-home patients. *Sleep* 1997;**20**:18–23.
14. Satlin A, Teicher MH, Lieberman HR, et al. Circadian locomotor activity rhythms in Alzheimer's disease. *Neuropsychopharmacology* 1991;**5**:115–26.
15. Frighetto L, Marra C, Bandali S, et al. An assessment of quality of sleep and the use of drugs with sedating properties in hospitalized adult patients. *Health Qual Life Outcomes* 2004;**2**:17.
16. Trompeo AC, Vidi Y, Locane MD, et al. Sleep disturbances in the critically ill patients: role of delirium and sedative agents. *Minerva Anesthesiol* 2011;**77**:604–12.
17. Khan BA, Zawahiri M, Campbell NL, et al. Delirium in hospitalized patients: implications of current evidence on clinical practice and future avenues for research – a systematic evidence review. *J Hosp Med* 2012;**7**:580–9.
18. Skjerve A, Nygaard HA. Improvement in sundowning in dementia with Lewy bodies after treatment with donepezil. *Int J Geriatr Psychiatry* 2000;**15**:1147–51.
19. Martin J, Marler M, Shochat T, Ancoli-Israel S. Circadian rhythms of agitation in institutionalized patients with Alzheimer's disease. *Chronobiol Int* 2000;**17**:405–18.

20. Caregiver- and patient-directed interventions for dementia: an evidence-based analysis. *Ont Health Technol Assess Ser* 2008;**8**:1–98.

21. Cohen-Mansfield J, Thein K, Marx MS, Dakheel-Ali M, Freedman L. Efficacy of nonpharmacologic interventions for agitation in advanced dementia: a randomized, placebo-controlled trial. *J Clin Psychiatry* 2012;**73**:1255–61.

22. Inouye SK, Bogardus ST, Jr., Charpentier PA, et al. A multicomponent intervention to prevent delirium in hospitalized older patients. *N Engl J Med* 1999;**340**:669–76.

23. Grace JB, Walker MP, McKeith IG. A comparison of sleep profiles in patients with dementia with Lewy bodies and Alzheimer's disease. *Int J Geriatr Psychiatry* 2000;**15**:1028–33.

24. Forbes D, Culum I, Lischka AR, et al. Light therapy for managing cognitive, sleep, functional, behavioural, or psychiatric disturbances in dementia. *Cochrane Database Syst Rev* 2009:CD003946.

25. McCurry SM, Gibbons LE, Logsdon RG, Vitiello MV, Teri L. Nighttime insomnia treatment and education for Alzheimer's disease: a randomized, controlled trial. *J Am Geriatr Soc* 2005;**53**:793–802.

26. Gehrman PR, Connor DJ, Martin JL, et al. Melatonin fails to improve sleep or agitation in double-blind randomized placebo-controlled trial of institutionalized patients with Alzheimer disease. *Am J Geriatr Psychiatry* 2009;**17**:166–9.

27. Mahlberg R, Kunz D, Sutej I, Kuhl KP, Hellweg R. Melatonin treatment of day-night rhythm disturbances and sundowning in Alzheimer disease: an open-label pilot study using actigraphy. *J Clin Psychopharmacol* 2004;**24**:456–9.

28. Cohen-Mansfield J, Garfinkel D, Lipson S. Melatonin for treatment of sundowning in elderly persons with dementia – a preliminary study. *Arch Gerontol Geriatr* 2000;**31**:65–76.

29. Jansen SL, Duncan V, Morgan DG, Malouf R. Melatonin for the treatment of dementia. *Cochrane Database Syst Rev* 2006:CD003802.

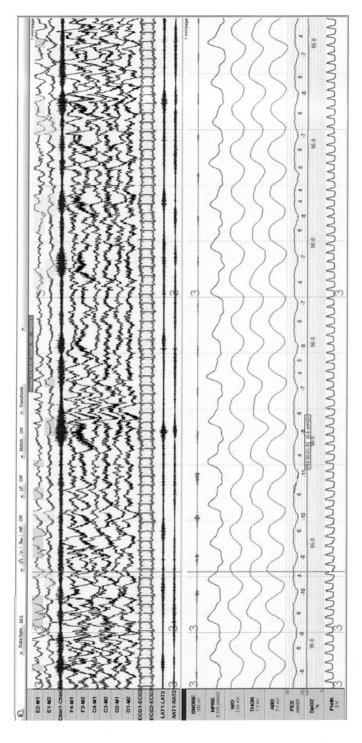

Figure 2.1 Baseline polysomnogram with esophageal pressure (Pes) monitoring. The Pes values suggest increased resistance of the upper airway, with pressure swings up to 15 cm of water shown. Pressure swings greater than about 10 cm of water often raise concern. The recording montage includes the following leads: central (C3-M2, C4-M1), frontal (F3-M2, F4-M1), and occipital (O1-M2, O2-M1) electroencephalograms; left and right eye electrooculograms (E1-M2, E2-M1); mental/submental electromyogram (Chin1-Chin2); electrocardiogram (ECG1-ECG2, ECG2-ECG3); left and right eye electromyograms (LAT1-LAT2, RAT1-RAT2); snore volume (SNORE); nasal pressure transducer (NPRE); nasal/oral airflow (N/O); thoracic (THOR) and abdominal (ABD) effort; esophageal pressure (PES); arterial oxyhemoglobin saturation (SpO2); and plethysmography (Pleth).

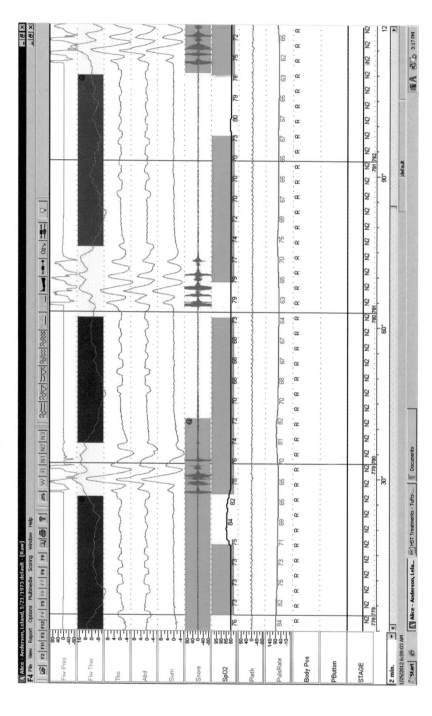

Figure 8.1 This 2-minute epoch from an in-home sleep apnea testing device (PDx, Philips Respironics) demonstrates significant obstructive sleep apnea. Three scored apneas are indicated by the shaded orange and gray boxes; note absent airflow, accompanied by continued respiratory effort for the majority of these events. The top two channels are nasal pressure and nasal–oral thermistor, followed by thoracic and abdominal effort bands with a combined sum effort channel. Below is a snore channel, oximetry, plethysmography, pulse rate, body position, patient event button, and "scored" sleep stage.

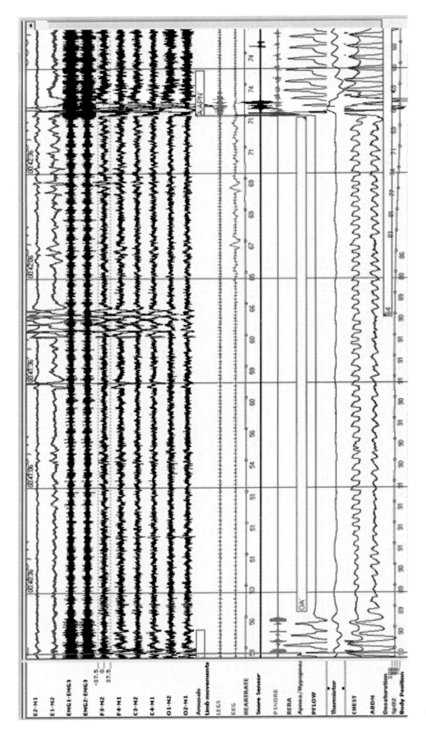

Figure 13.2 A prolonged apneic episode lasting 143 seconds in duration and occurring during REM sleep. (This frame represents a 3-minute epoch.)

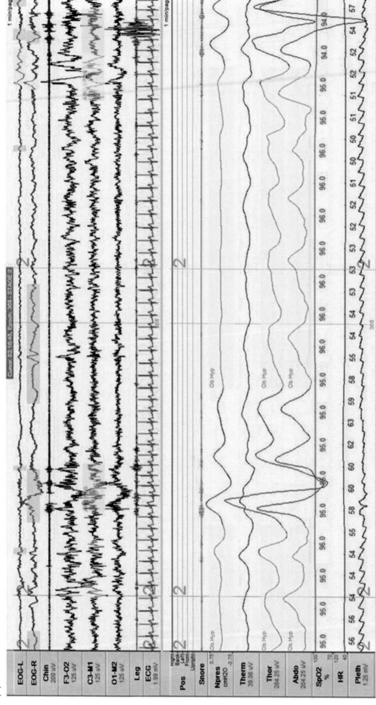

Figure 15.1 (a) Two epochs from the patient's level II sleepy study. (b) The same two epochs from 1 (a) as recorded in a level III study. (c) The same two epochs from (a) as recorded in a level IV study measuring a single parameter. (d) The same two epochs as 1 (a) recorded in a level IV study measuring three parameters.

Abbreviations used in figure: Abdo, abdominal effort; Chin, chin electromyogram; ECG, electrocardiogram; C3-M1, left central −> left mastoid electroencephalogram; F3-O2, left frontal −> right occipital electroencephalogram; HR, heart rate; Npres, nasal pressure (uses pressure as a measure of airflow); O1-M2, left occipital −> right mastoid electroencephalogram; Pleth, inductance plethysmography; Pos, body position; SpO2, oxygen saturation; Therm, naso-oral thermistor (uses temperature as a measure of airflow); Thor, thoracic effort.

(b)

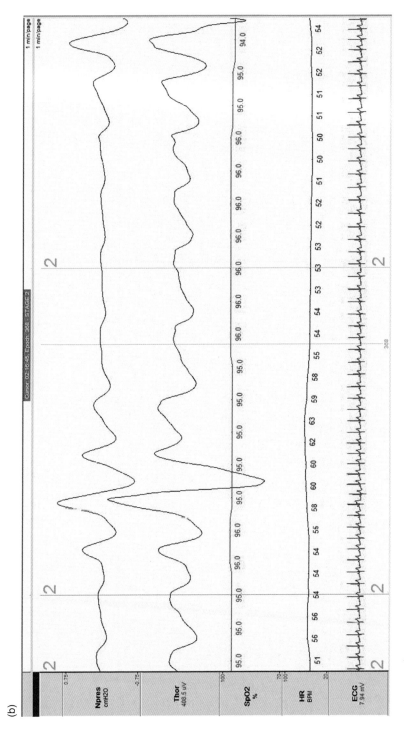

Figure 15.1 (*cont.*)

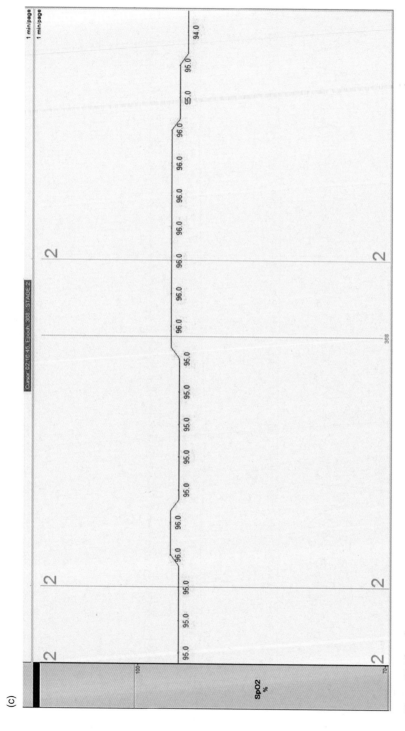

Figure 15.1 (*cont.*)

(d)

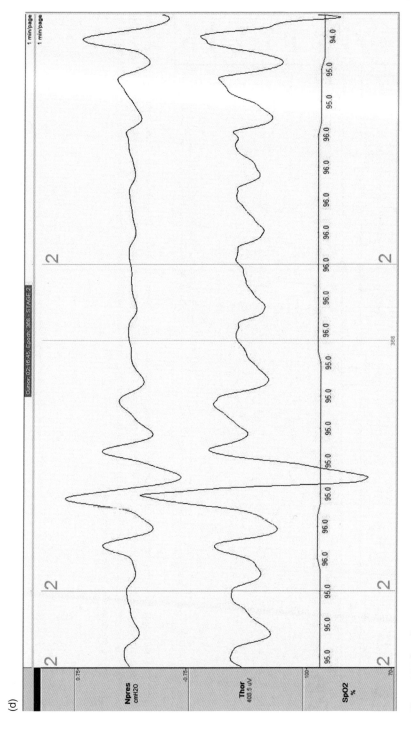

Figure 15.1 (*cont.*)

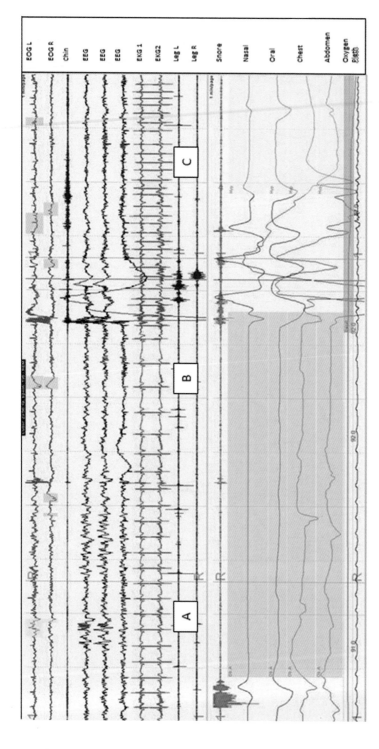

Figure 19.1 This figure highlights the electrocardiogram (ECG) changes observed during an obstructive apnea. Label **A**: Normal sinus rhythm; the rhythm that the patient maintained for the first 2 hours of sleep. Label **B**: Diving reflex is associated with an obstructive apnea and the associated oxygen desaturation. Label **C**: Atrial fibrillation, which began in association with the sympathetic surge that occurred at termination of this obstructive apnea. The patient remained in atrial fibrillation from this time through completion of the polysomnogram.

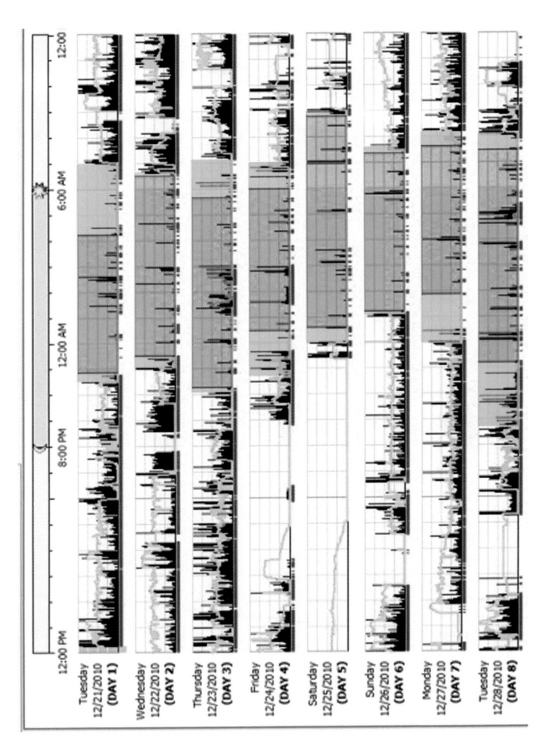

Figure 26.2 Sample 8 days of actigraphy from a patient with insomnia. Twenty-four hour activity data are presented from 12:00 PM on one day to 12:00 PM the following day. Black vertical bars represented activity and the yellow line represents light levels. Cyan shaded areas represent time in bed according to sleep diary information; blue shaded areas indicate estimated sleep periods according to the actigraphy analysis software. Note the variability in the bedtimes and rise times (particularly the early bedtime on the last day) and the significant wakefulness each day during the attempted sleep period.

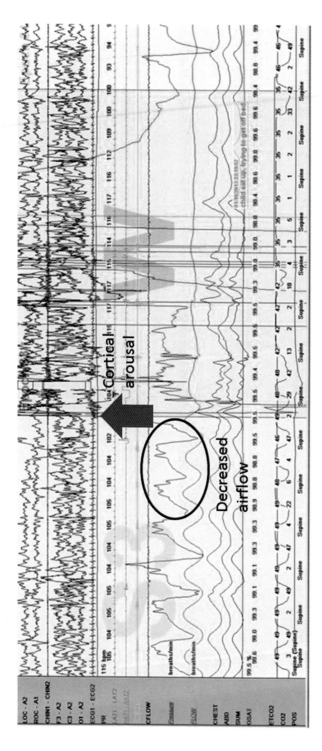

Figure 37.1 A 60-second epoch from the diagnostic polysomnogram of a 7-year-old child who was referred to the pediatric sleep center for evaluation of sleepwalking and was also noted to have snoring on clinical history. A typical episode of sleepwalking is shown as the child sits up and starts to get out of bed. Note the delta wave activity (large slow waves in the electroencephalographic channels) before, during (where legible), and after the cortical arousal that starts at the red arrow and continues through the duration of the child's movement. Channels are as follows: electrooculogram (left, LOC-A2; right, ROC-A1), chin electromyogram (EMG) (CHIN1-CHIN2), electroencephalogram (left frontal, F3-A2; left central, C3-A2; left occipital, O1-A2), electrocardiogram channel, pulse rate (PR), limb EMG (left, LAT-LAT2; right, RAT1-RAT2), snore channel, positive airway pressure signal (CFLOW), nasal pressure airflow (Pressure), nasal–oral airflow (FLOW), respiratory effort by respiratory inductance plethysmography (thoracic [CHEST], abdominal [ABD], sum channel [SUM]), oxygen saturation (OSAT), capnography value (ETCO2), capnography waveform (CO2), and position (POS).

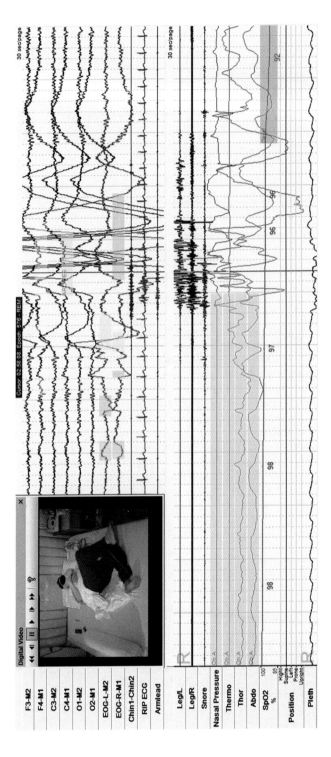

Figure 38.1 This 30-second epoch shows an example of an abnormal behavior observed during rapid eye movement sleep following a long obstructive apnea. The synchronized video recording demonstrates the patient to be aggressively moving his arms and legs during an arousal at the termination of the apnea. During the initial period without an arousal, normal chin atonia is observed. Figure abbreviations: F3-M2, left frontal electroencephalogram (EEG); F4-M1, right frontal EEG; C3-M2, left central EEG; C4-M1, right central EEG; O1-M2, left occipital EEG; O2-M1, right occipital EEG; EOG-L-M2, left eye electrooculography (EOG); EOG-R-M1, right eye electrooculography; Chin1-Chin2, chin electromyogram (EMG); RIP ECG, electrocardiographic leads; Armlead, extensor digitorum profundus surface EMG; Leg/L, left anterior tibialis surface EMG; Leg/R, right anterior tibialis surface EMG; Thermo, oronasal thermocouple; Thor, thoracic excursion; Abdo, abdominal excursion; SpO2, oxyhemoglobin saturation (%); Pleth, pulse waveform from oximeter.

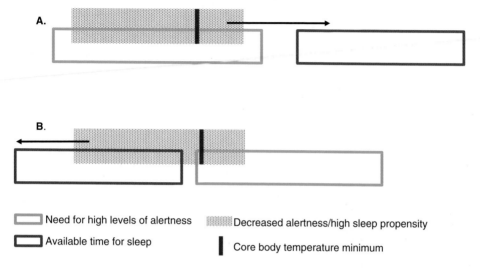

8 PM 10 PM 12 AM 2 AM 4 AM 6 AM 8 AM 10 AM 12 PM 2 PM 4 PM 6 PM 8 PM

A.

B.

☐ Need for high levels of alertness   ▨ Decreased alertness/high sleep propensity

☐ Available time for sleep   ▮ Core body temperature minimum

Figure 41.1 In patients with habitual sleep times of 11:00 PM to 7:00 AM, core body temperature minimum (CBT_{min}) is between 4:00 AM and 5:00 AM. Onset of melatonin secretion is approximately 7 hours before this time (9–10:00 PM) and peaks just prior to CBT_{min}. The time of peak melatonin secretion and CBT_{min} coincides with the nadir of circadian alertness. Label **A**: During a night shift condition, the intrinsic timing of high sleep propensity may result in somnolence during work and insomnia during the day sleep bout. Therapeutic goals include a phase delay (black arrow), such that sleep promoting factors fall within the available rest period rather than the work period. This could potentially be achieved with bright light during the first half of the shift, avoidance of bright light after the shift and on the commute home, and melatonin prior to day sleep. Label **B**: During early rise shift work, the intrinsic timing of high sleep propensity may result in somnolence during the first portion of the work period and insomnia at sleep onset. Therapeutic goals include a phase advance (black arrow), such that sleep promoting factors coincide with the available earlier rest period rather than the work period or morning commute. Use of a bright light box after arriving at work, avoidance of afternoon and evening bright light, and evening melatonin prior to bedtime may be beneficial.

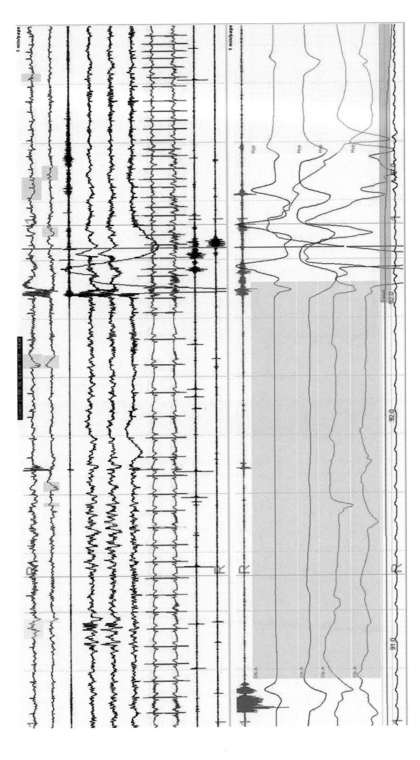

Figure 44.2 Polysomnogram of a patient in rapid eye movement sleep. It shows an obstructive apnea that is associated with bradycardia and desaturation. The apnea is followed by an arousal and atrial fibrillation with a rapid ventricular rate. Abbreviations used in figure: EEG, electroencephalogram; EKG, electrocardiogram; EMG, electromyogram; EOG, electrooculogram; NPT, nasal pressure transducer. Original content courtesy of Meredith Peters MD.

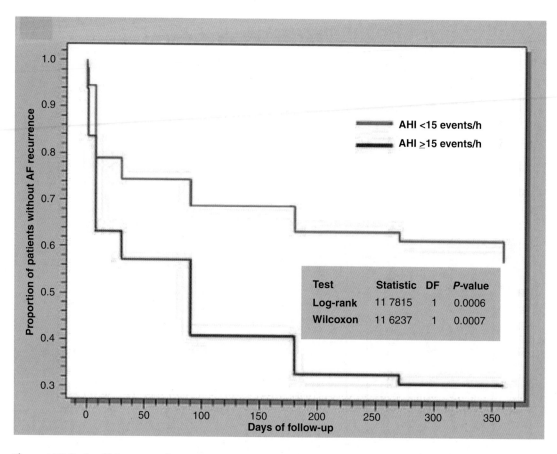

Figure 44.3 Kaplan–Meier curves showing survival free of atrial fibrillation recurrence according to dichotomized apnea/hypopnea index (< 15 / ≥ 15 events per hour). Abbreviations used in figure: AF, atrial fibrillation; AHI, apnea/hypopnea index. Data from Mazza A, Bendini MG, Cristofori M, et al.

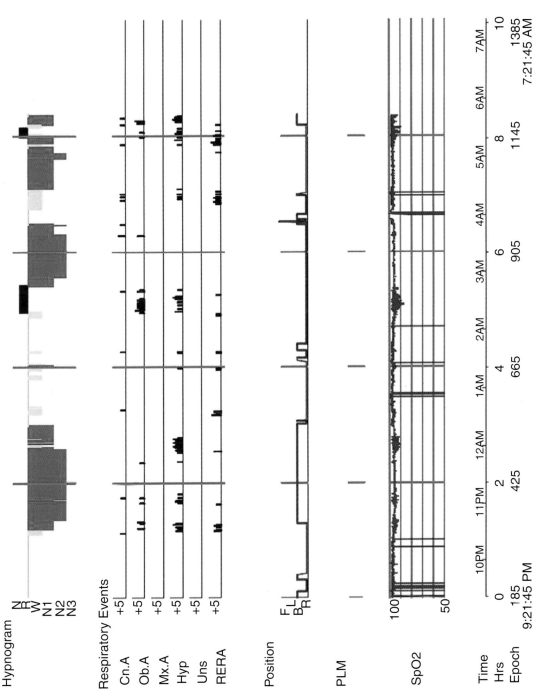

Figure 47.1 This hypnogram from the patient's baseline polysomnogram reflects sleep fragmentation and obstructive respiratory disturbances during rapid eye movement (REM) sleep in a child with obstructive sleep apnea (OSA). Abbreviations used in figure: N, unspecified non-REM; R, REM; W, wake; N1, N2, N3, non-REM stages N1, N2, N3; Cn.A, central apneas; Ob.A, obstructive apneas; Mx.A, mixed apneas; Hyp, hypopneas; Uns, unscored events; RERA, respiratory effort-related arousals; F, front; L, left lateral; B, back; R, right lateral; PLM, periodic leg movements; SpO2, oxygen saturation by finger oximetry; Hrs, hours.

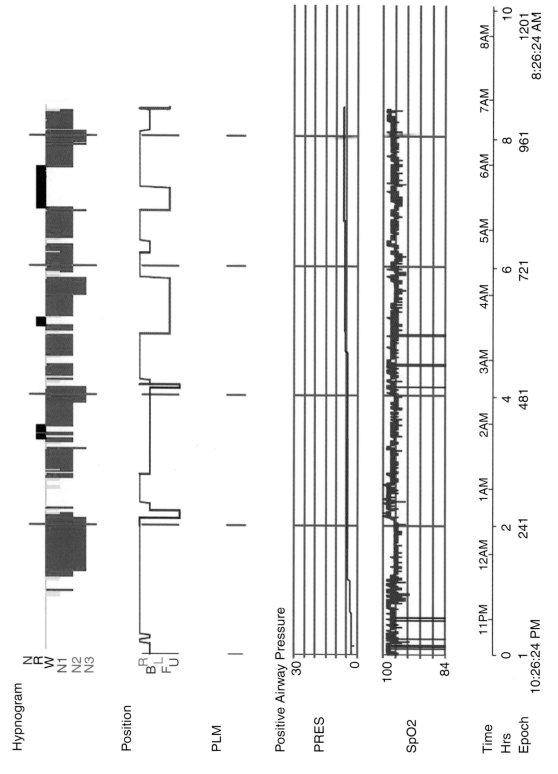

Figure 47.2 The patient's hypnogram, from the initial titration on continuous positive airway pressure (CPAP), reflects increased sleep and improved sleep when obstructive sleep apnea is treated. Abbreviations used in figure: N, unspecified non-REM; R, REM; W, wake; N1, N2, N3, non-REM stages N1, N2, N3; B, back; L, left lateral; F, front; U, undetermined position; PLM, periodic leg movements; PRES, CPAP pressure setting in centimeter of water; SpO2, oxygen saturation by finger oximetry; Hrs, hours.

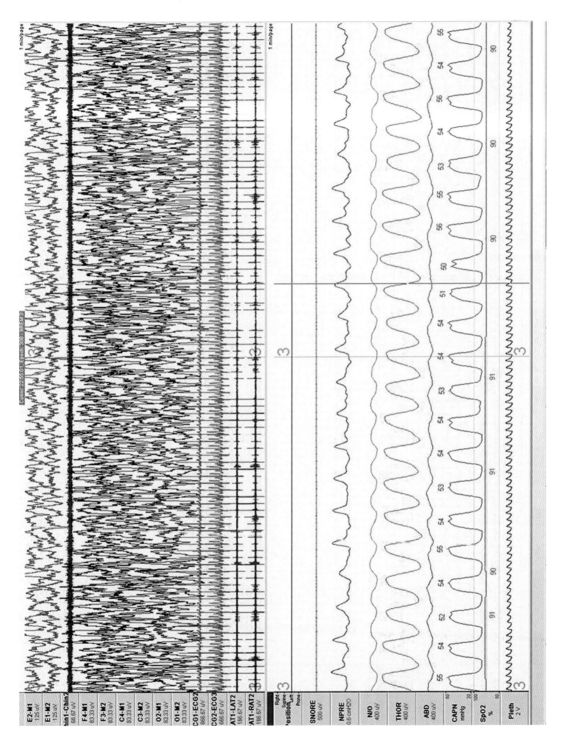

Figure 54.1 Hypoventilation noted during a diagnostic polysomnogram with end-tidal carbon dioxide monitoring. Abbreviations: E1 and E2, left and right eye leads; M1 and M2, mastoid leads; F, frontal electroencephalography (EEG) leads; C, central EEG leads; O, occipital EEG leads; ECG, electrocardiogram leads; LAT and RAT, left and right anterior tibialis leads; N/O, oro-nasal thermistor; NPRE, nasal pressure; THOR, thoracic belt; ABD, abdominal belt; CAPN, capnogram; SpO2, oxygen saturation; Pleth, plethysmography.

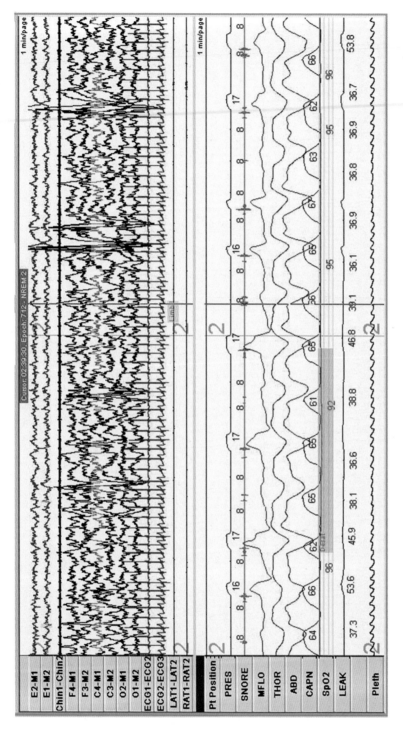

Figure 54.2 Bi-level positive airway pressure (Bi-PAP) with irregular, intermittent inability to trigger jump from expiratory positive airway pressure to a higher inspiratory positive airway pressure (IPAP). This is best reflected in the tracings marked PRES (mask pressure) and MFLO (mask flow). Abbreviations: E1 and E2, left and right eye leads; M1 and M2, are mastoid leads; F, frontal electroencephalography (EEG) leads; C, central EEG leads; O, occipital EEG leads; ECG, electrocardiogram leads; LAT and RAT, left and right anterior tibialis leads; NPRE, nasal pressure; N/O, oro-nasal thermistor; THOR, thoracic belt; ABD, abdominal belt; CAPN, capnogram; SpO2, oxygen saturation; Pleth, plethysmography; PRES, bi-level positive airway pressure; MFLO is mask flow.

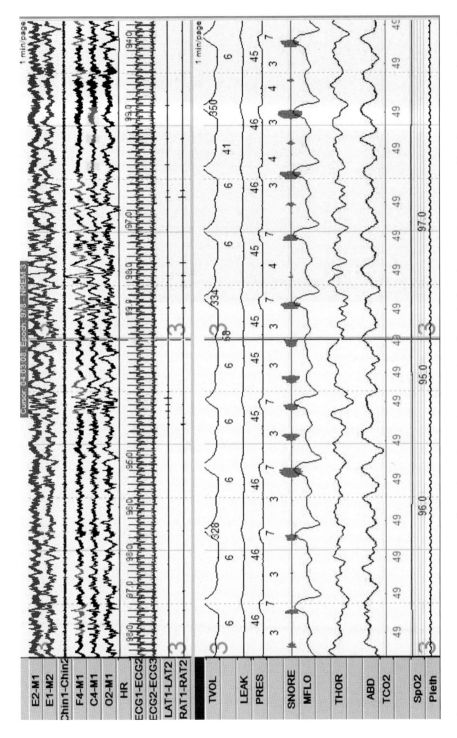

Figure 54.3 Bi-level positive airway pressure (Bi-PAP) with lower tidal volume (TVOL) noted when change to inspiratory positive airway pressure, from a lower expiratory positive pressure, does not occur. Abbreviations: E1 and E2, left and right eye leads; M1 and M2, mastoid leads; F, frontal electroencephalography (EEG) leads; C, central EEG leads; O, occipital EEG leads; ECG, electrocardiogram leads; LAT and RAT, left and right anterior tibialis leads; NPRE, nasal pressure; N/O, oronasal thermistor; THOR, thoracic belt; ABD, abdominal belt; CAPN, capnogram; SpO2, oxygen saturation; Pleth, plethysmography; TVOL, tidal volume; TCO2, transcutaneous carbon dioxide monitoring.

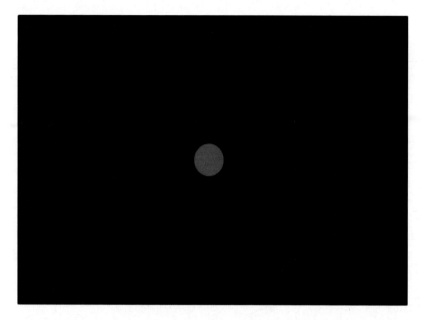

Figure 55.1 Test of sustained attention. Subjects are asked to press a button whenever the red dot appears on the screen.

58

Falls and hip fractures in the elderly: insomnia and hypnotics as unrecognized risk factors

Alon Y. Avidan

Case

For the past year an 82-year-old nursing home resident has suffered from middle of the night awakenings. While she had no difficulties falling asleep at 10:00 PM, with an alarm set at 5:00 AM, she would wake up nightly between 1:00 and 2:00 AM and would be up for "hours" until falling asleep again. She believes that she only gets 4 hours of sleep nightly. The patient was recently diagnosed with osteoporosis and hypertension and about 6 months ago she was placed on calcium and vitamin D supplementation, and was started on a beta-blocker. She described feeling depressed and "gloomy" during the day, due to the lack of good quality sleep. She also noted that she was more "lightheaded" for the last 6 months for an unknown reason. The patient denied snoring or restless leg symptoms. Her examination showed a body mass index of 23 kg/m². Her neck circumference was 12 inches (30 cm) and her oral airway showed a Mallampati Classification type I. Her general and neurologic examinations were completely normal except for reduced ankle jerk reflexes. Her physician referred the patient for a sleep consultation to address her insomnia. He wishes to start her on trazodone, but the nursing home medical director believes that this is a bad idea as hypnotics can cause falls and lead to hip fractures. Her primary physician asks for an official sleep medicine consult with the main question of whether it would be safe to treat the patient with a sleep aid.

Discussion

Background: insomnia and consequences in older patients

Insomnia is common in older adults and the prevalence increases with advancing age. Because of changes in sleep architecture, older adults are more likely than younger adults to experience increased nocturnal awakenings, interrupted sleep, and decreased sleep efficiency. The consequences of disrupted sleep in older patients are substantial and consist of poorer health, cognitive impairment, and mortality. Despite the high prevalence of insomnia, many older adults with complaints of insomnia do not seek treatment. A decade ago, the National Sleep Foundation conducted a poll about sleep patterns in older patients.[1] This was a national survey based on 1506 telephone interviews of older adults, aged 55–84 years, living in the United States. The data revealed that of the women sampled 34% had frequent middle of the night awakenings and 29% woke up feeling unrefreshed.[1] If fact, these sleeping difficulties are not just about lack of sleep or poor quality sleep, but in older women, regression analyses demonstrate that worse sleep is associated at subsequent follow-up with worsened health-related quality of life (even after adjusting for multiple covariates).[2] Important data about psychiatric consequences of untreated insomnia is derived from a 4-year, observational study of 3824 people aged $\geq$ 65 years from France. The

Common Pitfalls in Sleep Medicine, ed. Ronald D. Chervin. Published by Cambridge University Press. © Cambridge University Press 2014.

Table 58.1 Drugs and substances associated with insomnia

Drugs associated with insomnia

Antidepressants (MAOIs, occasionally SSRIs)

Asthma, COPD medications (theophylline)

Corticosteroids (oral prednisone and dexamethasone, IV hydrocortisone)

Nasal decongestants (pseudoephedrine)

Histamine antagonists (cimetidine)

Antihypertensives (beta-blockers)

Anticholinesterase inhibitors (donepezil)

Stimulants

Antineoplastic agents

Substances associated with insomnia

Alcohol

Caffeine

Nicotine

COPD, chronic obstructive pulmonary disease; IV, intravenous; MAOI, monoamine oxidase inhibitors; SSRIs, selective serotonin reuptake inhibitors.

study demonstrated that insomnia and daytime sleepiness are risk factors for depression in older adults.[3] At follow-up, specific predictors of new depressive symptoms in this study included insomnia (odds ratio [OR] of 1.23), poor sleep quality, difficulties initiating and maintaining sleep, excessive daytime sleepiness (OR 2.05), and the use of a sleeping medication(independent of insomnia symptoms [OR 1.62]).

What causes insomnia in older age?

When insomnia is present in older patients, the etiology may be multifactorial and is often related to underlying medical and psychiatric illnesses and polypharmacy. Given that sleep disturbances in older adults are often comorbid with an existing chronic medical condition, psychosocial morbidity, and overall poor physical health, it is important for clinicians to assess whether insomnia is a primary or secondary condition. Another key issue when searching for the etiology of insomnia in older adults is that the principal medical or psychiatric condition, as well as

medications used to treat it (e.g. antidepressants, dopamine agonists, cardiovascular medication), may cause sleep disruption and contribute to daytime sleepiness. Common causes of insomnia in the older patients are listed in Table 58.1.

Hypnotic use in older patients

Insomnia is characterized by insufficient or poor-quality sleep as a consequence of either difficulty initiating sleep, difficulty maintaining sleep, early morning awakening, or a sense that sleep is unrefreshing. Sleep disturbances are a common problem in older adults, with up to 40% of adults over the age of 65 reporting symptoms of insomnia. Data show that the medications used to treat insomnia have been associated with an increased risk of accidental events, including falls and fractures, which are of particular concern in older adults.

The treatment of insomnia includes both behavioral (e.g. cognitive behavioral therapy) and pharmacologic therapies (sedating antidepressants, long- and short-acting benzodiazepines, non-benzodiazepine hypnotics, and a selective melatonin receptor agonist). Although hypnotic medications effectively promote sleep, they may have a relatively long duration of action, which can be problematic as the therapeutic action of these medications can extend into the waking hours and induce daytime sedation. In fact, the US Food and Drug Administration issued a warning in January 2013 warning practitioners to exercise caution against excessive doses.[4]

Older patients experience the greatest use of hypnotic agents. A survey of 10216 members of the Swedish Pensioners' Association found that, overall, 13.5% of men and 22.3% of women reported they used hypnotics, and this use increased significantly with age.[5] Prevalence of hypnotic use in men aged < 70 years was 7.9%, 14.4% in those aged 70–80 years, and 21.8% in those aged ≥ 80 years ($P < 0.0001$). In women, the prevalence was 15.0%, 23.0%, and 34.9%, respectively ($P < 0.0001$). In this population, half of individuals treated with hypnotics reported a good night's sleep. Figure 58.1 depicts frequency of hypnotic use in older men and women.[5,6]

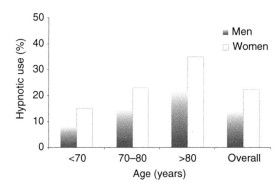

Figure 58.1 Use of hypnotics in older adults. The most significant use of hypnotic medications occurs in the older population in whom the prevalence and impact on quality of life of sleep disturbance is high.[6] A survey of 10 216 members of the Swedish Pensioners' Association found that, overall, 13.5% of men and 22.3% of women reported they used hypnotics, and this use increased significantly with age. Prevalence of hypnotic use in men aged < 70 years was 7.9%, 14.4% in those aged 70–80 years, and 21.8% in those aged ≥ 80 years ($P < 0.0001$). In women, the prevalence was 15.0%, 23.0%, and 34.9%, respectively ($P < 0.0001$). In this population, half of individuals treated with hypnotics reported a good night's sleep.[5] Average age (male) $= 73.0 \pm 6.0$ years. Average age (female) $= 72.6 \pm 6.7$ years.

What are the options for treatment of insomnia with hypnotics?

Pharmacologic treatment of insomnia in the older person may be complicated by age-related pharmacokinetics and pharmacodynamic changes. Some hypnotics, particularly those with longer half-lives, have multiple side effects in the older person, ranging from sedation, disruption of sleep architecture (reduction of stages rapid eye movement [REM] and slow-wave sleep [SWS]), to placing patients at risk for falls and accidents. A major concern with the long-acting sleeping pills is tolerance, which is the gradual need for higher drug dosages to achieve the same clinical efficacy, and rebound insomnia when the drug is discontinued.

If hypnotics are used in the older person, the advice is that they are administered at the lowest possible dose, for the shortest period of time. Shorter acting

hypnotics are preferable and patients need to be followed closely. Possible hypnotic-related side effects include anterograde amnesia and rebound insomnia. This is true for hypnotics with short to intermediate half-lives. Many different hypnotics are likely to improve insomnia if given at the appropriate doses. The goal for sleep specialists who use these agents is often to use the medication with the fewest side effects at the lowest dose that will achieve clinically efficacy until cognitive behavioral therapy gains momentum.

Hypnotics need to be dispensed with care to older patients especially when other comorbidities such as obstructive sleep apnea are suspected, since their use may potentially worsen nocturnal hypoxemia. Withdrawal from hypnotics may worsen insomnia and heighten anxiety, especially when the withdrawal is abrupt and from longer acting medications. The short-acting hypnotics may be safer in the older patient. Examples of these newer agents include zaleplon (selective for the benzodiazepine-1 receptor), zolpidem (selective for the type-1 GABA$_A$-benzodiazepine receptor), a melatonin receptor agonist, and a histamine-1 receptor antagonist (Table 58.2).

Arguments for hypnotics in the treatment of insomnia in older adults

The main argument for carefully tailored treatment management to improve insomnia is substantiated on data that untreated insomnia predicts poorer health, worsens psychiatric disease, or places patients at risk for injury. When the practitioner is asked to make a decision about leaving insomnia untreated versus selecting a hypnotic to treat insomnia, he or she is poised to make an important decision about risk–benefit ratio, as illustrated in Figure 58.2. The main contradicting view about hypnotic therapy is that not all hypnotics are safe in older patients, and their perceived benefit may not be justified due to the risk of falls and hip fracture. In fact, in one study, the greatest risk for falls among older persons living in the community (expressed as an odds ratio) was the use of psychotropics medications or sedative hypnotics (Table 58.3[7]). However, this study and many others that have

Table 58.2 Selected agents for the management of insomnia in older adults (>65 years old). The data are presented based on the indication (sleep initiation vs. sleep maintenance insomnia), half-life of the drug, recommended geriatric doses, and required period of inactivity prior to administration of the drug

Agent	Geriatric dose	Initiates sleep	Maintains sleep (*)	Sleep with limited opportunity	Required inactivity
Eszopiclone	Sleep initiation – 1.0 mg Sleep maintenance – 2.0 mg	√	√(*)		8+ hours
Zaleplon	5.0 mg	√		√	4 hours
Zolpidem tartrate	5.0 mg	√			7–8 hours
Zolpidem tartrate extended-release	6.25 mg	√	√(*)		7–8 hours
Zolpidem tartrate sublingual	1.75 mg		√(*)	√ (4 hours)	4 hours
Zolpidem tartrate sublingual	5.0 mg	√			4 hours
Zolpidem tartrate oral spray	5.0 mg	√			4 hours
Doxepin	3 mg		√(*)		7–8 hours
Ramelteon	8 mg	√			–

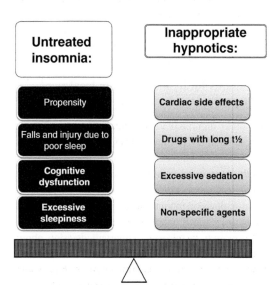

Figure 58.2 The main arguments for and against hypnotic therapy for older adult patients who complain of insomnia.

drawn attention to the potential risks of hypnotic therapy did not specifically control for the potential risk that disturbed sleep per se may drive this risk. In addition, many previous studies implicating hypnotics

Table 58.3 Does treating sleep disturbance with medications increase the risk of falls?

Risk factors for falls in a community population	Adjusted OR (95% CI)
Cognitive impairment	5.0 (1.8–13.7)
History of stroke	3.0 (1.5–6.1)
Arthritis	1.8 (1.0–3.1)
Balance/strength	3.8 (2.2–6.7)
Gait	1.9 (1.0–3.7)
Psychotropics/sedatives	*28.3 (3.4–239.4)

Data from Tinetti, Speechley and Ginter.[7]
*See text. Note: Disturbed sleep not used in model.
CI, clearance interval; OR, odds ratio.

as risky, may not have specifically adjusted effectively for multiple confounds such as severity of preexisting illness, an individual's degree of dependence, burden of illness, cognitive ability, and for a nursing home resident, direct care requirements.

Recent findings from the large study of osteoporotic fractures cohort of older women established a link between subjectively and objectively defined sleep problems and a greater risk of falls.[8] This risk was

Table 58.4 Insomnia, hypnotics, and falls in nursing homes: prediction of incident falls in the state of Michigan nursing homes ($N = 34{,}163$)

	OR	(95% CI)
Baseline insomnia without hypnotics	1.55	1.41–1.71
Baseline insomnia on hypnotics	1.32	1.02–1.70
No baseline insomnia on hypnotics (= effective treatment)	1.11	0.94–1.31
No baseline insomnia and not on hypnotics	Reference	Reference

Data from Avidan AY, Fries BE, James ML, et al.[10]
CI, clearance interval; OR, odds ratio.

present even after taking into account the use of insomnia pharmacotherapy in the form on benzodiazepines in this community-dwelling population of older women. The data imply that poor sleep itself, as opposed to hypnotic therapy, places patients at risk for falls and potential injury. Based on another recent study of 711 participants, untreated insomnia predicted worse treatment outcomes in depression (prolonged sleep latency alone [OR = 3.53] or in combination with insomnia [OR = 2.11]).[9]

While some clinicians may be apprehensive about prescribing a hypnotic due to the concerns of falls and subsequently hip fracture, this belief may not necessarily be correct. A study by the author and colleagues from the University of Michigan demonstrated that it may be untreated insomnia that could be a culprit in leading to falls. In this descriptive study utilizing the Minimum Data Set (MDS) of nursing home residents ($N = 34163$, aged > 65 years) hypnotic use did not appear to predict falls.[10] In fact, after adjustments for covariates, insomnia symptoms predicted future falls (OR = 1.52). Untreated insomnia (adjusted OR [AOR] = 1.55) and hypnotic-treated (unresponsive) insomnia (AOR = 1.32) predicted more falls than did the absence of insomnia or use of hypnotics without current insomnia (Table 58.4).[10] After adjustment for confounding variables, insomnia and hypnotic use were not associated with subsequent hip fracture. The adjusted models in this study imply that when

insomnia is not a clinically active issue, patients on hypnotic treatment do not have an increased risk for falls.

Our data from Michigan was among the first to suggest that current hypnotics may not confer risks to falls or hip fractures in nursing home residents. Indeed, antecedent data that implicated hypnotics as culprits in falls and injury did not carefully adjust for confounds, measure whether insomnia is a key confound, or utilize a longitudinal research approach. Previous data on hypnotics may have focused mainly on older benzodiazepines, which have inherently longer half-lives and more significant side effects. More recently released non-benzodiazepine hypnotics, such as zolpidem compounds and melatonin agonists, have short half-lives and may have less cognitive impact than older medications. In fact, in another study by the author, subjects who used a melatonin agonist showed a lower probability of experiencing an accidental event during the first 3 months following treatment initiation compared with subjects taking older and longer acting agents.[11]

A recent study from Japan was conducted to determine whether insomnia and hypnotic use are predictors of falls and bone fractures in older patients.[12] The authors evaluated clinical data for 599 late-stage elderly patients receiving home medical care over a 3-year period. As in the Michigan study, their conclusion demonstrated that hypnotic use was not associated with a greater risk of subsequent falls and bone fractures.

What do these data mean for the sleep practitioner? It may be important to rethink the widely held view that hypnotics are risky for geriatric patients. This is particularly true since newer, safer hypnotics have become more widely used since the original and perhaps older data were collected and analyzed. Now, appropriate control of insomnia is not only a quality of life issue, but perhaps a safety issue as well.

Argument for not using hypnotics

The main argument against the standard use of hypnotics is as follows: while the improvement in sleep with hypnotic use is statistically significant, the magnitude of effect may not be sufficiently strong to

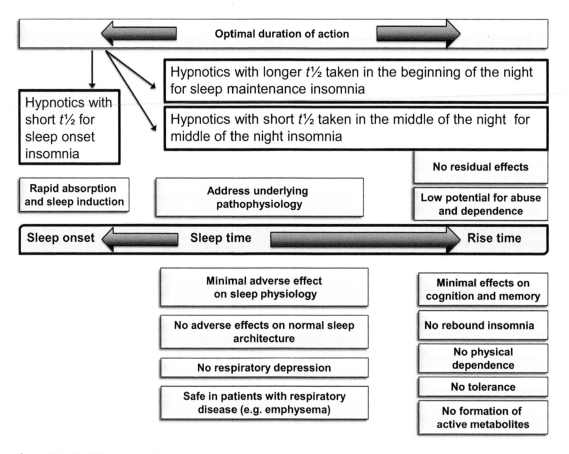

Figure 58.3 The "ideal hypnotic."

justify making a universal recommendation. Since the "perfect or ideal hypnotic" (Figure 58.3) does not yet exist, every hypnotic will pose a potential risk that may not justify its use. Data show that the increased risk of adverse events associated with hypnotics is statistically significant and likely clinically relevant in older people at risk of falls and cognitive disturbances.[13] The argument further suggests that in patients over age 60, the benefits of these drugs may not justify the increased risk, particularly if the patient has additional risk factors for cognitive or psychomotor adverse events.[13]

A historical cohort study from Tennessee showed that although the risk of falls among nursing home patients receiving short-acting benzodiazepines was less than that for the long-acting agents, these agents are correlated with an increased risk of nocturnal falls (Table 58.5).[14] However, this historical cohort study was a smaller study than the previously mentioned Michigan MDS study. The historical cohort study included 2510 residents of 53 Tennessee nursing homes and did not control for the fact that insomnia itself may be driving this relationship. Moreover, the majority of studies that have implicated hypnotics as risk factors for falls and injuries did not investigate the possibility that underlying insomnia, rather than medication, could be the main reason for the adverse outcomes. In fact, in a community-based cross-sectional survey of 1526 older adults, insomnia, but not psychoactive medication, was associated with falls within the

Table 58.5 Benzodiazepines increase the risk of falls in nursing home residents. The data depicted is based on a historical cohort analysis of 2510 residents in 53 Tennessee nursing homes

	Daytime falls (7:00 AM – 8:00 PM)	Nighttime falls (8:00 PM – 7:00 AM)
Any benzodiazepine	1.38 (1.25–1.51)	1.83 (1.55–2.15)
Short-acting* (half-life < 12 hours)	Not significant	2.19 (1.59–3.03)
Intermediate-acting (half-life 12–23 hours)	1.43 (1.29–1.59)	1.68 (1.39–2.02)
Long-acting (half-life ≥ 24 hours)	1.77 (1.38–2.26)	1.80 (1.14–2.83)

Data from Ray WA, Thapa PB, Gideon P.[14]

*Includes temazepam, oxazepam, zolpidem, and triazolam.

Rate ratios (95% confidence intervals); adjusted for age, gender, race, time since admission to facility and since zero time, body mass index (BMI), ambulatory status, activities of daily living (ADL) dependency, incontinence, cognitive impairment, physical restraint use, past falls, and use of anticonvulsants, antiparkinsonian drugs, antidepressants, antipsychotics, and other sedatives. Reference group is non-users, no benzodiazepines in the preceding 7 days.

past 12 months.[15] Furthermore, the use of psycho-active agents was infrequent in this Silicon Valley community cohort.

If one does contemplate using trazodone for this patient, what do the data suggest, specifically in older adults with insomnia?

In the case provided, consideration is given for the use of trazodone, which for several reasons has some safety concerns for older adults. Use of trazodone is associated with dizziness, oversedation, antiadrenergic effects with orthostatic hypotension, drug–drug interactions, and, infrequently, priapism. While the latter issue is not relevant here, the use of trazodone has been reported to induce or aggravate atrial and ventricular arrhythmias both in healthy individuals and in those with preexisting cardiac disease. In fact, trazodone although frequently used to treat insomnia due to its sedating property, had never been approved for insomnia by the US Food and Drug Administration. For our lightheaded and osteoporotic patient, the use of a sedative drug such as trazodone carried an unusual risk should she get up out of bed and experience hypotension (due to the beta-blocker and trazodone's inherent α_2-adrenergic blockade). A fall in our 82-year-old patient could be devastating, especially given that 30% of people with a hip fracture are

predicted to die in the following year, and many more will experience significant functional loss.

Recent data, from a small Brazilian nursing home community, suggested that trazodone was effective in as many as 65.7% of patients to manage sleep problems that arise in the context of dementia.[16] While the specific mechanism involved in the hypnotic effect of sedating antidepressants, including trazodone, remains unclear, it may be that the therapeutic effect of trazodone on sleep is independent of its antidepressant action.[17] Polysomnographic data on the use of trazodone in depressed insomnia patients demonstrate significantly increased total sleep time, improved sleep efficiency and sleep continuity, and reduced awakenings and stage shifts when compared to the baseline.[17] However, a large meta-analysis of trazodone concludes that "given the relative deficient data on efficacy in patients with insomnia and the adverse events associated with trazodone's use in general, it is uncertain whether the risk/benefit ratio warrants trazodone's use in nondepressed patients with insomnia."[18]

The consultant is therefore left to make a recommendation based on the risk of leaving insomnia untreated versus managing this patient with a sedative drug that is somewhat problematic given the conflicting data associated with its use. As falls are prevalent in the geriatric population, a thoughtful conclusion should be based on integrating knowledge of the data

concerning untreated insomnia and falls and a knowledge of desirable and undesirable hypnotic effects. The
medical decision-making should take into account the
patient's medication history, avoiding or minimizing
the use of high-risk drugs, and managing comorbid
diseases and disorders.

This patient's quality of life was disturbed given the
limited sleep duration, and the sleep consultant should
entertain specific therapy options. The sleep medicine
consultant provided the following plan, which resulted
in subsequent improvement:

1. Given the concerns with trazodone leading to
   orthostatic hypotension, it is not recommended to
   proceed with this treatment especially since the
   patient is on other drugs (beta-blockers) that can
   promote orthostatic hypotension. The underlying
   osteoporosis could also place her at an increased
   risk for a hip fracture if she were to accidently fall.
2. Consider management with a hypnotic specifically
   indicated for insomnia characterized by sleep maintenance difficulties. These are listed in Table 58.2 as
   noted by the asterisk (*). If zolpidem tartrate sub-
   lingual is selected, the patient is advised to ensure
   that 4 hours of additional sleep are available before
   taking the medication. The prescribing physician is
   to adhere to the appropriate dosing regimen for
   older adults and ensure that appropriate plans are
   in place for monitoring of side effects.
3. The patient may benefit from cognitive and behavioral therapy for insomnia.
4 Continue to assess progress with sleep diaries and
   have the patient return for follow-up in the sleep
   disorders clinic to evaluate treatment progress.

Main points

Older evidence and opinions of many clinicians hold
that hypnotics should be avoided in older persons with
insomnia, though more recent data suggest that
insomnia itself may be to blame for at least a significant portion of falls among patients treated with hypnotics. The clinician must consider available evidence,
the type of hypnotic, and the individual's complaints
and condition to derive the wisest choice for how to
approach insomnia in an older person. Fortunately,
non-pharmacologic approaches also can be highly
effective and may offer an alternative to hypnotics.
Insomnia in older persons is extremely common and
consequential, and should not be ignored.

REFERENCES

1. Foley D, Ancoli-Israel S, Britz P, Walsh J. Sleep disturbances and chronic disease in older adults: results of the
   2003 National Sleep Foundation Sleep in America Survey.
   J Psychosom Res 2004;**56**:497–502.
2. Lo CM, Lee PH. Prevalence and impacts of poor sleep on
   quality of life and associated factors of good sleepers in a
   sample of older Chinese adults. *Health Qual Life Outcomes* 2012;**10**:72.
3. Jaussent I, Bouyer J, Ancelin ML, et al. Insomnia and
   daytime sleepiness are risk factors for depressive symptoms in the elderly. *Sleep* 2011;**34**:1103–10.
4. US Food and Drug Administration. *FDA Drug Safety Communication: risk of next-morning impairment after use of
   insomnia drugs; FDA requires lower recommended doses
   for certain drugs containing zolpidem (Ambien, Ambien
   CR, Edluar, and Zolpimist)*. Rockville, MD: US Food and
   Drug Administration;2013.
5. Asplund R. Sleep and hypnotics among the elderly in
   relation to body weight and somatic disease. *J Intern
   Med* 1995;**238**:65–70.
6. Ancoli-Israel S. Insomnia in the elderly: a review for the
   primary care practitioner. *Sleep* 2000;**23**(Suppl 1):S23–30;
   discussion S36–8.
7. Tinetti ME, Speechley M, Ginter SF. Risk factors for falls
   among elderly persons living in the community. *N Engl
   J Med* 1988;**319**:1701–17.
8. Stone KL, Ewing SK, Lui LY, et al. Self-reported sleep and
   nap habits and risk of falls and fractures in older women:
   the study of osteoporotic fractures. *J Am Geriatr Soc*
   2006;**54**:1177–83.
9. Troxel WM, Kupfer DJ, Reynolds CF, 3rd, et al. Insomnia
   and objectively measured sleep disturbances predict
   treatment outcome in depressed patients treated with
   psychotherapy or psychotherapy–pharmacotherapy combinations. *J Clin Psychiatry* 2012;**73**:478–85.
10. Avidan AY, Fries BE, James ML, et al. Insomnia and
    hypnotic use, recorded in the minimum data set, as pre-
    dictors of falls and hip fractures in Michigan nursing
    homes. *J Am Geriatr Soc* 2005;**53**:955–62.

11. Avidan AY, Palmer LA, Doan JF, Baran RW. Insomnia medication use and the probability of an accidental event in an older adult population. *Drug Health Patient Saf* 2010;**2**:225–32.

12. Kondo S, Kitagawa C, Katsuta S, Kondo Y. [Assessment of the relationships between insomnia and hypnotic use with the risk of falls and bone fractures in late-stage elderly patients]. *Gan To Kagaku Ryoho* 2012;**39**(Suppl 1):113–14.

13. Glass J, Lanctot KL, Herrmann N, Sproule BA, Busto UE. Sedative hypnotics in older people with insomnia: meta-analysis of risks and benefits. *BMJ* 2005;**19**:1169.

14. Ray WA, Thapa PB, Gideon P. Benzodiazepines and the risk of falls in nursing home residents. *J Am Geriatr Soc* 2000;**48**:682–5.

15. Brassington GS, King AC, Bliwise DL. Sleep problems as a risk factor for falls in a sample of community-dwelling adults aged 64–99 years. *J Am Geriatr Soc* 2000;**48**: 1234–40.

16. Camargos EF, Pandolfi MB, Freitas MP, et al. Trazodone for the treatment of sleep disorders in dementia: an open-label, observational and review study. *Arq Neuropsiquiatr* 2011;**69**:44–9.

17. Kaynak H, Kaynak D, Gozukirmizi E, Guilleminault C. The effects of trazodone on sleep in patients treated with stimulant antidepressants. *Sleep Med* 2004;**5**:15–20.

18. Mendelson WB. A review of the evidence for the efficacy and safety of trazodone in insomnia. *J Clin Psychiatry* 2005;**66**:469–76.

Index